The International Medical
Relief Corps in Wartime
China, 1937–1945

The International Medical Relief Corps in Wartime China, 1937–1945

ROBERT MAMLOK, M.D.

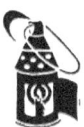

McFarland & Company, Inc., Publishers
Jefferson, North Carolina

LIBRARY OF CONGRESS CATALOGUING-IN-PUBLICATION DATA

Names: Mamlok, Robert, 1954– author.
Title: The International Medical Relief Corps in wartime China, 1937–1945 / Robert Mamlok, M.D.
Description: Jefferson, North Carolina : McFarland & Company, Inc., Publishers, 2018 | Includes bibliographical references and index.
Identifiers: LCCN 2018040516 | ISBN 9781476675831 (softcover : acid free paper) ∞
Subjects: LCSH: World War, 1939–1945—Medical care—China. | International Medical Relief Corps—History. | Chinese Red Cross Society—History. | Sino-Japanese War, 1937–1945—Medical care—China. | Physicians—China—Biography. | Internationalists—China—Biography.
Classification: LCC D807.C6 M37 2018 | DDC 940.54/750951—dc23

BRITISH LIBRARY CATALOGUING DATA ARE AVAILABLE

ISBN (print) 978-1-4766-7583-1
ISBN (ebook) 8-1-4766-3426-5

© 2018 Robert Mamlok. All rights reserved

No part of this book may be reproduced or transmitted in any form or by any means, electronic or mechanical, including photocopying or recording, or by any information storage and retrieval system, without permission in writing from the publisher.

Front cover images *from top* Dr. Erich Mamlok's Chinese Red Cross Medical Relief Corps identity card from 1941 (author's collection); the International Medical Relief Corps Unit 32 in Lukou (Hunan Province), China on August 4, 1940, unidentified Chinese medical volunteers with (front row center) Mrs. Mania Kamieniecki and (back row center right) Dr. Erich Mamlok (author's collection); Dr. Adele (Cohn) Wright, an American pulmonologist sent by the American Bureau of Medical Aid to China to the Chinese Red Cross Medical Relief Corps, circa 1940 (courtesy Max Wright)

Printed in the United States of America

*McFarland & Company, Inc., Publishers
    Box 611, Jefferson, North Carolina 28640
    www.mcfarlandpub.com*

Table of Contents

Acknowledgments   vii
Preface   1
Introduction   7

PART I: THE PHYSICIANS' FIGHT AGAINST THE GLOBAL RISE OF FASCISM

1. The Call of Spain: 1936–1939   11
2. The International Medical Response of 1939   21
3. The Call of China: 1936–1939   35
4. The Journey to the Chinese Red Cross Headquarters   60

PART II: THE INTERNATIONAL MEDICAL RELIEF CORPS IN WARTIME CHINA

5. Political and Cultural Conditions at the Chinese Red Cross Medical Relief Corps Headquarters   83
6. Medical Conditions in Wartime China   98
7. Travel to and from China's Battlefields: 1939–1940   112
8. The Forced Restriction of Healthcare Delivery: 1941–1942   129

PART III: THE INTERNATIONAL MEDICAL RELIEF CORPS AND THE CHINESE EXPEDITIONARY FORCES: 1943–1945

9. The International Medical Relief Corps and the Chinese Expeditionary Force in Burma and India   147
10. The International Medical Relief Corps and the Chinese Expeditionary Force in China   167

11. The International Medical Relief Corps' Epilogue:
    1945–2012 186
 12. What Did the International Medical Relief Corps
    Members Accomplish? 193

Appendix A: International Medical Relief Corps Timeline 197
*Appendix B: The International Medical Relief Corps' Memorial
 Dedication (September 1, 2015, Tuyunguan, China)* 201
*Appendix C: Other International Volunteers of the Chinese
 Red Cross* 204
Chapter Notes 209
Bibliography 231
Index 235

Acknowledgments

The present work is not only a tribute to the men and women who fought fascism for the freedom of all, but it is a way for younger people to understand why freedom is very important and how their ancestors stood up against all forms of tyranny because they understood that freedom requires fighting for ideals. All the International Medical Relief Corps doctors were imbued with ideals that motivated them in the fight against the rise of fascism and imperialism. They were fighting for your freedom and their own. And, in so doing, we acknowledge this history of goodwill between the people of North America, Europe, and China. We have a strong proud heritage to celebrate and on which we can build for the future.

Some of the International Medical Relief Corps' members carefully chronicled their travels but much of this information is not available in English or Chinese; thus, many people—especially young people—do not know about the adventures of this unique group of doctors who risked their lives to help the Chinese during the Japanese invasion. However, it is important to acknowledge the works of Dr. Walter Freudmann, who published his memoir of China, *Qi lái! (Arise!)*: *A Physician's Adventures in China and Burma 1939–1945* (German) in 1947, and Dr. Fritz Jensen, who published his memoir of China, *China Siegt (China Wins)*, (German), in 1949. Dr. Rolf Becker wrote *Als Arzt in China (As a Doctor in China)* (German) in 1972. Tania Iancu, daughter of Dr. David Iancu, published her father's 1979 memoir, *9 Ani Medic Pe Front Spania—China (1937-1945) (9 Years on the Front: Spain—China (1937-1945)*, (Romanian) in 2008; and Ulrike Unschuld published *You Banfa—Es Findet Sich Immer ein Weg: Wilhelm Mann's Erinnerungen an China 1938-1966 (There Is Always a Way: Wilhelm Mann's Memories of China, 1938-1966* (German), in 2014.

This work reflects memoirs, letters, and diaries from Drs. Rolf Becker, Carl Coutelle, Erich Mamlok, and Adele (Cohn) Wright. Other International Medical Relief Corps' members, including Drs. Wolf Jungery, Bedřich Kisch,

Frantisek Kriegel, Heinrich Kent, György Somogyi, and Wiktor Taubenfligel shared additional information with their families and friends about their period in China.

However, this project would not have been possible without the generous support, camaraderie, and hundreds of emails with the International Medical Relief Corps' descendant families. Bernard Becker, Dr. Charles Coutelle, Nadia and Tania Iancu, Peter and Dr. Joseph Somogyi, and Max Wright were particularly tireless in sharing their linguistic and historic knowledge and editorial assistance.

In addition, the editors, Kelli Christiansen and Alice Heiserman helped Anglicize this first-time author's diction while the historians Caroline Reeves and the late Theodore Bergmann's encouragement and help were needed to bring this project to fruition. In addition, Yang Yongxuan, Yuan Huimin, Sunny Liu, Chen Guode, and Raye Wang of the Guizhou Provincial Foreign Affair Office and the Guiyang People's Association for Friendship with Foreign Countries were the most gracious of hosts as they commemorated these shared memories with us. Kelong Wang helped to launch this book with his tireless Mandarin translations while Mohammad Shaheen Qureshi provided the finishing touches with his photo editing skills. Finally, my multilingual and loving wife, Dr. Viviane Mamlok and computer savvy son Michael endured endless historic reflections with just the right combination of help, humor, and encouragement. Thank you. Thank you. Thank you.

Preface

On August 31, 2015, I traveled the last six miles of a long journey to the thickly forested hills around the village of Tuyunguan in southwest China. The muggy summer morning mist half hid this sleepy hamlet. A military band, officials from the Chinese Foreign Affairs Office and Consulate Generals awaited our arrival. Tucked in the corner of the park and veiled in crimson silk was a rectangular marble memorial to the twenty-seven foreign volunteers who began joining the Chinese Red Cross Medical Relief Corps in 1939.

Their progeny and I traveled to Guizhou Province to celebrate a new national holiday commemorating the end of the Sino-Japanese War. This war was won, in part, through the efforts of our ancestors. The story of these volunteers and their families, pieced together through their diaries and archives, is an exhilarating tale that shines a spotlight on some of the unsung heroes of World War II.

My father, Dr. Erich Mamlok, was one of the twenty-seven foreign volunteers who joined the Chinese Red Cross Medical Relief Corps in 1939. On that hot August day in 2015, I found myself with three improbable generations of physicians, fashion models, psychologists, and retirees from seven countries. The People's Association for Friendship with Foreign Countries of the Guizhou Foreign Affairs Office had invited us to celebrate their new national holiday marking the end of the Sino-Japanese War. Our Chinese hosts carefully fastened commemorative pins to our lapels, uniting us as a group who could keep alive the memory of our intrepid ancestors.

We spent a week sharing the musty multigenerational memories and faded photos of the work of this courageous group of friends of China. We forged a linguistically tentative yet emotionally earnest friendship connected by the English, German, Romanian, and Polish oral histories of our parents and grandparents. Members of the group narrated adventures and recreated the thrills of the exploits of our families so that we could pass this sliver of history on to the next generation. With each shared story and photo, our questions grew: What were these physicians really like, what hardships and conflicts had they endured, and what legacy had they left behind? This book related their tale.

After the military salutes, a well-orchestrated file of Chinese dignitaries paid their homage to this distant memory. Then, I climbed up to the Tuyunguan memorial podium. I bowed deeply and awkwardly to the rectangular marble memorial. As I spoke, my translated words flashed in Mandarin onto the projection screens I was sandwiched between: "I too am truly honored and humbled to be at this great site. I thank you for the opportunity to share a few of these doctors' words while they were here, in Tuyunguan more than seventy years ago."

As I spoke, I looked out on the thickly forested hills that had once shielded the woefully undermanned remnants of the Chinese Red Cross Medical Relief Corps from the onslaught and horror of the Japanese invasion. The thatched roofs of the bombed Orthopedic Center, the student and faculty dormitories of the Emergency Medical Service Training School, and the 1,000-bed Base Hospital 167 were long gone. Crumbling concrete and newer marble memorials to the Chinese Red Cross stood in their place. I glanced back at the audience and continued:

As many of you know, they appeared with no money, very, very weak Chinese and very, very strong convictions. What were their convictions? Dr. Flato had one written on a flag he had just fought under. It was written in Yiddish and Polish on one side and Spanish on the other. The message was simple and strong: "For your freedom and for ours." It was the reason why he was here. For your freedom and for ours.

His comrade, Dr. Iacob Kranzdorf, paraphrased words from the poet Emma Lazarus and said: "Until we are all free, none of us are free." It is with this world view that his wife Gisela Kranzdorf, Barbara Courtney, and Teddy Wantoch gave their lives in China.

Dr. Becker asked the question: "Was it not also our struggle, which was carried on in China?" and added: "A great country, which did not have sufficient forces to fight back, had been invaded by a conquest-addicted colonial power. China urgently needed help." And so, he came.

Dr. Carl Coutelle came, too. He wrote that "China's war is part of the world war against fascism. By resisting the Japanese aggression, we can stop the advance of fascism and it will allow us to return to our homes and build a better society." And that is just what he did.

Fighting against fascism was the highlight of many of their lives. Dr. Wolf Jungermann wrote: "We worked with an élan and purpose very rarely experienced in life." Dr. Erich Mamlok said that the fight against fascism gave him a clear purpose, too: "Survival is never enough. Rats survive. Humans need to strive for something more."

When journalists in China tried to make sense out of these doctors, they struggled to do so. Some referred to them as "premature anti–Fascists." They meant that these doctors saw the dangers of fascism before others did and that they had the strength and the will to confront it head on. Agnes Smedley, an American journalist, came to Tuyunguan in 1941 and wrote: "These men were entirely different from any other foreigners I had met in China. Despite definite political differences, they were united as anti–Fascists. Unlike several other foreign doctors whom I had known, they dressed, ate, and lived like the Chinese. They saw the conditions in their proper perspective, and responded by shouldering whatever burdens they could."

When Dr. Fritz Jensen was later killed, his friends said: "He showed the strength and bravery of a man who fights for a just cause." The same could be said for all the International Medical Relief Corps' members and those friends in China who shared their vision. And now that I may have embarrassed my friends enough, let us take a moment to recognize the International Medical Relief Corps' families that are with us: Dr. Rolf Becker, Dr. Carl Coutelle, Dr. Stanislaw Flato, Dr. David Iancu, Dr. Wolf Jungermann, Dr. Ianto Kaneti, Dr. Iacob Kranzdorf, Dr. Erich Mamlok, Dr. Wilhelm Mann, and Dr. Wictor "Julio" Taubenfligel.

As the applause for each standing attendee ended, my thoughts drifted back to how this gathering began two years earlier in the attic of the house where my mother had enjoyed the last years of her life. There, I had found a well-traveled trunk with musty memoirs and letters, like what many parents preserve yet often shelter from their children. These were memories that were kept rather than discarded—perhaps in the hope of sharing thoughts that may have been too difficult to tell.

Among the no-longer-important legal and financial statements that littered my parents' attic was a frayed and frustratingly incomprehensible folder of Chinese documents. It included a 1940 identity card of my father, a twenty-six-year-old, German-born, newly minted Jewish physician now with the Chinese Red Cross, voluntarily thrust into the furnace of wartime China. The pictures of his medical colleagues told of their youth and East European origins. They included: Drs. Taubenfligel, Iancu, Kamieniecki, Kaneti, Kranzdorf, and Volokhine along with the more recently renamed Drs. Kent and Jensen.

As I examined these documents and photos, I wondered what I should do with this distant yet compelling very personal information. Was this an important story in need of some personal and historical reflection? Or, by my telling this story, would my parents have just worried that I did not have anything better to do with my time? As I pondered these thoughts, I hoped that trying to understand their lives and perhaps preserving a small piece of the past would outweigh the worries of opening a Pandora's box of emotional baggage. Yet, upon reflection and further research, I realized that their struggles and persistence in the face of major tribulations and bureaucratic political red tape and conditions of war offer a legacy of which all the families and friends of these doctors can be proud.

A few weeks later, Dr. Janny Chen, a Chinese postdoctoral student, rang my doorbell. An underpaid computational biologist working at Texas Tech University, she had answered my request for some Mandarin translations. As

I glanced at her immaculate work and fumbled for my wallet, she stepped backward. Her lovely black eyes forwarded a no-argument look: "No take money. This is a friend of China. China never forgets its friends." My feeble insistence fell far short of her too rapidly departing footsteps.

I was hooked. I knew that I needed to compile this story to discover more details about the motivations and the personal ways that this disparate group fought fascism both during the Spanish Civil War and during the war of Japanese aggression in China, Burma, and even in India. What intrigued me was how much each of the participants hated being sidelined and resented being unable to be useful as medical professionals.

Based on the hints I received from my parents' attic, the hunt for the other International Medical Relief Corps' descendants was on. Some of them were well known and easy to locate. Dr. Charles Coutelle, the British-born, Emeritus Professor of Gene Therapy at Imperial College, London, was my first contact. He, in turn, located Bernard Becker, the Shanghai-born son of Dr. Rolf Becker, and he got in contact with the nieces of Dr. Wilhelm Mann in Italy. Just as the doctors had been from many countries, so too were their descendants. The children and grandchildren of Dr. Taubenfligel were in Canada, and the daughters and son of Dr. Iancu were in Romania and Canada, respectively. Karin Kleiner, the surviving daughter of Dr. Jungermann, and cousins of Drs. Kisch and Kriegel were in the United States.

Genealogical websites also provided help, along with obituaries, to locate the Polish-born children of Dr. Stanislaw Flato in Sweden. Dr. Robert Lin's granddaughters were in Jamaica and England, and Dr. Kaneti's granddaughters were in America.

To discover details about the lives of the members of the International Medical Relief Corps, we exchanged hundreds of emails and shared diaries and letters. We visited archives of the Hoover Institute, Columbia University, Arizona State University, New York University, The League of Nations and Guiyang, China, as well as the National Archives of Great Britain, the United States, and the Czech Republic. We researched and gathered existing German, Romanian, Polish, Mandarin, and English literature about the International Medical Relief Corps and its members.

The International Medical Relief Corps included twenty-one physicians, one biochemist, two nurses, one laboratory technician, one administrative assistant, and one medical student. Although born in ten different nations, their love of medicine and the fight against fascism united all of them.

During their time in China, three of them (Dr. Barbara Courtney, Dr. Arno Theodor Wantoch, and Mrs. Gisela Kranzdorf) gave their lives and were buried in China. Ten of them got married in China—Dr. Rolf Becker and Joan (Staniforth) Becker, Dr. Adele (Cohn) Wright, Dr. Heinrich and Edith (Marens) Kent, Dr. Fritz Jensen, Dr. Ianto Kaneti, Dr. Iacob Kranzdorf

[Bucur Clejan], Dr. George Schön [György Somogyi], and Dr. Władyslaw "Wolf" Jungermann [Jungery]—and several of their children were born in China. Nineteen of the twenty-seven International Medical Relief Corps' members had served previously with the Republicans in the Spanish Civil War, and ten of them went on to serve with the Chinese Expeditionary Force in Burma.

All told, these twenty-one men and six women spent between four and twenty-five years of their lives caring in China for the Chinese. They were a young, idealistic group of healthcare providers ranging from twenty-four (Dr. Wilhelm Mann) to forty-five (Dr. Bedřick Kisch) years of age. They shared great pride in their slow but progressive command of Chinese and their ability to live, eat, and serve together with their Chinese medical colleagues.

They spoke out strongly against the horrors of war and could not ignore whatever corruption, inhumanity, and inequality they saw. The International Medical Relief Corps' members harshly denounced those who tried to limit their opportunities to help the Chinese people they had come so far to serve. They developed a keen and practical sense of public health needs, and they contributed to the recognition and management of infectious diseases and nutritional disorders and to the improvement of the military medicine strategy.

Theirs is a story worth telling—although it remains an incomplete one. Despite our best efforts, the story told in these pages suffers from the fog of war, time, and language. However, the story shares many of the motivations that led the International Medical Relief Corps' members along the path to serving with the Chinese Red Cross. This book presents their fate through the first-hand voices from International Medical Relief Corps' members and the friends and foes they encountered from 1938 to 1945. This tale relates their personal convictions and dogged determination to provide medical help to the people of China and simultaneously fight oppressive menaces of fascism and corruption thousands of miles away from home.

Introduction

In the 1930s, the global voice of tolerance fell to a whisper as the strident calls of fascism rose to a roar. European nations, families, and friends scurried to find shelter and answers: "What to do?" "Where to go?" and "Who and what to fight with?"

At the same time, Japanese imperialism scorched the soil and soul of China. The same questions of, "What to do?" and "Where to go?" trembled off millions of lips as Japan forced China into a world at war. Pacifists, warmongers, and bystanders shared their competing visions and created unique international alliances. Among them was a group of two dozen Western and fifteen dozen Chinese physicians who would be bound together in the newly formed Medical Relief Corps of the Chinese Red Cross, deep in the interior of wartime China.

The improbable story of the Chinese Red Cross/Medical Relief Corps began with the clash between strong-willed individuals and the global political conflicts that engulfed them. In Europe, young, predominantly Jewish physicians faced tough questions that often placed them at odds with friends and family. You can imagine the family arguments, the hysteria, the tears. The times were perilous. Each day the Jewish community saw new encroachments on their liberties. Many wondered whether they would survive if they ignored the rise of fascism and kept a low profile. Surely, the insanity of the politics of the day would resolve and reason would again prevail.

Or, would their survival be better insured if they rallied to the cause of communism, an ideology that most directly opposed the rise of fascism in Europe in the 1930s? Had the time now come to take up arms and give their lives in the most righteous of fights? Finally, were they striving for something more meaningful than their personal survival?

In 1936, when Hitler and Mussolini backed the Nationalist forces of General Franco and attempted to overthrow the democratically elected and Soviet Union backed Republicans in Spain, more than 30,000 international volunteers rallied to the Republican side. Fighting for Spain's freedom from fascism was something these volunteers all sought. The Spanish Civil War quickly became a testing ground of the international resolve to confront the rise of fascism in Europe.

Most European and North American nations did not yet see the value of joining the fight against fascism and maintained a strict non-intervention policy. They would not send troops nor allow their citizens to go to fight as volunteers, and they would not supply any help including medical aid. The Communist International, or Comintern, was an exception. They coordinated the clandestine enlistment and transport of volunteers from different national communist parties and the International Brigades of the Republican Army were born. However, the German tanks and Italian aircraft of the Nationalists routed the outgunned and overmatched Republicans. The surviving International Brigade volunteers retreated to the border of Spain and France where confinement in primitive internment camps awaited them.

These volunteers arrived in Spain as healthcare providers without borders but had now become men and women without countries. Most of them could not go back to their country of origin due to the Nazi hatred of Jews and others could not return because of their alliance with the communists. They were truly people without a country and their options of where to go and how to survive were very limited.

At the same time, other, younger European physicians, who were just finishing their medical studies in 1939, had broader options. Should they pursue applying for visas to England, Shanghai or South America with their friends and families? And, if they did, would they still be able to fight in the war against fascism?

International turmoil was not restricted to Europe. On September 18, 1931, the Kwantung Army of the Empire of Japan invaded Manchuria and set up a Japanese state called *Manchukuo*. Thus, what became World War II descended earlier on the Chinese. The war in China escalated into full-scale conflict in July 1937, when both sides—on the pretext of an incident at the Marco Polo Bridge near Beijing—embarked on open war. The Imperial Japanese Army quickly swept through and occupied the large eastern coastal cities of China where most modern ethnic Chinese doctors practiced in the universities and medical clinics.

Much as the International Brigade physicians were trapped in internment camps on the Spanish border, many Chinese physicians were now trapped in the Japanese occupied coastal cities of eastern China. The options for physicians in China to resist the Japanese occupation were limited and further complicated as there were two opposing forces within China—the Chinese Nationalists led by General Chiang Kai-shek who virulently opposed the Chinese communists led by Chairman Mao Zedong. While they both actively resisted the Japanese invasion, they hated each other. This distrust and lack of cooperation between them led to many unnecessary deaths as the staff and supplies could not freely travel between the areas of the Chinese Nationalists and the communists.

By 1938, the Imperial Japanese Army had forced General Chiang Kai-shek's battered Chinese Nationalist, or Guomindang government to retreat westward, nearly two thousand miles into the interior of China. In the 1930s, the backwater southwestern Chinese cities of Chongqing and Guiyang were not places that urbanites from Shanghai and Beijing could easily reach. The headquarters of the Chinese Communist Party was as remote. Chairman Mao Zedong had barely survived his prior Long March and battle with Chiang Kai-shek's Guomindang Nationalist Party in 1935. The northern Chinese city of Yan'an became the home base of the Chinese Communist Party, almost one thousand miles northwest of Shanghai. The Chinese Communist Party kept separate control from the Guomindang Nationalist Party over its Eighth Route and New Fourth Armies that waged guerrilla campaigns in Japanese occupied China.

Unity between the Chinese Communist Party and the Guomindang Nationalist Party in the fight against Japan would remain a hope that was tentative and temporary. In addition, the Chinese Army did not have an effective medical service. Corruption and lack of centralized control reduced the services of the Chinese Army Medical Administration to its bare bones. A loose network of warlords kept a tentative alliance with the Guomindang Nationalist Party and the Army Medical Administration gave medical care to the millions of conscripted soldiers that was little more than an afterthought.

However, the German bombing of Guernica, Spain, and the Japanese Rape of Nanjing, China, shocked a world engulfed in humanitarian crises. Putting aside the politics of the day and liberating the underutilized and endangered physicians in Europe and China was the task at hand. English, Norwegian, American, and Chinese Medical Aid Committees came together. In China, the responsibility of providing medical aid to the Chinese Army fell on the Army Medical Administration and, ultimately, on the newly created Chinese Red Cross/ Medical Relief Corps and its charismatic leader, Dr. Robert Lin.

Most of the ethnic Chinese who were practitioners of modern biomedicine remained in the relative safety of the occupied universities and clinics in the large coastal cities and only a small and brave minority of these Chinese physicians answered Dr. Lin's call for help. The China Medical Aid Committees in Europe had to overcome a distrusting Comintern to get the release of the European physicians to serve China while Dr. Robert Lin had to overcome a distrusting Guomindang Nationalist Party to allow his Chinese Red Cross/ Medical Relief Corps to serve all the Chinese; particularly those in the areas of China controlled by the Chinese Communist Party. The competing wish of most of the European physicians to serve in the Chinese Communist Party-controlled areas and the Guomindang Nationalist Party's wish to restrict medical aid to the Chinese Communist Party-controlled areas would inevitably place these physicians again in an endangered role. In this cauldron of catastrophically unmet medical needs and political divisions, these young physicians would learn how to strive for both their patients' survival and their medical and political conscience.

I. THE PHYSICIANS' FIGHT AGAINST
THE GLOBAL RISE OF FASCISM

1. The Call of Spain: 1936–1939

The rise of fascism in the mid-1930s in Europe had forced many of the twenty-seven future members of the International Medical Relief Corps out of their medical schools and practices and into exile. Only the uncertainty of their individual survival united them. The Nazis revoked or restricted medical degrees of several physicians because of their ethnicity or political convictions. Then, by the late 1930s, most of the future International Medical Relief Corps' physicians were displaced persons or asylum seekers from ten separate countries who had fled their homelands due to political or religious persecution.

For example, the "non-Aryan" medical diplomas earned by the Jewish graduates of the University of Vienna, Austria, such as Drs. Fritz Jensen (严斐德医生 Yan Feide) and Arno Theodor Wantoch (王道医生 Wang Dao), either forbade them from practicing medicine or overtly revoked their licensure.[1] Other medical schools placed strict limits (*numerus clausus*) on the admission of Jewish students, forcing many future International Medical Relief Corps' physicians to study abroad. German medical schools, such as the University of Berlin (*Friedrich-Wilhelms Universität zu Berlin*), classified student transcripts based on a student's membership in fascist organizations such as the German Student Union (*Der Deutschen Studentenschaft*). The German Student Union became best known for its overt anti-Semitism and book-burning campaigns until the Allied command declared it an illegal organization in 1945.

While fascism and its ominous forebodings had yet to reach everyone, Jewish-German medical students, such as Dr. Erich Mamlok, (孟乐克医生 Meng Leke), understood its potential. Not only were non-Aryan and newly graduated physicians reeling from persecution, but all the future International Medical Relief Corps' physicians already practicing medicine in Europe were also feeling the repercussions of fascism. Some of them, such as Dr. Fritz Jensen, were arrested and placed in concentration camps (KZ Wöllersdorf);

others, such as Dr. Carl Coutelle (顾泰尔医生 Gu Taier), were forced to flee their native lands because of their political views. Almost all would endure an endless stream of refugee, internment, and concentration camps. The distinction between these types of camps is not always clear. The term "refugee camp" describes mass voluntary detention while the "internment camps" and "concentration camps" denote mass involuntary detention. The term *concentration camp* is most associated with the German National Socialists who used these camps to confine millions of Jews and others to be purged from the German state.

Several of the future Jewish International Medical Relief Corps' members changed their names in an attempt to escape the pervasiveness of anti-Semitism. Dr. Friedrich Jerusalem became Dr. "Fritz" Jensen. Dr. Heinrich Kohn became Dr. "Carner" Kent (肯德医生 Kende). Dr. Wladyslaw Jungermann became Dr. "Wolf" Jungery (戎格曼医生 Rong), Dr. George Schön (Schoen) became known as Dr. György Somogyi (沈恩医生 Shen En) and the Romanian Dr. Iacob (Jacob) Kranzdorf became Dr. Bucur Clejan (柯让道医生 Ke Rangdao).

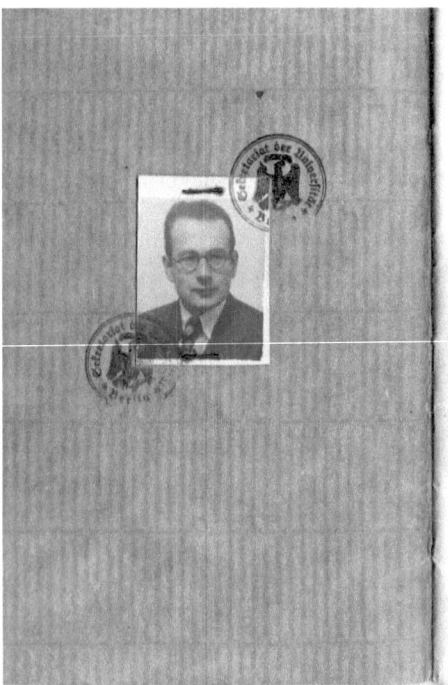

Dr. Erich Mamlok's University of Berlin (*Friedrich-Wilhelms-Universität zu Berlin*) medical student book of 1936 ominously branded as: "*Nicht mitglied der Deutschen Studentenschaft*" (Not a member of the German student union) (author's collection).

On July 18, 1936, when the Spanish rightwing General Francisco Franco headed a revolt against Spain's elected leftist Republican government, these doctors saw a path to joining the struggle against fascism. Twenty of the future International Medical Relief Corps' physicians rallied to the Republicans side. They were part of almost 30,000 men and woman who ignored their native government's neutrality and joined the Spanish Republicans.

These medical volunteers became part of the International Brigades, which the Comintern organized in 1936. The number of physicians who reached the International Brigade is unknown. This lack of documentation is not surprising, as their journey was clandestine to protect them from arrest for attempting to join the armed forces of a foreign country. The Comintern gave each country's communist party a specific number of volunteers to recruit. The Comintern also sent several leaders to help the French Communist Party coordinate the creation of the International Brigade.

These physicians fled their homelands in central and east Europe. When they arrived as volunteers in Spain, the Spanish Republicans hailed them as heroes. Dr. Walter Freudmann (富华德医生 Fu Huade), an Austrian International Brigade and future International Medical Relief Corps doctor, captured the palpable excitement of their newfound camaraderie: "I was now among thousands of raised fists that had welcomed us."[2]

After their warm welcome, the International Medical Relief Corps' physicians quickly became close comrades as they developed their linguistic and military skills in the International Brigades. They were among the more than 250 physicians from 25 countries who had volunteered to serve with the International Brigade. The multinational medical corps of the International Brigade included forty-two Polish doctors, the largest national group of volunteer physicians in Spain. Among the Polish medical volunteers was twenty-nine-year-old Dr. Wiktor Taubenfligel (陶维德医生 Tao Weide). He left Poland to complete his medical studies at the University of Padua, Italy, and rose to the rank of captain and battalion doctor in the predominantly Polish Dabrowski or XIIIth Brigade.[3] The affable Taubenfligel was known to all as "Julio."

In the International Brigade, Spanish slowly replaced Yiddish, Polish, English, and a multitude of other foreign tongues. The multilingual International Brigade doctors would often sign letters they wrote to their friends and families with a valiant, but less than prophetic, "*Salut y Victoria!* (Greetings and Victory!)"

Dr. Wladislav ("Wolf") Jungermann, another Polish-born future International Medical Relief Corps' physician, was forced to flee his native land. He completed his medical studies in Serbia at the University of Belgrade. When the Comintern began to recruit an International Brigade to help the Spanish Republicans in their fight against the Spanish Nationalists, scores of

Jewish Communist Party volunteers welcomed the privilege of fighting against the anti–Semitism of fascism and for the ideals of the Communist International. By 1935, the Comintern had broadened its appeal with the creation of the Popular Front (1935–1939), which united moderate socialists and other forces resisting fascism.

These medical volunteers never questioned that they were fighting for a just and right cause. Dr. Jungermann later reflected: "We worked in Tarancon [Spain] with an élan and purpose very rarely experienced in life."[4]

Like Drs. Jungermann and Taubenfligel, the Polish-born Dr. Stanislaw (Moishe) Flato (柯理格医生 Fu Ladu) had to complete his medical studies abroad. Dr. Flato, who came from a small middle-class family, became active in left-wing student and Jewish worker organizations. While attending the Sorbonne University Medical School in Paris, France, Flato became a member of the French Communist Party. He was one of the first International Medical Relief Corps' physicians to head south in December of 1936 to answer the call of Spain.[5] Dr. Flato's medical colleagues shared memories of his charismatic and down-to-earth character:

> In all the ceremonies and gatherings there can be found a young thirty-year-old major who mixes with the troops whom he speaks to in a juicy Yiddish, which has the barely noticeable trace of a Polish accent. If the Major stands out from those around him by his rank, he overcomes this through his simplicity and lively interest in the Jewish boys in such a manner that he is considered just another Jewish volunteer as the rest of us. The older members of the Botwin Company will say to you that is Dr. Flato, the head of the medical service, formerly in charge of the 13th Brigade and lately head of the 35th Division…. Flato's face lights up when he talks about the impression the Botwin company has made on the staff of the Brigade and the division. The doctor has many friends especially among the wounded [whom] he has taken care of and healed.[6]

Information about the pre- and postwar experiences of the fourth Polish born physician, Dr. Leon Kamieniecki (甘理安医生 Gan Lian), and his wife Mania (甘曼妮 Gan Manni) is scant. Both came from the then–Polish part of Lithuania. They went separately to Spain to join the International Brigade, he as a doctor and she as a bacteriologist. Dr. Kamieniecki and Mania were married in Spain, sharing a close professional and personal relationship throughout the war in Spain and China.

In addition to the Poles Drs. Taubenfligel, Jungermann, Flato, and Kamieniecki, three German-born physicians—Drs. Herbert Baer (贝尔医生 Beier), Rolf Becker (白乐夫医生 Bai Lefu), and Carl Coutelle, as well as Edith Marens (马绮迪 Ma Kusi)—would serve in both Spain and China. These German nationals had taken a path that relatively few of their German and Italian compatriots followed. In fact, most of the foreigners who took part in the Spanish Civil War, fought with Franco's Nationalists. More than 70,000 Italian and 14,000 Germans soldiers fought against the Republicans.[7]

Dr. Baer was born to a Jewish family in the then-Prussian province of Posen on April 2, 1898. As a member of the German Communist Party, he needed to flee to Czechoslovakia in 1935. As the chief inpatient physician of the 45th Division of the International Brigade, his commanders spoke highly of his political acumen and mature organizational skills.[8] Dr. Baer's more youthful German International Medical Relief Corps friends, Drs. Becker and Coutelle, would later refer to Dr. Baer as *Der Alte* ("old man"). In 1936, at age thirty-eight, he was six years older than Dr. Becker, who had completed his medical studies in Tubingen, Germany, before answering the call of the Spanish Republicans. Dr. Becker traveled across Western Europe to reach the Spanish Pyrenees that year. Once in Spain, he served throughout the battlefront as a brigade and battalion physician, based in the hospital at Benicassim.

Dr. Becker's compatriot, Dr. Coutelle, was twenty-eight years old in 1936. Born in Elberfeld, Germany, Dr. Coutelle had completed his medical training in Freiburg, Germany. His membership in the German Communist Party resulted in the loss of his medical license in 1933, and he immigrated to the Soviet Union. Dr. Coutelle joined the International Brigade and arrived in Spain in 1937.[9]

The twenty-nine-year old Edith Marens, the fourth German healthcare provider to serve in both Spain and China, hailed from Hannover, Germany, where she was born on November 17, 1908. Some historians reported that Marens was married to the Spanish Civil War Veteran Fritz Marcus, but most sources refer to her by the name, Edith Marens.[10] In 1937, as a medical student, she was forced to emigrate from Germany to present day Yugoslavia before she arrived in Spain. Marens worked as a radiology technician together with Dr. Jungermann in Taragon, Spain.[11]

Two additional, and arguably the most gifted of the International Medical Relief Corps' physicians, Drs. Frantisek "Franta" Kriegel (柯理格医生 Ke Lige) and Bedřich Kisch (纪瑞德医生 Ji Ruide) are best identified with Czechoslovakia. However, Dr. Kriegel was born in Stanislau, Ukraine, which became part of Poland between the two World Wars. The Nazis forced him to immigrate to Czechoslovakia, where he completed his studies at the University of Prague Medical School in 1934. He, too, became a member of the Communist Party, and the Comintern approved his wish to volunteer for service with the International Brigade in Spain in 1936. He became the chief physician of the XIth Division of the International Brigade and led a group of twenty-one physicians serving six thousand men. People praised Dr. Kriegel's medical and military skills as much as they recounted his faults. The French Communist Party shared concerns in 1938 about his authoritarian character and his individualistic tendencies.

One of Dr. Kriegel's International Brigade medical colleagues and future biographer, Dr. Gabriel Ersler, quoted Dr. Taubenfligel's opinion: "Kriegel is sure of himself and sometimes behaves in a brutal manner towards others ... despite all this, he is probably the most gifted among us." Dr. Flato also shared Dr. Taubenfligel's concern: "Franta Kriegel is an energetic and capable man, but with a very strong personal ambition that sometimes leads to serious mistakes and even a lack of discipline to the Party."[12]

Dr. Bedřich Kisch, a highly respected trauma surgeon, was the other Czechoslovakian physician who served in both Spain and China. Dr. Glaser, the head of the International Brigade medical command, described Kisch in 1938 as a "good surgeon with broad experience, conscientious of his responsibilities and able to get good results with his interventions. He is easy to get along with and his character is frank and clear with his comrades."[13] Later, Kisch would serve with future International Medical Relief Corps physicians: Drs. Volokhine, Iancu, and Kent. In addition, Dr. Norman Bethune (白求恩 Baiqiuen), a Canadian, would serve briefly under Kisch.[14]

Drs. Fritz Jensen, Walter Freudmann, and Heinrich Kent were three Austrian physicians who also would serve in both Spain and China. Dr. Jensen joined the Spanish Republicans in August 1936 and became the chief physician of the XIIIth Brigade. He received wounds in the Battle of Brunete in 1936 in Spain, and separated from his second wife, Ruth Domino Jerusalem (RN), in 1937.[15] He was fortunate to have escaped from Franco's forces to Paris in 1938. Dr. Jensen's International Medical Relief Corps friend, Dr. Becker wrote:

> I knew him [Jensen] since the spring of 1937 under the burning sun of Andalucía, where the XIIIth International Brigade was actively resisting the assault of the Fascist bands of Franco.... He was a good and wise doctor that the French, German, Spanish, Czech, and Austrians all submitted to, in the mountains of Teruel, in the hills of Andalucía, in the fiery combat for Madrid, in the abysses of Ebro, everywhere where the blood of Spanish and international fighters flowed, Fritz risked his life thousands of times as the brigade doctor and later as the chief doctor of the division. Not just a few times was it necessary to admonish him to be more careful when he himself carried a stretcher in order to take a wounded comrade out of the line of fire. He showed the strength and bravery of a man who fights for a just cause.[16]

Writing with "Antifascist greetings from Barcelona in March 1938," Dr. Jensen summarized his reasons for going to Spain:

> I wanted to do everything I could to fight against those who threaten the life and existence of my own compatriots and myself.... We feel extremely thankful to the Spanish folk for giving us the possibility of this sort of fight against fascism. This possibility should be used wherever and however it exists.... We ourselves are in a difficult situation. My own country was occupied by Nazi Fascism while I was working here in Spain. A lot of my comrades, because in their land fascism is in power, are in the same situation. There is no land that wants to accept us.[17]

Dr. Jensen's fellow University of Vienna Medical School alumni, Drs. Freudmann and Kent, left Austria and joined the Spanish Republicans in 1937. Dr. Freudmann's initial joy at "being among thousands of raised fists of like-minded progressives" was soon replaced by his "hard work at the military hospital on the Jarama front, the dramatic days of the battle of Teruel, the joyous victory at Brunete, the temperamental songs of the Spanish village girls and the bitter retreat over the Pyrenees to France."[18]

Dr. Kent had been working in a tuberculosis clinic in Vienna for three years prior to the start of the Spanish Civil War, and it is probable that he contracted tuberculosis in this setting. With the help of the Austrian Communist Party, he joined the International Brigade in 1938 and became the hospital director in Mataro, 30 kilometers northeast of Barcelona. He fell in love and married the Spanish nurse Maria Rodriquez, a thirty-one-year-old Galician who had worked as a dressmaker in the small town of Boveda in northwest Spain before completing her training in nursing school.[19] Dr. Kent's friend, Moses Ausubel, described him as a strict Stalinist and a man who rarely showed his emotions at that time.[20] However, Dr. Kent's calm outward demeanor covered a troubled and conflicted soul tormented by bouts of depression.

Dr. Alexander Volokhine (何乐经医生 He Lejing) and the German nationals Drs. Becker and Coutelle were the only so called "Spanish doctors" in the International Medical Relief Corps not born to Jewish parents. The Asian press coined the term "Spanish doctors" to acknowledge these International Brigade physicians' Spanish Civil War experiences prior to their service in China. At the same time, many "Spanish journalists" would report from both Spain and China. Their ranks included W.H. Auden, Robert Capa, Martha Gellhorn, Ernest Hemingway, and John Rich.

The son of White Russians living in exile in France, Dr. Volokhine's family remained politically divided by the Russian Civil War (1917–22). His parents had fled from Russia to France as members of the White Russian movement that had opposed the "Red," or Soviet, rule. His International Brigade medical colleague Dr. Ersler wrote, "He [Volokhine] hoped that his services in Spain would make up for his parents turning their backs on the Soviet Union and permit him to rehabilitate himself and be allowed to live there. He desired to separate himself from his parents and not be blamed for their flight from and attitude toward the Soviet Union. As a French citizen, he was placed in the French section [of the International Brigade] and labeled [as being of] White Russian descent."[21]

The Spanish Civil War mirrored the Russian Civil War as several hundred Russian advisors fought with the Republicans and less than a hundred White Russians joined Franco's nationalist side. The irrevocable division of many families occurred when their children chose to take on an early role in the fight against fascism. As Drs. Volokhine, Becker, and Coutelle strove to realize their communist and anti-Fascist convictions, their families chose to disown them. Several of the International Medical Relief Corps' physicians were willing to pay this painful price.

Dr. George Schön, the only Hungarian physician in the International Medical Relief Corps, was born into a Jewish family in Szeged, Hungary, in 1912. He completed his medical studies at the University of Bologna in Italy. Much like many of the Jewish International Brigade members, Dr. Schön's attraction to the communist party came from the hope that they would end the persecution of Jews in his native land.

Dr. Schön left Hungary with the plan to travel by sea from Marseille to Barcelona in the spring of 1937 with the steamship, *Ciudad de Barcelona*. Fortunately, he missed the embarkation as an Italian submarine sank the *Ciudad de Barcelona* off the coast of Barcelona on May 30, 1937. Dr. Schön subsequently succeeded in reaching Spain where he joined the Spanish Communist Party in 1937 and became a medical captain in the XIVth Division of the International Brigade.[22]

The twenty-seven-year-old Romanian-born physician Dr. David Iancu (杨固医生 Yang Gu) arrived in Spain in April 1937. He had graduated from the University of Iasi, Romania, Medical School and responded to the Romanian Communist Party's plea for volunteers for the International Brigade. Dr. Iancu served with the medical headquarters of the XIIIth Division on the Andalusian Front in southern Spain together with Drs. Jensen and Becker. As with many of the International Brigade Divisions, they bore much of the frontline action and a disproportionately high number of casualties. Dr. Iancu survived the decimation of the XIIIth Division and joined the XVth Division where he fought with Dr. Freudmann in the battle of Teruel.

Other physicians in the XVth Division, such as the American, Dr. Edward Barsky, were to survive this conflict but ultimately also lose their medical licenses because of their political convictions. After the war, Dr. Barsky was subpoenaed when he refused to release financial records from the Joint Anti-Fascist Refugee Committee. He was held in contempt of Congress and imprisoned. Upon his release, the New York State Board of Regents suspended his medical license. After years of appeals, the U.S. Supreme Court upheld a six-month suspension of his license. In a dissenting opinion, Judge William O. Douglas asserted, "When a doctor cannot save lives in America because he is opposed to Franco in Spain, it is time to call a halt and look critically at the neurosis that has possessed us."[23]

Dr. Iancu later joined his compatriot, Dr. Iacob Kranzdorf in Barcelona.[24] Dr. Kranzdorf was born in Bucharest to a Jewish family, the eighth of twelve children. He too, studied abroad, and graduated from the University of Parma, Italy, medical school. He practiced dermatology in Bucharest and married his neighborhood sweetheart, Gisela Goldstein (柯芝兰 Ke Zhilan). Her family was very active in underground revolutionary activities.[25] Dr. Kranzdorf credited Gisela with his participation in the Communist Party and subsequent travel to Spain: "Fortunately, she led me on the right track, or else my life would have been meaningless."[26]

Dr. Kranzdorf described his harrowing trip from Romania to Spain as a clandestine journey through the Pyrenees where,

> If we got lost, we might encounter wolves, but even more frightening was to encounter the French border police—a catch, a hit, and then to be returned home. As doctors, we had never before endured hunger, braving the cold and wet, and finally barely being able to move our legs forward. And in our hearts, we have only one goal, that is, for our own and for other people's national struggle for freedom.[27]

In winter 1938–39, Dr. Kranzdorf belatedly reached Spain—just as the civil war was coming to its fiery end.

Robert Jordan, Ernest Hemingway's fictional American International Brigade protagonist in *For Whom the Bell Tolls*, captured what many of these young physicians' likely felt about the Spanish Civil War at that time:

> You felt, in spite of all bureaucracy and inefficiency and party strife, something that was like the feeling you expected to have and did not have when you made your first communion. It was a feeling of consecration to a duty toward all the oppressed of the world which would be as difficult and embarrassing to speak about as religious experience and yet it was authentic…[28]

The passion of fighting for a just international cause united many of these young healthcare providers in more than medical and military ways. Love and marriage abounded. In addition to Leon and Mania Kamieniecki (a Lithuanian/Polish couple), Carl Coutelle and Rosa Sussman (a German/Polish couple), Wolf Jungermann and Edith Marens (a Polish/German couple), and the Austrian/Spanish couple Heinrich Kent and Maria Gonzales Rodriquez all wed in Spain.

Despite the strength of their common conviction and heroic medical efforts, the Spanish Civil War did not go well. With the fall of Barcelona, the International Brigade fell back into the ranks of the retreating Republican army near the French border. Dr. Jensen described the International Brigade's retreat in his 1955 memoir:

> They threw themselves into gaps that emerged on the front and a few hours later, the German tanks were at their backs, the Italian aviators over our heads and the Moroccan machine guns on all sides. This final battle was about crossing over the border. Positions were held until they had to be abandoned. One withdrew, moved to new positions, which again were bypassed by the enemy, until finally the French Spanish border was reached. Then the crossing to France … where you finally hoped to find a way to rest, to treat the wounded and after the hunger of the last months in Spain, to eat.[29]

Dr. Iancu marked this solemn occasion:

> In Spain there was no longer cheering, just the police and a concentration camp. We retreated into the Pyrenees Mountains and in February 1939 crossed into France.... We were all overcome by the great pain of departing from a land and a people to whom we felt tied, a land under whose soil many of our brothers lay forever as witnesses of the Romanian folk's love of liberty and justice.[30]

Although overcome by pain, the physicians of the International Brigade could take some solace in knowing that they had "evolved from an improvised medical service to a highly regulated medical organization of a modern army" Dr. Jensen wrote. "It was a remarkable fact that this was brought about by the combined efforts of doctors from various countries. The final form was a product of collaboration combining features of the German, French, and British medical services."[31]

This international cooperation resulted in such military medicine innovations as mobile, frontline surgical and transfusion services, in addition to numerous surgical and medical triage innovations.[32]

The American Quaker, John Rich, who would later follow the International Medical Relief Corps' members to China, shared the resolute convictions of many of the Republicans in Spain in 1939: "I am glad to have been involved in this Spanish War and to have contributed something to its pacification. If I died today, I could at least say I've done something worthwhile."[33] Six other anti-fascist physicians would soon join these fifteen Spanish Doctors in the fight against Japanese imperialism in Asia. Despite the pain and sorrow of the Spanish Republicans' military defeat, it was already clear that the future International Medical Relief Corps members' and their multi-denominational friends' spirit would be hard to crush.

2. The International Medical Response of 1939

As the remnants of the Spanish Republican army and their International Brigade supporters fled across the Spanish border to France in 1939, the French government reacted to the Spanish Civil War refugee crisis by establishing primitive internment camps in the towns of Gurs, Argeles, and St. Cyprien at the foot of the Pyrenees Mountains near the Mediterranean Sea. Heavily armed French soldiers and their colonial Senegalese mercenaries quickly gathered tens of thousands of refugees to these sites. This included the battered remnants of the Republican Army, and most of the International Medical Relief Corps physicians who served in Spain. International Medical Relief Corps physician, Dr. Iacob Kranzdorf, described his detention in camp Gurs:

> Gurs was several kilometers long. It was divided into several small partitions with barbed wire, and guarded by police and military troops stationed there.... The camp has large tents arrayed in columns ... they are made to accommodate 80 people each, and everyone is lying side by side.... The concentration camp diet is sorely lacking; hard beans every day, sometimes with smelly salted fish ... everyone is infested with lice and fleas, we are hungry, yellow and bone thin.... Due to the adverse conditions many of the people are buried in the desert next to the camp ground. However, even in this environment, we still secretly hold party meetings and have organized a secret published mimeographed newspaper.[1]

The futility of trying to establish a medical clinic without supplies from the French authorities dismayed many International Brigade physicians, such as the strong-willed Dr. Franta Kriegel. In February 1939, Dr. Kriegel fell out of favor with Eduardo "Edo" d'Onufrio and the other communist leaders of the camp because he refused to oversee the health service of this Brigade. This refusal to go along with the Comintern's directives kept him at odds with the Polish Communist Party cell. His defiance excluded him from all political activities of the Communist Party and work in the medical camps.[2]

The International Medical Relief Corps physicians based in Barcelona, Drs. Kisch and Jensen, were fortunate to avoid internment and travelled to Paris with the help of the British nurse Patience Darton whom they had befriended on the Ebro front.[3] Dr. Jensen later wrote of his colleagues' collective misery after he secured permission to visit the camp in Gurs.

> The camps were a sandy desert, not far from the sea. A cold, sand-laden wind blew without interruption day and night. Sand was everywhere. In the clothes, the food, the bedding. The sand penetrated the comrade's eyes, they breathed it in, it filled the spaces between their teeth and sat firmly imbedded in their nasal mucosa.... Immense flat squares, surrounded by barbed wire were guarded by black colonial troops. Within the barbed wire there was just sand and a cold sky, and between the sky and sand was the spring wind: these were the camp in southern France, where three hundred thousand soldiers of the Spanish Republic lived.... Many were wounded, more suffering from dysentery and typhoid, and all suffered from the hunger and cold.... I saw in the faces of my comrades the tiredness of the last struggles and in their bodies the leanness that comes from rigors and hunger. In their clothes they bore the dust of the earth and their eyelids were inflamed by powdery sands. But in their eyes was the steadfastness of fighters against Fascism, the discipline that belongs to the cause of progress, and their confidence in their class and party.[4]

This internment was another test of the strength of the International Medical Relief Corps members' convictions. It would not be their last battle against hunger and infectious disease.

The International Medical Relief Corps' physicians viewed their defeat in Spain as just an early battle in the global fight against fascism. With unshaken passion, Dr. Iacob Kranzdorf paraphrased the poet Emma Lazarus[5] from Camp Gurs in 1939: "Unless all human beings are to be free, no one is free."[6] However, they realized that there were no guarantees for their personal freedom and safety. In the process of acting as physicians without borders, they had become men and women without countries. Their political convictions and/or ethnicity made them *persona non grata* who could not return to their native lands. Trapped in limbo, they anxiously awaited their destiny in what they now referred to as the "Spanish waiting warehouses."[7]

Fortunately, and unknown to the interned International Brigade physicians, several organizations were being formed with the goal of helping these doctors continue their fight against fascism. When the International Brigade physicians learned that the Comintern was planning to help with China's anti–Fascist war against Japan, more than forty physicians volunteered to leave the internment camps and go to China. The Comintern decided to allocate the few available Chinese Red Cross positions for foreign physician volunteers in proportion to the number of each nationality's concentration camp internees.[8] Drs. Carl and Rosa Coutelle explained:

> With the dismissal of the International Brigade in Spain, everyone had to name the country in which he hoped to get asylum. We chose China, in the belief that the fight

against Fascism was now worldwide, and that we could apply our "Spanish experience" best in the anti–Japanese struggle. So naïve that sounded at that time, but it turned out to be a lifesaving decision.[9]

Dr. Becker echoed the logic of continuing the international fight against fascism by helping China:

> We did not live in Spain isolated from world politics, and the shadow of a new war was visible everywhere. Even in the hospital of the International Brigades in Benicasim, I had given a lecture on the development in China and the aggression of the Japanese imperialists. Was it not also our struggle, which was carried on there in the Far East? A great country had been invaded by a conquest-addicted colonial power, which did not have sufficient forces to fight back. China urgently needed help, not the least of which was their [the people's] medical needs.[10]

Not everyone shared that enthusiasm. The English International Brigade nurse, Patience Darton, wrote from Paris that Drs. Jensen and Kisch were less than enthralled with the prospect of leaving Europe and going to China:

> I was in the company of six doctors with the Interbrigades, among them "Fritz" Jensen and "Caspar" Kisch-poor old sweetheart; he was a very good physician, very nice, a real dear.... The French Government was also not very fond of these six physicians, and because they wanted to escape the infamous internment camps, they decided with a heavy heart, to go to China to work in the Guomindang troops.[11] My friends were very sad to have to leave Europe. And they knew not what was in store for them in China. Their bad anticipations ... were not mistaken![12]

Writing to their Spanish friends from the Maison de Convalescence de Vouzeron, France,[13] on October 6, 1939, newlyweds and asylum-seekers (Austrian) Dr. Heinrich and (Spanish) Maria Kent similarly shared the uncertainty of the time: "The only thing that we plan to do is to go to England and probably later to China. If Maria can go with me to China, if I go or if she can stay in England or as a Spanish subject perhaps go to Mexico, it is not clear.... For the moment we are more happy here than in the camps."[14]

In 1939, thousands of refugees from the Spanish Civil War were able to stream more than 600 kilometers north of the Spanish border to the Loire Valley district of Cher. They were transported to Vouzeron Castle, which was owned by the French metalworker's union. The options for expatriation from France were very limited. Travel to Mexico was common, and a Mexican diplomat in France, Gilberto Bosques, became known as the "Mexican Schindler." He is credited with saving over 40,000 lives from the Nazis through his diplomatic efforts to expedite visas and passports. The Kents were very fortunate to stay briefly in the French Loire Valley before continuing their journey, with temporary asylum in England.

In addition to the Comintern, other international anti–Fascist organizations were shocked into action by the rising escalation of global atrocities.

This carnage included the German bombing of Guernica, Spain, in April 1937, followed by the Japanese Rape of Nanjing, China, in December. The widow of Sun Zhongshan (孫中山 / 孫逸仙 Dr. Sun Yat-sen), Song Qingling, (宋庆龄 Madame Sun Yat-sen) formed the China Defence League in June 1938 with the mission of "stimulating all lovers of peace and democracy throughout the world to do still greater efforts in the provision of medical and other relief to China in her present struggle against Japanese aggression."[15]

At the same time, Mme. Sun Yat-sen's younger sister, and bitter rival, Song Meiling (宋美龄 Mme. Chiang Kai-Shek), provided patronage for the Foreign Auxiliary to the National Red Cross Society of China. The hostility between the Song sisters stemmed from China's simmering Civil War. Mme. Chiang loyally supported her husband, the Generalissimo's Guomindang (Nationalist Party), while the left-leaning Song Qingling put her support behind the Chinese Communist Party.

The need to shield the refugee physician volunteers from these dangerous political differences was apparent from the beginning. Mrs. Hilda Selwyn-Clarke served as the diplomatic British Secretary of both the Chinese Defence League and the Foreign Auxiliary of the Chinese Red Cross. She was the wife of Sir Percy Selwyn-Clarke (司徒永觉) the British Director of Medical Services in Hong Kong. Hilda Selwyn-Clarke wrote to Mildred Price of the China Aid Council in January 1940: "The Chinese Defence League was not involved in the arrangements for the foreign doctors. This responsibility has been accepted by the Foreign Auxiliary [of the Chinese Red Cross]."[16]

However, the political boundaries of the different relief organizations in China were not clearly drawn. On the one hand, Hilda Selwyn-Clarke saw the need to distance the Foreign Auxiliary of the Chinese Red Cross from allegations of Chinese Communist Party support. On the other hand, Ronald Hall, the Bishop of Hong Kong, led the Foreign Auxiliary of the Chinese Red Cross. His clear support for the Chinese Communist Party earned him the nickname, "the Pink Bishop." Much as the Comintern was striving to create a united popular front with socialists and others against fascism in Europe, the Chinese Defence League, and the Foreign Auxiliary of the Chinese Red Cross were striving to create a united front against Japanese imperialism in China. This need for anti–Japanese unity swayed several philanthropic, political, and religious organizations to downplay their political preferences.

In 1938, Norwegian war correspondent Tor Gjesdahl visited Chiang Kai-shek in China, along with Selwyn-Clarke, Mme. Sun Yat-sen, and Dr. Robert Lin, the future leader of the Chinese Red Cross' Medical Relief Corps.[17] Gjesdahl's reports helped to convince the Norwegian Relief Committee for Spain to fund the reassignment of the Spanish doctors to the Chinese Red Cross/Medical Relief Corps.[18]

In London, a China Medical Aid Committee sprang into action. The London-based China Medical Aid Committee included some of the leading physicians in England such as Chinese missionary physician Dr. Harold Balme (巴慕德 Ba Mude); the physician to the King, Sir Maurice Allen Cassidy; and their chairman, the Oxford professor. Dr. Millais Culpin.[19] The China Medical Aid Committee of London wrote that one of its initial aims would be to transfer the Spanish, Czech, and Austrian doctors to China to help the Chinese Red Cross.[20]

Despite the early unanimity of support from the English, Chinese, and Norwegian relief organizations, distrust and political bickering between the Comintern and the China Medical Aid Committees erupted. The political complexity of how to seek asylum for these interned physicians without countries mounted. As all the International Brigade physicians were members of different national Communist Parties, the Comintern wanted the political commissar of the International Brigade, Andre Marty, to decide how to best use the service of these doctors.

Marty was, at best, a controversial figure, known by most as the "Butcher of Albacete" because of his cruelty. He was responsible for the execution of hundreds of men in the International Brigade for their alleged lack of resolve or "ideological soundness." The Spanish Party Politburo would ultimately try to limit his autocratic rule.[21] In 1938, a wary and paranoid Marty wrote to the Comintern about the danger of sending to China physicians who might not prove to be loyal to the Communist Party. Despite his concerns, the Comintern proceeded with the task of assessing the fifty detained physicians who had volunteered to go to China. This was not an easy undertaking, as Marty continued to share with the Comintern his concerns of sending physicians to China under the auspices of the Norwegian and British China Medical Aid Committees. The major fear was a deep distrust of the leadership of the Norwegian and British China Medical Aid Committees. For example, an anonymous informer in the Gurs camp wrote (with communist greetings) to Marty on June 13, 1939, that the Norwegian China Medical Aid Committee leader, Dr. Max Hodam, was a dangerous Trotskyist and a traitor.[22]

The impressions that the French Communist Party shared with the Comintern about these volunteer physicians ranged from paranoia concerning their possible political impurity to the realization that it would be more valuable to have some of these doctors continue their service in the French internment camps. The French Communist Party compiled lists of physicians and harshly subjective views as to their suitability for travel to China. The following are the verbatim quotes of the French Communist Party members who Marty approved in July 1939:

> Dr. Wolf Jungermann [Jungery] (Polish): As a doctor, medium. Good organizer. Member of the party. With a tendency to use the party for his personal desires.

In general, he is considered a good comrade. He is a worker who can go to China.

Dr. Victor Taubenfligel (Polish): Limited ability as a general physician. Worker and member of the Party. Sometimes he is not very good with his comrades. He can go.

Dr. George Schoen [Somogyi] (Hungarian): He finished his studies in Italy in 1937. General medical skills: average. He does not have a great capacity. He is a member of the Party. Politically inactive. *Petit bourgeois*, not very clear. Health is weak.

Dr. Alex Volokhine (Russian immigrant): Is not a member of the Party. Cannot be trusted. Can work as a general practitioner.

Dr. Jacob Kransdorf [Iacob Kranzdorf] (Romanian): Dermatologist, capable in his specialty. A good worker in the Camp from day one. May go to China.[23]

The French Communist Party created and Marty approved another list of physicians who they could not authorize for travel to China. This included several scathing political assessments:

Dr. Frantisek Kriegel: Works in medicine and is a member of the party. It would be very dangerous for him to go because he is very clever, has enough personality and has the ability to influence and deviate good comrades who are politically weak.[24]

Dr. Fritz Jensen: Andre Marty wrote specifically to Harry Pollitt, leader of the British Communist Party, in May 1939 that Jensen was among several other doctors he considered "bad elements, Trotskyites, a divisive influence." He wrote that the Aid Committee for Spanish refugees in France had, therefore, "refused to accept them, or to recommend them for service in China, whatever their professional competence."[25]

Other physicians, such as Drs. Flato and Kamieniecki, did not initially receive permission to go to China because of the need for their medical services in the internment camps:

Dr. Leon Kamieniecki: Regarding medicine in general, he is capable. He worked well in the Camp. In time he became a member of the party. Behaves well enough and works well. Does not have great political strength. His work is needed in the camp.

Dr. Moishe [Stanislaw] Flato: General practitioner. Capable enough. Limited political skills. His work is needed here as a hospital director and he works well.[26]

Finally, some of the other future International Medical Relief Corps physicians who did not appear on Marty's lists had received the following less-than-favorable reviews from their commanders:

Dr. David Iancu: Dr. Glaser, the chief medical officer of the International Brigade, wrote that Dr. Iancu had "little knowledge and experience. [He was] proud, passive without interest. Reserved and retired."[27] Perhaps this evaluation reflected Dr. Iancu's wish to be fighting at the front lines instead. After the evacuation to Catalonia, he [Dr. Iancu] asked for front line duty but was sent to surgical service at the hospital in Vich.[28]

Edith (Marcus) Jungermann [Marens]: In Spain since September 10, 1937, [she] was a radiologist in the state of Murcia. After her evacuation to Mataro, Dr. Franek proposed in March that she be repatriated. The information we have is that she acted in a demoralizing manner in front of the wounded and showed defeatist practices. Politically she is not good.[29]

The mechanism by which these last six physicians could reach China and prevail over the concerns of the Comintern is not well known. In the case of Dr. Franta Kriegel, help clearly came from his International Brigade colleague, Dr. Len Crome.[30] Dr. Crome had already made it to London, and helped Dr. Kriegel get on the list of physicians liberated from Gurs and sent to the Chinese Red Cross.

However, Dr. Kriegel, in contrast to the other Polish International Medical Relief Corps' members, never obtained permission from the Comintern to go to China. Because of this, Dr. Flato, the secretary of the International Medical Relief Corps communist party cell, released Dr. Kriegel of all responsibility to the party in China.[31] Dr. Kriegel's non-acceptance of the dictates of the upper echelons of the communist party had been born. Another twenty-three International Brigade physicians who volunteered to go to China were not able to escape internment in France. However, the reasons for prohibiting these physicians' travel to China remain unclear.[32]

Despite the French Communist Party's concerns, the London China Medical Aid Committee in the summer of 1939 received temporary asylum in Great Britain for several of the interned physicians who could no longer return to their native lands. These included the German doctors Herbert Baer and Carl Coutelle (with his wife Dr. Rosa [Sussman] Coutelle), the Austrian doctor Heinrich Kent and his Spanish wife Maria Rodriquez Gonzales, and the Bulgarian doctor Ianto Kaneti (甘扬道医生 Gan Yangdao). In addition, doctors Jensen, Becker, Kisch, Freudmann, and Iancu stayed briefly in England prior to journeying to China.

How these doctors escaped further internment and peril in the internment camps of southern France and reached England is not well known. Their close camaraderie with fellow International Brigade members may again have been at play. For example, when Patience Darton's newlywed husband, Robert Aaquist, was killed in combat in Spain, she thanked Dr. Jensen for transferring her to a small unit with future International Medical Relief Corps physicians Becker and Kisch. Robert Aaquist was another German Jewish brigadier who emigrated in 1934 from Hamburg, Germany, to Palestine. He was among several hundred Palestinian Jews who came to fight against fascism in Spain. Darton wrote: "It was Jensen who saved me." A few months later, Darton reciprocated this good will by initiating plans for some of the doctors to go to China. She sympathetically summarized the Spanish doctors' dilemma:

Where could they go and what could they do anyway? They wanted to go on fighting—they wanted to go—on doing something, and China of course, we all knew about, we had read *Red Star over China*,[33] which was one of the books being passed round in Spain. We knew all about Mao and the rest of them. And there was this group of seven doctors,[34] who wanted to go to China, because at least it was somewhere to be—they didn't particularly want to leave Europe but they wanted to go on being somebody in something. So we were starting to organize a committee and they wanted me to get people to get them to England. In those days it was fairly easy if you had somebody who'd say they'd look after them and they were only going through anyway.[35]

The physicians who obtained temporary asylum in England celebrated their good fortune and worried about their uncertain future as they traveled north through France in a heavily guarded train. In Paris, the French Communist Party accepted the asylum requests of the English China Medical Aid Committee, and small groups of refugee physicians crossed the English Channel and steamed into London's Victoria Station by train. Drs. Becker, Jensen, and Kisch arrived first on a gloomy and rainy night. Drs. Kaneti, Freudmann, Baer, and Iancu followed them in the summer of 1939. Drs. Charles and Rosa Coutelle and Dr. Heinrich and Mrs. Maria Kent would be the last of the International Brigade physicians to arrive in England prior to their service in wartime China.

The Kents had spent a month in Paris and had registered for an immigration visa to the United States, where Dr. Kent's sister Edith had immigrated. Although the Spanish Catholic, Maria Rodriquez Kent, could immigrate to the United States or Mexico, Dr. Heinrich Kent, an Austrian Jew, faced a quota that would make his immigration impossible for at least three to four years. Despite an appeal for immigration help to their American International Brigade medical colleague, Dr. Francis Vazant, the Kents settled on securing temporary asylum in England.[36]

Dr. Francis Vazant was a thirty-five-year-old Texan who served with the medical services in Murcia, Spain. She was the only American female physician known to have fought in the Spanish Civil War.

Dr. Alex Tudor Hart, a tall, Cambridge-trained Welch orthopedist and member of the British Communist Party was instrumental in helping them.[37] Because Dr. Tudor Hart had completed his medical training in Vienna and served with the International Brigade in Spain, he could clearly communicate in German and understand his medical colleagues' needs. Hart provided the financial guarantee needed to permit temporary asylum in Britain during their brief stay in London.

Dr. Mary Gilchrist, secretary of the China Medical Aid Committee of London, became another close friend of the refugee physicians. She helped to coordinate housing during their brief asylum in England. Other English physicians and friends who had fought with the International Brigade refugee physicians in the Spanish Civil War similarly answered the call for help. For example, Dr. Tudor Hart also assisted Drs. Iancu, Kent and Freudmann.

The President of the Socialist Medical Association of Great Britain, Dr. Somerville Hastings, sheltered Dr. Becker during his asylum in London (March-April 1939).[38] He also helped Dr. Becker obtain inpatient care at the Tropical Institute of London for treatment of the malaria he had been trying to fight off in Spain. Dr. Hastings denounced Britain's acquiescence to Japan's embargo of medical goods to China through the closure of the Burma Road in 1940. After the war, he championed the development of socialized medicine in England.

Patience Darton persuaded her parents to support Dr. Jensen's application for asylum in England and they also helped Dr. Jensen obtain a Spanish passport and Spanish nationality.[39] Although Darton shared the International Medical Relief Corps physicians' will to serve in China, being a female nurse, she could not obtain approval to go to wartime China. Both the China Medical Aid Committee and the Chinese Red Cross/Medical Relief Corps would not accept female foreign healthcare providers. Fortunately, the Chinese Red Cross/Medical Relief Corps would soon be able to bend these rules.

While Gilchrist, Hart, Darton, and others were working with the China Medical Aid Committee of London to secure temporary asylum in England for some of the refugee International Brigade physicians in 1939, the China Medical Aid Committee of Norway continued its negotiations with the French Communist Party. The Norwegians eventually obtained permission for the direct release from the camps in France of an additional group of ten refugee physicians from the International Brigade.

Other European International Medical Relief Corps' members, who did not serve in Spain, were viewing an equally uncertain future. Drs. Erich Mamlok and Arno Theodor "Teddy" Wantoch, both of whom had recently completed their medical training, and Dr. Wilhelm Mann (孟威廉医生 Meng Weilan) who was still studying biochemistry, knew that their prospects for remaining alive in Europe were poor. Dr. Mamlok wrote to his family from the University of Basel, Switzerland, in December 1938 that the time had come to leave Europe:

> Four weeks ago there appeared, (before the vom Rath murder by Grynspan),[40] an article in the *Schwarze Korps* that the Jews (1) should be expropriated, (2) should be chased from the quarters of the Aryans, and (3) even when they were later driven to destitution as a result of their crimes, they should be "physically exterminated with fire and sword." Since the *Schwarze Korps* is the Journal of the SS, the police and the Gestapo, this article must be taken very seriously. Meanwhile, the first two points are understood to be already in implementation; these are the reasons why I absolutely plea for our parents' immigration. I know also that immigration preparations take months (e.g., to get a passport or visa somewhere); but you must start now to get something in the foreseeable

future. The outlook in all countries I see rather gloomy, and am aware of the huge and not foreseeable difficulties as well. On the other hand, I'm convinced that by staying in Germany our parents are in great danger of being killed. It was just proclaimed in the last issue of the *Schwarze Korps*, that an attack by a Jew or a Jew servant on a leading German personality would have the effect that "no Jew would live any longer on the same day in Germany." That's clear enough, and who can guarantee that tomorrow, through some unfortunate incident that somewhere a second Grynspan incident will not occur?[41]

Dr. Walter Lurje (罗益医生 Luo Yi) was another Jewish-German-born physician who had managed to reach the Chinese Red Cross/Medical Relief Corps in wartime China. He had a diverse medical career that included pediatric service during World War I, post-graduate study in psychiatry at the University of Frankfurt Medical School, and worldwide service as a ship's doctor. He published on such diverse topics as music composition, autism, and Buddhism.[42] Lurje also recognized the growing threat of the rise of fascism in the mid–1930s. He was forced to give up his German medical license in 1934 due to his Jewish faith and fled to Italy. Dr. Lurje became one of several Jewish physicians who then applied to the League of Nations to travel to China as part of the League's anti-epidemic work in 1935. However, in 1937, the League of Nations' Secretary, Dr. Smets, "regretted to inform him that all the personnel to fight the epidemics in China had already been chosen."[43] However, Dr. Lurje remained adamant in his desire to serve with the Chinese Red Cross and made the journey to China without known institutional help.

Although Drs. Lurje, Mamlok, Wantoch, and Mann heeded the warnings signaling the rise of fascism, six million other European Jews, including many of the International Medical Relief Corps participants' family members, would eventually perish—in some cases hanging on to the belief that genocide could never happen in their native lands.

Other members of the International Medical Relief Corps headed to China without the immediate threat of anti-Semitism. For example, Dr. Barbara Courtney (高田宜医生 Gao Tianyi) was the only International Medical Relief Corps physician who was neither born in the Jewish faith nor a member of a national communist party. She was, by all accounts, an outgoing, petite, perpetually smiling English physician. Dr. Courtney was one of only two female foreign volunteer doctors to serve with the Chinese Red Cross/Medical Relief Corps. She graduated from the London School of Medicine for Women and became interested in both tropical medicine and the mystical spiritualism of Theosophy. She was drawn to this complex philosophy that seeks direct knowledge of the mysteries of being and nature, particularly concerning the nature of divinity. These interests took her to India, before she joined the Chinese Red Cross/Medical Relief Corps in China.

Many Chinese were frustrated with North American isolationism and

2. The International Medical Response of 1939

a general lack of interest in the war in China against Japan. Journalists in China lamented that North Americans remained interested only in the fates of the missionaries and in tales of the mysterious East. "Even in the middle of the Pacific War, a story that got headlines in much of the American press was that the clever Chinese in Chungking [Chongqing], during the Lunar New Year, could make eggs stand on their small ends."[44]

Despite North Americas' anemic interest in China, however, a few North American physicians served in Spain and China. Among these was the Canadian International Brigade surgeon Dr. Norman Bethune[45] and the American surgeon Dr. Leo Eloesser.[46] Some of Dr. Bethune's first encounters with the future International Medical Relief Corps' physicians were less than cordial. On November 3, 1936, he arrived in Madrid and reported to General Kleber, who was in command of the International Brigade defending Madrid. Kleber directed Dr. Norman Bethune to Dr. Bedřich Kisch, already one of the chief medical officers of the International Brigade. Kisch had recently replaced Eloesser when Bethune arrived. "A weary Kisch had been operating continuously in Spain for two months. He welcomed Bethune enthusiastically and, in broken English cried, 'We must put you to work at once!' Bethune asked a few more days to make up his mind and the interview ended coldly."[47] Although he chose not to relieve Dr. Kisch, Dr. Bethune established a mobile Canadian blood-transfusion service in 1936 before he returned to North America.

In 1938, Dr. Bethune would also travel to China. It is there that Drs. Kisch and Bethune's personal need for medical relief became tragically reversed. A reunion of the European Spanish doctors and Dr. Bethune did not occur in China. However, Dr. Bethune's service to China in 1938–39 became legendary. Chairman Mao subsequently glorified Dr. Bethune's medical efforts with the Chinese Communist Party's Eighth Route Army in his *Red Book*. Dr. Bethune remains the most well-known Canadian in China and his name continues to be linked to most diplomatic gestures of Sino-Canadian goodwill.

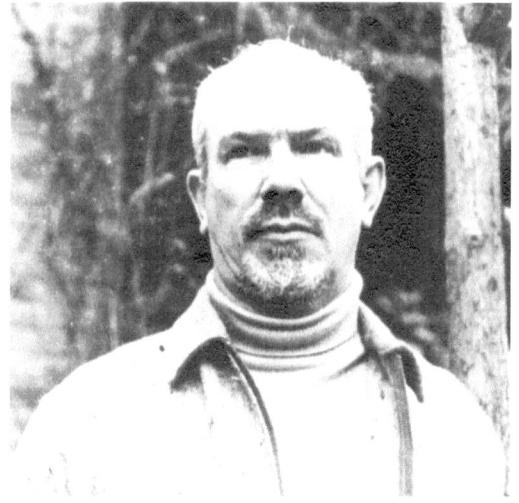

Dr. Norman Bethune, the iconic Canadian physician who served with the Chinese communists Eighth Route Army medical services in northern China from 1938 to 1939 (National Archives: 208-FO-OWI-18).

Another North American International Medical Relief Corps physician, Dr. Adele Cohn (科恩医生), was a strong-willed and idealistic woman making her own way in the male-dominated world of medicine of the 1930s. She was a pulmonologist who specialized in tuberculosis (TB). In the 1940s, TB or "the white death," was an incurable, infectious disease that posed grave risk to both patients and caregivers. She wrote that very few of her colleagues, male or female, chose to specialize in TB work at that time as it invariably was poorly paid and potentially dangerous and did not have the glamour of other procedure-driven specialties.

Dr. Cohn, who was born in Rochester, New York, completed her residency in pulmonary medicine at Sea View and Montefiore Hospitals in New York City in 1936–39. In November 1940, she shared with Dr. Louis R. Davidson, her mentor at Montefiore Hospital, her wish to combat TB in war-torn China:

> For some time, I have been considering the possibility of going to China to do medical work, and now I am sure that I want to go. Dr. Max Pinner tells me that you are in touch with the committee for medical aid to China, and that sort of thing. Can you take time out to write me and let me know the best person with whom I can get in touch and get started with the necessary arrangement?[48]

Dr. Max Pinner, Chairman of Pulmonary Medicine at Montefiore Hospital in New York, was a pivotal inspiration in Dr. Adele Cohn's professional life. Her lifelong admiration for Pinner included later naming her son, Max, in his honor.

Dr. Cohn wrote to her brother, Jerry Cohn, at about the same time:

> I have some news that will shock you but I must tell you because my mind is made up. I am going to China! The American Bureau of Medical Aid to China is paying my round-trip passage and I have been invited by the Chinese Red Cross to teach TB to the Chinese doctors, the latter will pay my salary. It will be for one year and it will be my part in helping China overcome fascism in the East. I can see no other way out in this world with fascism everywhere and I could not sit by and not do my part. (I would be of no use in England, as much as I would like to go there.)
> I sail from San Francisco July 25th and I finish here July 1st. What do you advise I should do about Mother and Father? I wish they could see it as I do—and I will not be in the war zone naturally. Let me hear from you soon.
> Love,
> Adele.[49]

Despite Dr. Cohn's impeccable credentials and an overwhelming shortage of medical specialists in China, she received a lukewarm, conditional approval from Dr. Robert Lin, the Director General of the Chinese Red Cross/Medical Relief Corps in March 1941. He would accept Dr. Cohn's medical services only if she met all the Chinese Red Cross/Medical Relief Corps' foreign physician volunteer conditions:

2. The International Medical Response of 1939   33

1. Physically fit male (preferably not over forty).
2. Politically pro–Chinese and have necessary papers approved by the Waichiaopu, or Chinese Diplomatic Office, abroad.
3. Technically qualified surgeon, recommended by a competent authority.
4. Willing to accept Chinese rates of pay (maximum NC$200/month for Unit Surgeon) and to live under Chinese conditions and on Chinese food.
5. Prepared to go anyplace ordered and [to] abide by the regulations of the Chinese Red Cross.
6. Travel to and from the Chinese frontier cannot be provided by the Chinese Red Cross. Besides travel to China, foreign volunteers are advised to obtain a guaranteed return passage, which should be deposited with their Consul or a bank or a shipping company.
7. Travel within China will be provided by the Chinese Red Cross according to regulations.[50]

Since the Chinese Red Cross/Medical Relief Corps specifically excluded all female medical volunteers, Dr. Cohn requested further clarification about the first condition. Given the shortage of qualified doctors in China, Dr. Lin was willing to overlook his preference to exclude female physicians. In addition, Dr. Lin had already been willing to overlook the fact that Drs. Baer and Kisch were both over the age of forty. However, Dr. Lin warned Dr. Cohn that conditions were hard in wartime China and that she too would first need to obtain all government and financial support before he could welcome her to the Chinese Red Cross.[51] Despite these forewarnings, Dr. Cohn succeeded in joining the Chinese Red Cross/Medical Relief

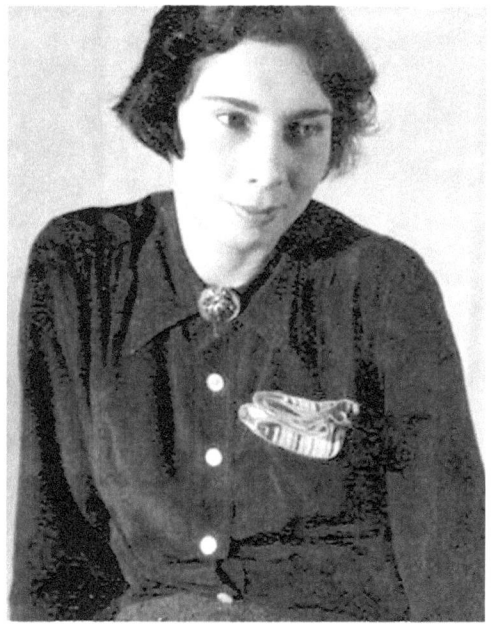

Dr. Adele (Cohn) Wright, an American Pulmonologist sent by the American Bureau of Medical Aid to China to the Chinese Red Cross Medical Relief Corps. Circa 1940 (courtesy Max Wright).

Corps. She became the only American physician sent to wartime China by a medical relief organization.

However, another American tried to serve with the Chinese Red Cross/Medical Relief Corps with less than altruistic intentions. The American Bureau of Medical Aid to China needed to report the American Dr. Torrance's application to serve in China to the Federal Bureau of Investigation. Torrance was under indictment for the murder of his wife in Mexico and had recently forfeited bail. An astute executive secretary recognized his name from the tabloids and kept him from escaping justice.[52]

An eclectic, improbable band of urban, intellectual physicians slowly came together in the summer and fall of 1939. At an average age of thirty-one years, they became early medical responders to the global menace of fascism and wanted to continue that fight wherever it would take them. The path to China was unpredictable, but logical for physicians who had no prospect of returning home and little long-term hope of surviving in what they now called the "Spanish waiting warehouses." At the same time, China was reeling from the Japanese invasion and needed more modern medical assistance. As the International Medical Relief Corps headed east, they must have envisioned that they would soon be serving together with thousands of raised Chinese fists in the global war on fascism.

3. The Call of China: 1936–1939

Asia was neither more peaceful nor less complicated than Europe. The Chinese had been fighting foes since 1931, when the Japanese invaded Manchuria under the pretext of the Mukden (Manchurian) Incident (柳条湖事变 Liutiaohu Shibian). However, the ongoing civil war between Mao Zedong's Chinese Communist Party and Chiang Kai-shek's Guomindang Nationalist Party often overshadowed China's fight against Japan.

The duality of the domestic conflict between the Chinese Communist Party and the Guomindang Nationalist Party and their conditional coalition in the fight against Japan was the political reality that dominated wartime China. So, besides the question of fighting Japan, a civil war was raging in China and Russia was playing a self-serving role.

Both Chairman Mao and Generalissimo Chiang were fortunate to have survived so far. Mao had barely lived through the long and epic march to Yan´an in November 1935. This circular trek from southeast to northcentral China lasted over a year and covered 4,000 miles as the embattled and outnumbered Chinese Communists evaded the pursuit of the Guomindang Nationalist Party army. The Generalissimo was equally fortunate to have endured his abduction, in Xi´an on December 12, 1936, by General Yang Hucheng and the "Young Marshal," Zhang Xueliang.[1]

The anti–Japanese needs of the Soviet Union strongly affected the subsequent Zhou Enlai (周恩来)-mediated negotiations of the Xi´an Incident (西安事变). Zhou Enlai served as the representative of the Chinese Communist Party to the Guomindang Nationalist Party in Chongqing and became the first Premier of the People's Republic of China in 1949. The Soviet leader, Joseph Stalin, wanted to avoid a two-front war against Japan and Germany. While Stalin was a political ally of Chairman Mao's fledgling Chinese Communist Party in 1936, the Russians also believed that Chiang Kai-shek was the best man to ensure that China's Guomindang Nationalist Party would continue the fight against Japan and thus protect the Soviet Union's interests in China. These negotiations resulted in the reinstatement of Chiang Kai-shek as the head of the Guomindang Nationalist Party and the arrest of the Young Marshal. Reconciliation ensued as the Guomindang Nationalist Party and Chinese Communist Party formed an uneasy Second United Front against Japanese aggression. In 1923, the Guomindang Nationalist Party and Chinese Communist Party had formed the First United Front. This was an alliance against regional warlords rather than the Japanese invaders.

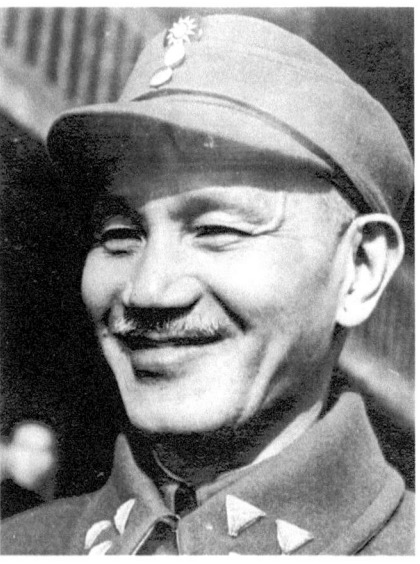

Generalissimo Chiang Kai Shek, Kunming China, April 26, 1945 (National Archives: 111-SC-11134).

Despite China's new, and ultimately fleeting unity, Japanese aggression burst into general warfare in July 1937. Japan invaded China under the false pretext that China had abducted a Japanese soldier at the Marco Polo Bridge near Beijing. The ensuing assault wrought by the modern, mechanized Imperial Japanese Army on a defenseless population resulted in incalculable carnage and the displacement of millions of people from east to central China, leading to one of the largest forced migrations in history.

The trauma of what became the Imperial Japanese Army's policy of "kill all, burn all, loot all" continued as its forces marched into central China. Nanjing fell in December 1937. The ensuing Rape of Nanjing resulted in the loss of more than three hundred thousand lives.[2] Six months later, in an attempt to slow the Japanese advance into central China, the Generalissimo ordered the destruction of the dams of the Yellow [Huanghe] River near Zhengzhou. Thus, four thousand villages were flooded, two million people became homeless, and the Japanese advance bogged down for a mere three months.[3]

The cities of central China fell like dominos to the West as the Imperial Japanese Army pushed inland. Wuhan and Canton [Guangzhou] fell first. Then Changsha, the capital of Hunan province, burned to the ground. A swarm of shaken, starving, and wounded refugees snaked toward the sunset. They fled to the west from the occupied eastern coastal regions toward Chongqing, the capital of Free China in the Szechwan [Sichuan] basin, more than 1,000 miles away.

3. The Call of China, 1936–1939

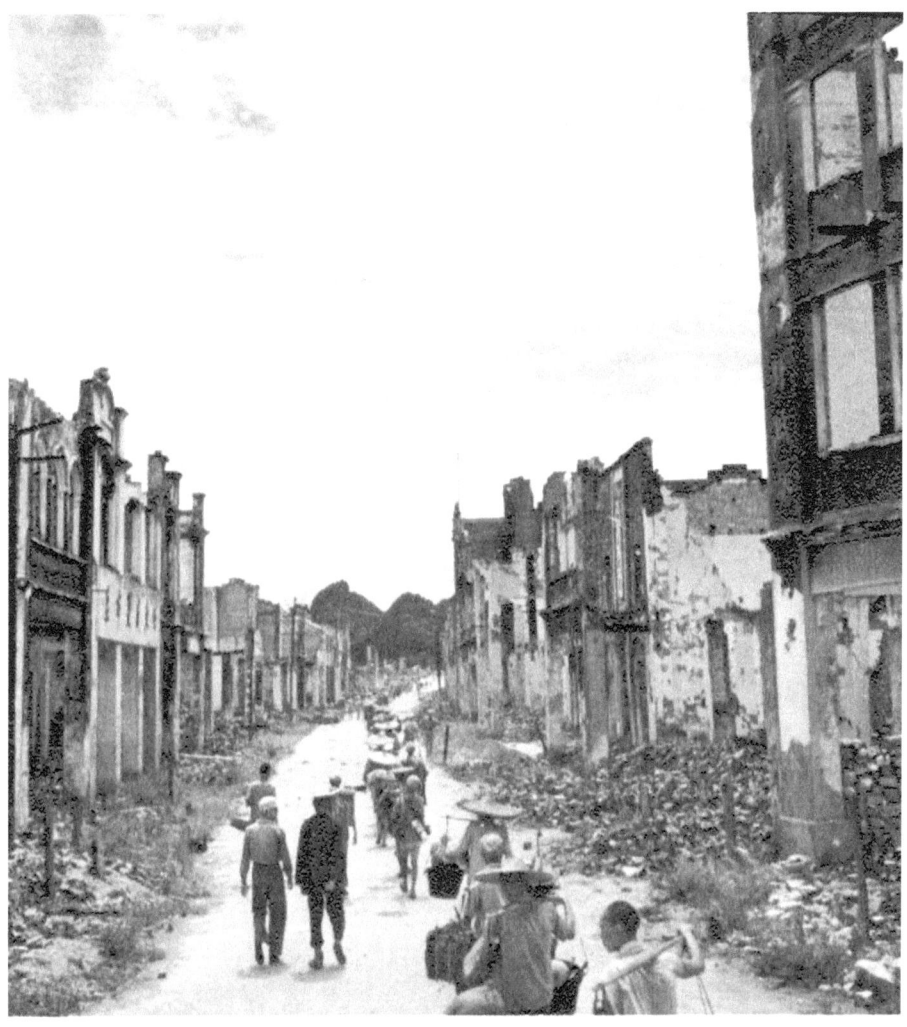

Chinese refugees fleeing from the Japanese onslaught in central China (undated) (National Archives: 208- FO-OWI-6749).

Much as in Spain, the under-armed Chinese military and unprotected civilian population reeled from the horror of modern warfare. In contrast to Spain, and unknown to the International Medical Relief Corps physicians, China's army did not have a functional, modern biomedical service in the 1930s. During the Spanish Civil War, more than 200 physicians served 30,000 men in the International Brigade, while in China, there were about the same number of physicians in the Chinese Red Cross/Medical Relief Corps serving 3,000,000 soldiers and many fold more civilians. However, the relative absence of biomedical care in rural China in the 1930s was not solely due to a lack of resources.

Prior to the onset of the Japanese invasion, China had been striding to improve the healthcare of its large, agrarian population. Numerous international organizations, such as the church mission hospitals, the Rockefeller Foundation, and the League of Nations Anti-Epidemic Units were providing assistance. In addition to these international organizations, the domestic healthcare services were divided between the civilian healthcare services of the National Health Administration and the military healthcare services of the Army Medical Administration. This complex of international and domestic medical organizations remained united by well-intended humanitarian efforts; yet, often they were separated by the politics of allocation of the very limited medical resources.

By the mid-1930s, the failure of these international and national organizations to meet rural China's basic medical needs became increasingly apparent. An amalgamation of international and national organizations scrambled to create a better organization from the embryonic and battered biomedical system's remnants in wartime China. At the same time, a few thousand predominantly urban, well-trained Chinese physicians wondered what they should do as their occupied medical facilities ceased to function in their prewar capacity.

International Medical Organizations in Wartime China

MISSION HOSPITALS

The mission hospitals in China had provided an infrastructure of faith-based outpatient and hospital services since the 1830s. The Rev. Dr. Peter Parker, a thirty-year-old Yale graduate, was the first full-time Protestant medical missionary in China. He believed that he could "open China to the gospel at the point of a lancet."[4] In some quantitative ways, he succeeded. By the 1930s, there were more than 250 mission hospitals in China. However, the faith-based nature of their medical services had its limitations. Their concurrent mission of religious salvation and conversion favored a curative, personal medical approach and few efforts to tackle the enormous needs of public health were forthcoming.

However, the quality of the mission's curative biomedical services in China were excellent. Some of the future International Medical Relief Corps' physicians, such as Dr. Franta Kriegel, would describe the mission hospitals as "the best and only medical care in rural China."[5] But, as the Japanese control of China grew, the missions' resources shrank. By 1941, John Rich, public relations director of the American Friends Service Committee, noted that, "the church committee for China relief was very shaky because it had lost its channels for distribution in China."[6] Although there had been several hundred missionaries in Henan Province in 1941, only a handful remained operative in 1945.

Rockefeller Foundation

Biomedical education in China developed in the early 20th century with the help of international aid. The China Medical Board, created in 1914 by the Rockefeller Foundation aimed to modernize medical education and improve the practice of medicine in China. This aim resulted in the creation of the Peking Union Medical College in 1919. It focused on research and the development of a small cadre of well-trained Chinese physicians.

Although it produced only 381 doctors, this elite group became key leaders and proponents of bioscience and public health.[7] By the 1930s, the Peking Union Medical College's academic mission evolved as it tried to become an integral part of the Chinese medical system. Significant differences in opinion on how to approach China's enormous healthcare needs ensued. Chiang Kai-shek was a backer of the Anglo-American faction at the Peking University Medical College while others, such as Chen Guofu and his younger brother Chen Lifu, backed the larger German-Japanese trained health care providers.[8]

Several public health visionaries saw the limitations of funding centralized, urban medical institutes. Dr. John Grant (兰安生 Lan Ansheng), the Chinese-born and American-trained head of the Rockefeller Institute's China Program, argued that China's future development required more public health resources. Specifically, he envisioned integrating preventative and acute care medicine into rural community-based models. He argued for resources to be directed from large, urban research centers such as the Peking University Medical College toward these goals.[9] Dr. Lin and others similarly pressed upon Peking Union Medical College the need for a state-supported medical system that would include the mass education of healthcare providers.[10]

This need became more pronounced in 1938 as the Japanese invasion disrupted China's medical education system. Very few of the medical, pharmacy, and dental colleges continued to operate as before the war. The majority were destroyed, inactivated, or forced to relocate in a reduced capacity to the interior of China. The Rockefeller Institute's China program was an early casualty and closed its doors in 1939. However, a vision of how to deal with China's medical and public health needs had been born.

LEAGUE OF NATIONS ANTI-EPIDEMIC UNITS

The League of Nations' Health Organization had worked closely with Chinese health officials since 1928, under the leadership of Dr. Ludwik Rajchman, a Jewish, Polish-born public health expert. Dr. Rajchman had been the Medical Director of the League of Nations' Health Organization and a strong proponent of extending the League of Nations' Health Organization's efforts to East Asia.

An outspoken critic of Japanese military aggression in China and Nazi support for Franco's forces in the Spanish Civil War, he was forced to resign from the League of Nations' Health Organization in 1939. After the war, he was instrumental in founding the United Nations Children's Emergency Fund (UNICEF) when the United Nations Relief and Rehabilitation Administration ceased its activities.

A primary mission of the League of Nations' Health Organization was to develop strategies to improve national health systems. As such, Dr. Rajchman and his colleague, Dr. Berislav Borčić were more interested in adequately addressing rural public health needs, rather than creating large, urban biomedical research and education institutions.

The League of Nations' Health Organization sent several internationally acclaimed public health experts to China through the mid–1930s. Among them were the Austrian plague and cholera experts Drs. Robert Pollitzer and Heinrich Jettmar, the Scottish pathologist Dr. R.C. Robertson, the German epidemiologist Dr. Erich Landauer, the French Inspector General Dr. A. Lanset, and the Swiss typhus expert Dr. Hermann Mooser.[11] Pollitzer worked with the Manchurian Plague Prevention Service in the 1920s and the League of Nations' anti-epidemic cholera units in the 1930s.

Much as in Europe, the League's efforts in China were limited by the political neutrality of the League's charter and by the disruption of warfare. However, the League of Nations' Health Organization's public health experts in China did not always feel compelled to avoid helping combatants; and they did engage in some measures of curative rather than preventative medicine. For example, Dr. Hermann Mooser gave Dr. Bethune all his surgical supplies to help the Eighth Route Army. Dr. Bethune thankfully recognized the unofficial circumstances of Mooser's help: "Geneva is an awful long way from Sian [Xi'an] and Mooser is in full charge east of the Lake of Lucerne."[12]

The League of Nations' Health Organization succeeded in working with the Nationalist government to establish laboratories for vaccine production and biomedical sanitary and health services. However, much like the missionary experience, the Japanese invasion of China and the focus on the war in Europe rapidly depleted the ranks of the League of Nations' Health Organization representatives in China. By 1940, only two League experts remained and the entire program was terminated in 1941.[13]

However, several League of Nations' medical experts, such as Drs. Hermann Mooser, Erich Landauer, and Robert Pollitzer chose to remain in China. They continued to help China and their International Medical Relief Corps colleagues through several public health initiatives throughout the war. For example, Dr. Pollitzer aided the Chinese Red Cross/Medical Relief Corps by lending his expertise in cholera and plague epidemiology.[14]

INTERNATIONAL RED CROSS COMMITTEE FOR CENTRAL CHINA

While many of the pre-war international medical relief efforts, such as those of the mission hospitals, Rockefeller Foundation, and League of Nations declined in wartime China, others, such as the International Red Cross Committee for Central China and the Society of Friends (Quakers) rose in an attempt to fill the growing gaps in access to medical care. The International Red Cross Committee originated in Wuhan in September 1937 in response to the humanitarian crisis brought on by the Japanese invasion and subsequent refugee crisis.

Medical missionaries obtained funding through donations from abroad. Dr. Robert "Bob" McClure (麦克卢尔医生), born in China to Presbyterian missionary parents, became the International Red Cross Committee's first field director. The English poet, W.H. Auden, described him as "a stalwart, sandy, bullet-headed Canadian Scot, with the energy of a whirlwind and the high spirits of a sixteen-year-old boy. He wore a leather blouse, riding breeches and knee-high boots with straps."[15]

The American Quaker public relations director, John Rich, who previously wrote from the Spanish Civil War, added that, "[h]e [McClure] is an amazing man, full of vigor and crackling with ideas. He has been all over the Northwest and comes back bursting with plans for men to work on sanitation, delousing of refugees, engineering and establishing new communities for refugees, agricultural schemes. His ideas are not all workable and must be checked to verify the connections he wants to establish. It is invigorating to deal with him."[16] Drs. McClure and Lin, the future head of the Chinese Red Cross/Medical Relief Corps, would develop a rocky relationship despite sharing similar dress, personalities, and training (at the University of Edinburgh Medical School). It was inevitable that "When Lin and McClure got together, voices rose, arms raised and before long people were taking sides and shouting."[17]

The Chinese Red Cross made it very clear that the International Red Cross Committee's mission was restricted to the mission hospitals in China through the accrual of medical supplies that were not readily available in China. In 1938, Dr. Li Shu-Pui, director of the National Red Cross Society of China, described his concern with the International Red Cross Committee's nomenclature:

> The International Red Cross Committee is misnamed, as it has no direct connection with the Geneva body. It is in fact a committee of the Chinese Red Cross and works through a charter conferred by the latter body.... It consists predominantly of missionary medical men who place the facilities in their mission hospitals at the disposal of civilians and soldiers wounded in the war."[18]

Indeed, in 1941, the International Red Cross Committee changed its name to the International Relief Committee.

United China Relief

Henry R. Luce, was another so called "Mish Kid"—a Tengcho, China-born son of poor Presbyterian missionaries. He became a *Time Inc.* media mogul and was a strong supporter of Chiang Kai-shek and vocal salesman for an Americanized China. Luce envisioned a Christianized and democratic China and championed for a special relationship between China and America. He used the economic and political might of his media empire to educate Americans about wartime China and to unite the fundraising activities of different American organizations. He recruited a Board of Directors that included such luminaries as the author Pearl S. Buck, the philanthropist John D. Rockefeller III, and the Republican Presidential candidate Wendell Wilkie.

In 1941, he succeeded in uniting the diverse humanitarian efforts of the American Bureau for Medical Aid to China, The American Committee for Chinese War Orphans, the American Committee in Aid of Chinese Industrial Cooperatives (Indusco), the American Friends Service Committee, the Associated Boards for Christian Colleges in China, the China Aid Council, the China Emergency Relief Committee, and the Church Committee for China Relief.[19] Under the banner of the United China Relief, he raised millions of dollars for broad medical, industrial, and political initiatives in wartime China. The American Bureau for Medical Aid to China and the Society of Friends (Quakers) were most directly involved in humanitarian medical aid with the Chinese Red Cross/Medical Relief Corps. The Society of Friends included both the United China Relief's American Friends Service Committee and the British Friends Service Council. The American Bureau for Medical Aid to China was jointly-founded in 1937 by Drs. Farn B. Chu, Frank Co-Tui, and Mr. Joseph Wei. Dr. Co-Tui was Professor of Surgery at New York University prior to becoming President of the American Bureau for Medical Aid to China.

It was the first American organization that responded to the health needs in wartime China. The large material contributions of the American Bureau for Medical Aid to China have been extensively reviewed.[20]

THE SOCIETY OF FRIENDS (QUAKERS) FRIENDS AMBULANCE UNITS

The Friends Ambulance Units was an independent Quaker charity established during World War I. It provided an alternate service for pacifists who conscientiously objected to military service. The demobilization of the Friends Ambulance Units occurred after World War I as it had fulfilled its mission of providing emergency ambulance services to British and French troops on the Western front.

In 1939, there again was a need to create an outlet for conscientious objectors to war who wished to provide humanitarian aid and the Friends Ambulance Units was re-established. The Friends Ambulance Units included a China Convoy that worked closely with the leadership of the British Friends Service Council and received funding largely from the American Friends Service Committee through their parent organization, the United China Relief. The Friends Ambulance Units' China Convoy provided a means for Quakers to participate in a war effort that was consistent with their testimonies to pacifism and social equality. The sole qualification for service in the Friends Ambulance Units was to be a pacifist, and only a minority was in fact Quakers. Recognition of the efforts of the Friends Service Committee and the American Friends Service Committee came later when they received the 1947 Nobel Peace Prize on behalf of all Quakers for their desire to help others without regard to nationality or race.

The Friends Ambulance Units' core activity was to develop a network for transporting medical supplies along the Burma Road. This mountainous 717-mile road provided a vital lifeline between Burma and the southwest of China. In addition, two mobile surgical vehicles were imported, and a constantly

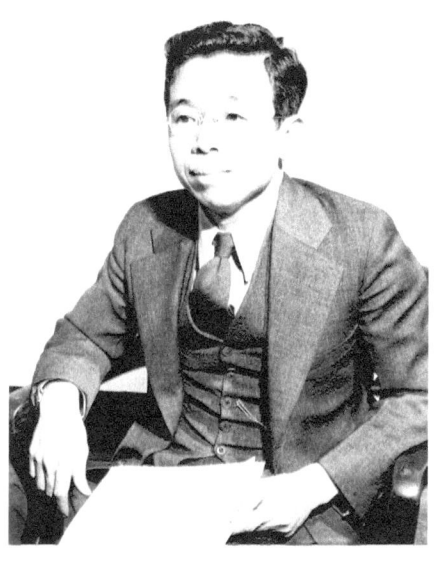

Dr. Frank Co-Tui, New York University Professor of Surgery and co-founder of the American Bureau of Medical Aid to China (courtesy the American Bureau of Medical Aid to China archives, Rare Book & Manuscript Library, Columbia University's Butler Library).

changing series of medical teams were established. The Friends Ambulance Units transported most of the civilian drugs and medical supplies imported into west China during the war.[21]

John Rich wrote to his family in April 1943 that the Friends Ambulance Units had a tough hard job:

> [They were] tearing trucks apart, rebuilding them with no spare parts, and taking them out on the roads on runs that may last from four days to three months. The roads are incredibly bad and fuel consists of charcoal, alcohol and mixtures of wretched stuff concocted from vegetable oils. Travel is impeded by endless red tape and the meanness of petty officials. It takes fourteen different permits to get a load of supplies from here [Kutsing][22] to Chungking [Chongqing].[23]

The ethical and moral quandaries for these conscientious objectors in wartime China would follow an equally tortuous path. Dr. McClure's biographer wrote:

> They would in no way assist to wage war but they would assist in every way possible to alleviate suffering. The crunch time came in deciding what actions would do the one and not the other. If they hauled non-medical supplies, what constituted relief? Was medicine and food the same for wounded soldiers and civilians?[24]

Maintaining qualified medical staff was, as in all the relief organizations, extremely difficult in wartime China. Dr. McClure noted that the Friends Ambulance Units' small medical staff became largely depleted. By 1943, the two remaining American Quaker physicians with the Friends Ambulance Units, Dr. Ernest Evans and Dr. Louderbough, "spoke of the disillusionment resulting from inadequate support, hostility to foreign doctors, inefficiency of the members of the mobile surgical teams and lack of facilities in which to work."[25] Although their direct medical mission fluctuated in scale and was constantly adapting to changing needs and circumstances, the Friends Ambulance Units continued to serve a critical role in the transport of medical goods to many relief organizations. Even when the Japanese invaded Burma in early 1942 and closed the Burma Road, the Friends Ambulance Units continued to distribute medical supplies. However, the supplies then needed to be flown over the Himalayan Mountains to the city of Kunming, and distributed throughout China by truck.

Cooperation and Conflict Between the International Medical Organizations in China

The interactions between the secular medical aid organizations and the church-based missions in wartime China were complicated. As Dr. Franta Kriegel and others had pointed out, the mission hospitals earned an excellent reputation as the best-equipped hospitals in China in the 1930s. However, Mme. Sun Yat-sen wrote that despite this, their rural location, jealousies, and conflicts made use of mission hospitals by the Chinese people very difficult. As Chinese troops retreated to the west, an increasing number of mission hospitals fell into the hands of the Japanese, further reducing their utility.[26]

Mme. Sun Yat-sen (宋庆龄 Song Qingling) was one of the three influential Song sisters. The other two sisters were Mme. H.H. Kung (宋蔼龄 Song Ailing, married to the wealthy finance minister of China, H.H. Kung), and Mme. Chiang (宋美龄 Song Meiling, married to Generalissimo Chiang Kai-shek). The Song sisters are often now recognized by the Chinese as the one who loved China (Song Qingling), the one who loved money (Song Ailing), and the one who loved power (Song Meiling).

Although individual physicians shared common goals and frustrations, their parent organizations continued to differ in the scope of their medical mission. For example, the mission hospitals refused direct medical care to the military and to indigent civilian refugees. The pragmatic Dr. McClure explained this "no margin, no mission" policy: "Many mission hospitals had learned from bitter experience that the arbitrary dumping of the wounded could seriously impede the hospital's ability to finance its services to the community at large."[27]

This strategy of the International Red Cross Committee and many of the Chinese mission hospitals raised considerable ire in other relief organizations. In September 1938, Dr. Erich Landauer of the 1st Unit of the League of Nations' Epidemic Commission to China wrote of his displeasure with the International Red Cross Committee's narrow medical mission in a memorandum to the Chinese Defence League:

> The International Red Cross Committee is more concerned in maintaining mission hospitals than in carrying out the Red Cross work expected of it by a public that is pro Chinese, but not necessarily pro missionary.... The International Red Cross Committee does not allow the missionary doctors to use their resources freely and without bias.... The charge has been made and I believe proved that profiteering is the result of the International Red Cross Committee policy of pouring money into the mission hospitals. The Committee, which is purely a local organization, sails under the flags of the IRC [International Relief Committee] and one cannot help gaining the impression that when soliciting help, it intentionally conceals its strong bias in favor of the missions.... The International Red Cross Committee exists for the relief of missions rather than the relief of refugees in the mind of many missionaries.... They are missionaries first and hospital physicians second, and not in a single instance has this writer found any of them interested in activities to be carried on beyond their compound walls. It has never published any statements as to the channels through which its resources flow. It has received and spent over $1,000,000 and this writer knows of only three instances when [any of this money] has been given to strictly non–Christian organizations.[28]

Some of Dr. Landauer's observations appear overstated. For example, the Canadian Missionary, Dr. Richard Brown, served patients well outside his mission walls. He was an Anglican missionary whose home base, the mission hospital in Kweiteh, Henan, was overrun by the Japanese. Agnes Smedley had been instrumental in getting him to join Dr. Norman Bethune in the Chinese Communist Party's Eighth Route Army. Dr. McClure was another well-traveled and energetic proponent of the Friends Ambulance Units' efforts throughout China and Burma. Indeed, Brown countered Landauer's observation of missionary misappropriations by writing that the League of Nations' Health Organization had wasted much of the money allocated for anti-epidemic work in China. Brown praised the work done by Dr. Mooser, the Swiss typhus expert, and the League of Nations' anti-epidemic commissioner for North China. However, Brown also wrote that sending high-salaried European specialists to China was a poor allocation of resources. With the salary of one such foreign specialist, he argued, he could maintain a whole hospital in China for the best part of a year: "The salary of the anti-epidemic commissioner came to NC$60,000 a year, whereas NC$100,000 was all that he [Dr. Brown] needed to run his 'International Peace Hospital' for a whole year."[29] In many ways, Dr. Brown was an exceptional missionary physician as he echoed the public health views of Drs. Grant and Lin at the Peking Union Medical College.

Many other individuals argued that China would be much better served by allocating resources for public health infrastructure rather than urban biomedical "Ivory Towers" and mission-based hospitals. For example, the

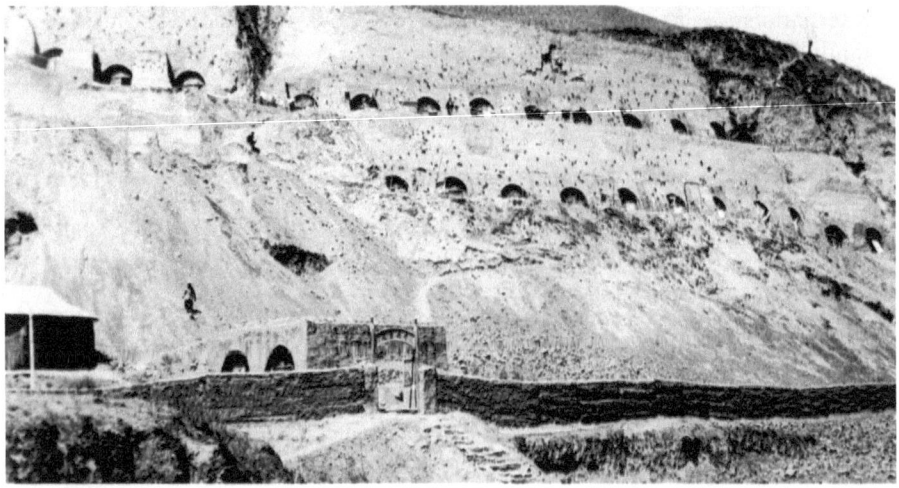

A pockmarked north China mountainside facade belies its name: The 8th Route Army's International Peace Hospital (National Archives (208-FO-OWI-8313).

American journalist Agnes Smedley (史沫特莱 Shi mo te lai), who later befriended several Chinese Red Cross/Medical Relief Corps and International Medical Relief Corps' members, was another candid critic of the mission hospital's practices. Despite her outspoken nature, "[it] is impossible not to like and respect her," the English poet W.H. Auden wrote of her, "so grim and sour and passionate; so mercilessly critical of everyone, herself included ... as if all the injustice of the world were torturing her bones like rheumatism."[30] In November 1939, Smedley shared her widespread observation of the missions' practice of charging wounded patients for acute medical care:

> This is occurring in the Seven Day Adventist Hospital in Loho in Honan [Henan] Province and the Lutheran Hospital at Lochan on the Pinghan Line. The International Relief Committee in Hankow [Hankou] is giving free supplies to these mission hospitals. While in the Hwangchan Lutheran Hospital I saw the same problem.[31]

She later wrote about what she saw as the hypocrisy of combining theology and medical relief in wartime China:

> Honan [Henan] and Hupeih [Hubei] are one great American Lutheran bible belt in which some missionaries are industriously harvesting souls, some of them preaching that the war, like the countless sicknesses that inflict the Chinese people, is due to sin. But I also found some missionary doctors conducting modern hospitals, and none of them seemed to regard the malaria mosquito, the relapsing fever louse, or the dysentery germ as messengers of the Almighty to punish the "heathen" for their sins.[32]

The Friends Ambulance Units continued in the difficult task of maintaining its members' roles as pacifists while juggling their relationships with their sponsors and the other international medical aid organizations they worked with. John Rich of the American Friends Service Committee wrote:

> Dr. Flowers, head of the British Red Cross, wants to cooperate more closely with the Friends of the Ambulance Units, but it struck me that he wanted secretly to trade in on our stronger position and had little to offer us. He admitted that China did not want him to bring more personnel into China and wondered how we are being encouraged to do so. I could not tell him that it was probably because he never cooperated with the Chinese but tried to run his own show.[33]

Rich also shared his concerns regarding Dr. Robert Barnett, the Chongqing based representative of the American Bureau for Medical Aid to China:

> He does not understand our principles. I don't like the way he is ready to jettison the British Quaker work just because it is British. I don't believe that he reflects the true mind of the United China Relief in this respect.... Helen Stevens [the president of the American Bureau for Medical Aid to China] wants us to work closer with the American Bureau for Medical Aid to China. Undoubtedly we are trespassing on their field of work.[34]

Throughout the war, variances in the core missions of the international medical aid organizations limited their optimal cooperation with each other. These differences dealt with the questions of how to co-exist with the Guomindang Nationalist Party—Chinese Communist Party conflict during the Sino-Japanese War, and how to determine the best mechanism to allocate and develop medical resources and personnel. Similarly, the institutional politics and self-interests of China's national medical healthcare organizations limited their ability to work with each other and the international organizations that tried to serve them.

National Medical Organizations in Wartime China

Even with optimal international assistance, modern health care remained in an embryonic state in wartime China. It was painfully clear that China's domestic medical organizations were woefully unprepared to deal with the humanitarian crisis of war. The political controversies that surrounded the distribution and access of their relatively meager medical resources further limited their potential value. Much like the international associations, each of the domestic Chinese medical organizations had to confront unique challenges and inherent limitations.

National Health Administration (Wei Sheng Shu)

China's National Health Administration was created in 1931 when the Ministry of Health was abolished and the National Health Administration was placed within the Ministry of the Interior. Chinese biomedical proponents in the Ministry of Health, such as Drs. Liu Ruiheng, (刘瑞恒 J. Heng Liu), and Jin Baoshan (金宝善 P.Z. King), had already focused on the need to create a centralized health administrative system.

Dr. Liu Ruiheng was a graduate of the Harvard Medical School and former head of the Peking Union Medical College. He was appointed head of the National Health Administration from 1933–1938. Dr. Jin Baoshan was a medical graduate of Chiba Union in Japan and received an advanced degree in public health from Johns Hopkins University. He was a strong proponent of public health and anti-epidemic measures.

In his broadcast from Chongqing on October 14, 1938, the subsequent director general of the National Health Administration, Dr. Yan Fuqing (颜福庆 F.C. Yen), elaborated on its wartime mission:

> Unhygienic living, unsanitary environment, [and] undernourishment are [an] inevitable accompaniment of war, hence war spells disease. Furthermore, with large numbers of soldiers gathered together, and refugees in overcrowded centers, epidemic diseases, when they exist, are bound to spread with great rapidity and intensity.[35]

Dr. Fuqing was a Chinese-born son of an Episcopalian minister who trained in St. John's College in Shanghai and Yale University Medical School. He headed the National Health Administration in 1938 but resigned in 1940 amid charges of corruption.

To meet its goals, the National Health Administration needed to serve several domestic medical organizations from China's wartime capital of Chongqing. This included the anti-epidemic organizations, the National Red Cross Society and its Medical Relief Corps, and the National Institute of Health. The National Health Administration's public health mandate depended on promoting rural reconstruction and basic literacy, areas of political controversy for the conservative Guomindang Nationalist Party.[36] Despite these administrative and political challenges, the National Health Administration succeeded in overseeing many joint efforts on immunizations, vaccine production, and infectious disease surveillance that affected millions of lives.

To highlight the wartime growth of the National Health Administration, Dr. Baoshan noted that its budget increased from $2 million to $10 million between 1938 and 1941 and from $11 million to $31 million between 1941 and 1942.[37] In wartime China, the National Health Administration contributed to many improvements in public health despite limitations in the support from the Guomindang Nationalist Party. Most historians agree that the potential of the National Health Administration was tempered by a nationalist government that remained more interested in eliminating the Chinese Communist Party than in health construction.[38]

ARMY MEDICAL CORPS

In contrast, the Army Medical Corps, which was responsible for the healthcare of the military, did not receive many accolades. In 1938, Mme. Sun Yat-sen wrote that,

> [t]he Chinese Army was built up without an existing medical service and consequently the existing skeleton organization is totally incapable of even tackling the care of the enormous number of wounded. The doctors have little specialized training, the nurses even less, and the patients are left in Army Hospitals under the care of dressers of the soldier-coolie variety.[39]

Although the amount of training given to the Army Medical Corps physicians is difficult to measure, less than 10 percent of the Army Medical Service's two thousand members were medical college graduates.[40]

The International Medical Relief Corps' physicians, who had taken great pride in developing an international medical service in Spain, would find the relative absence of military healthcare appalling. Dr. Heinrich Kent wrote:

> In one division there may be one or two doctors who've graduated from a medical school. The others have a short training program after nursing in the Army or the best may have had some official nursing training in a hospital. Those who have worked in Mission hospitals may know some English.[41]

The main organizational problem in the Army Medical Corps was the relative absence of a central command, a vestige of the semiautonomous and fragile alliances of warlords that had supported the Guomindang Nationalist Party armies of Chiang Kai-shek. In 1937, Chiang Kai-shek appointed Dr. Zhang Jian (张建) as the dean of the Army Medical School.[42] Dr. Zhang, an alumnus of the University of Berlin, was a very pro–German Guomindang Nationalist Party general. It is clear that the Jewish-German International Medical Relief Corps physician, Dr. Mamlok and ethnic Chinese Army Medical Corps physician Dr. Zhang left the University of Berlin medical school in the 1930s under very dissimilar circumstances and with opposing political views.

The Army Medical Corps' continued dependence on local command resulted in poor and often nonexistent military medical services. Each general had the task of appointing the chief medical officer of a division, without consulting the Army Medical Corps' central command. The quality of the appointed healthcare providers varied considerably from division to division and from army to army. The English Journalist Freda Utley[43] wrote:

> A modern-minded man, like General Li Han-yuan [李汉魂], would appoint as good a man as he could find, realizing the importance of good care of the wounded in maintaining the morale of the army. But a more feudal-minded General would think only of giving jobs to his relatives and friends, and not consider the lives of his soldiers as of much importance.[44]

Within the Army Medical Corps' regionalized and often self-serving system of loosely knit military alliances, the International Medical Relief Corps members' future goals of standardizing medical and surgical care and setting up a system of checks and balances would prove untenable. Indeed, military commanders often saw "their" recruits as sources of personal income and power, which they could not afford to lose by fighting. Dr. Carl Coutelle noted that:

> [t]he officers and the "doctors" were frequently transported on the march by paramedics on the stretcher. The sick, often in an acute attack of malaria, had to walk. Contempt for ordinary people was noticed throughout. There were enough coolies, so why make any effort for their health? Some officers let the nail of their little finger grow to a centimeter-long claw in order to demonstrate their belonging to the non-working class. Cruel beatings resulting in injuries requiring treatment were common.[45]

In addition to the Army Medical Corps' organizational problems, the absence of sustainable funding troubled the healthcare providers. One patriotic but economically challenged Chinese physician shared his dilemma:

3. The Call of China, 1936–1939

The scale of pay for technical men like doctors, social workers etc. is NC$60/month for fresh graduates. For experienced [physicians], they take off 20% of what they last received. So it is very difficult for married people, especially to work for a very long period of time in the Chinese Red Cross.... Although I feel it is my duty to work for my country especially at this time, I must confess I cannot feel happy when I have to hear of my family's suffering from financial difficulties. The kids are not going to school and my wife cannot find any suitable work.... What to do?[46]

The official exchange rate was listed in 1939 by Agnes Smedley as NC$6.30 = U.S.$1. The value of NC$60/month in 1939 is estimated at U.S. $163/month in today's dollars. The contract surgeon's salary of NC$200/month is similarly estimated as U.S. $543/month. Converting the purchasing power of the NC$ to U.S.$ is problematic as there was a period of hyperinflation between 1939 and 1945 in China that quickly eroded the purchasing power of the cash- strapped Chinese government. Dr. McClure wrote that in 1942, he would take a 1937 price and multiply it by a 100 to estimate the price in 1942.

Dr. Fritz Jensen would later share the same economic sentiments:

No medical student or physician can afford to serve with the Army medical service unless he can be assured of supplemental pay for himself and his family. Hence the various requests to foreign organizations for supplemental pay.... Even the Surgeon General, [Dr.] Loo Chih-The [卢致德 Lu Zhide], on his resignation sent a report to Madame Chiang Kai-shek stating that remedies lay at more attention at the top; with a need for clearer responsibility of the various branches, a very much larger budget and higher pay for the personnel.[47]

Mrs. Susanne Wantoch (Wang Daodi) an International Medical Relief Corps' member who traveled to China with her Austrian husband, Dr. Theodor Wantoch, summarized the moral dilemma of the poverty and corruption of the Army Medical Corps' medical staff with her story of Dr. Schiau:

Slowly the life of the young physician, Dr. Schiau, changed in military hospital 125. It started with the fact that his colleagues wanted to include him in their get-togethers—to costly meals at the restaurant, where you had delicious food instead of the miserable military food; to nightly Mahjong games in doctor's rooms; excursions to Loyang to the bathhouse, where not only hot baths were issued, but also varied girl's company—and that his rejection was very resented. The rejection had valid reasons. If a meal for a small company cost almost as much as a whole month's salary—how can a poor military physician join in there? However, there were resourceful ways and means to supplement the meager salary, and each of us somewhat cunningly made use of such methods. For example, the Red Cross medicines. Was it not a sin to waste these beautiful, expensive foreign preparations on dirty, lice-ridden soldiers who would be lying tomorrow or the next day under the grass? Was it not more reasonable to put a small portion aside and in this way to improve one's own miserable life? Patients died every day. You had to put all of these deaths on a list. Could not a few, pro forma, remain alive and could we not reap the military wheat for them? Who can harm them? The poor devils were dead anyway, the wheat was also there, and if I do not take it, another will who does not necessarily need it more than me. Dr. Schiau rationalized that he must by all means preserve the friendship of his colleagues, otherwise he would lose his authority in the hospital, and the few reforms that he, due to his better professional qualifications, had introduced to the medical service would all go back to hell. Stealing—Pooh, who calls it stealing? Everyone does it in China, except the stupid peasants and some ridiculous university professors. Who does not, starves as do their family.[48]

The Army Medical Corps remained as an underpaid, understaffed, and undertrained entity that was unable to meet the basic medical care needs of the Chinese Army. Very few graduates of the up-to-date Chinese medical schools of the period would consider joining the military and working with peasants for low pay under terrible and often corrupt conditions. In the mid-1930s, most modern doctors stayed in urban centers to secure lucrative practices. Shanghai alone had 22 percent of China's doctors of Western medicine.[49]

It is not surprising that when the Japanese occupied Beijing in 1942, more than three-fourths of the Peking Union Medical College community remained in Beijing. Some joined the staff of local hospitals while others retreated into private practice or research.[50] It would take forced physician conscription in 1944 to get most Chinese physicians to come to the aid of the Army Medical Corps.[51] Fortunately, however, a small number of Chinese and foreign physicians did find a way to come to wartime China's medical aid, at its moment of greatest need.

The National Red Cross Society of China and Medical Relief Corps

During 1937–39, a time when many of the future International Medical Relief Corps' members had been gathering to fight the rise of fascism in Europe, a cadre of equally frustrated and idealistic Chinese medical students and physicians was looking for a similar path to fight against the Japanese invasion of China. The overseas Chinese physician, A.W. Chung wrote of the concerns of Chi, a Chinese medical student, at that time. The term "overseas Chinese" refers to people of Chinese birth or descent who live outside the People's Republic of China, the Republic of China (Taiwan), Hong Kong, and Macao:

> Chi's worried expression belied his confidence: "]Don't you feel frustrated, not being able to take an active part in the war? How can we justify ourselves, serenely attending class every day as if nothing out of the ordinary was happening?" Chi's steps slowed and he was silent for a moment. "What would you have us do? We'd make poor soldiers. Our training so far is less than that of medical orderlies. Sure, what could be more gratifying than to say let's throw ourselves against the enemy! Practically, that would be as wise as an egg testing itself against a stone wall." Chi chuckled.[52]

This group of young and idealistic Chinese physicians and their overseas colleagues were looking for credible leadership in the fight against fascist military aggression. The obstacles were well recognized. There were public health experts sent from the League of Nations' Health Organization and additional assistance from the International Red Cross societies, but both stipulated that their direct medical intervention could only extend to the civilian population.

To serve the soldiers that the Army Medical Corps could not adequately care for, a new program and leadership were needed. Dr. Robert Lin was the man chosen to lead this new organization above the constraints of caring only for civilian or military personnel or caring only for the Guomindang Nationalist Party-aligned personnel. The Chinese Red Cross' newly created program, the Medical Relief Corps, became the medical home of the International Medical Relief Corps from 1939 to 1945.

Lin's initial success was due to his appeal to the Chinese, the overseas Chinese, the foreign diplomats, and the international relief organizations. Dr. Liu Ruiheng, director of the National Health Administration and a fellow Peking Union Medical College professor, spearheaded the drive to recruit Dr. Lin. He implored Dr. Lin to cut short a sabbatical, as he was in route to Singapore and return to China.[53] By all accounts, Dr. Ruiheng chose the right man at the right time. Dr. Lin was a well-recognized investigator and clinician, and he was one of the few Chinese professors at the prestigious Peking University Medical College. In addition, he had served in France as a medical officer with a British Gurkha Regiment of the Indian Expeditionary Army in World War I.

However, one of Lin's greatest attributes was his charismatic ability to lead by tireless example. His patriotism was unquestionable as he strove to place China's medical needs above politics and petty per-

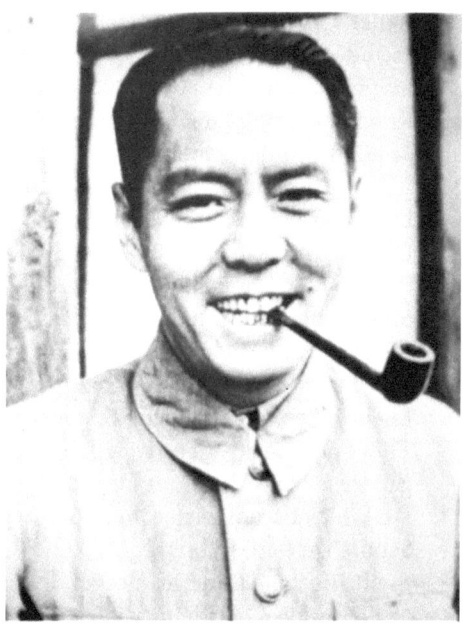

The charismatic director general of the Chinese Red Cross Medical Relief Corps, Dr. Robert Lin (林可胜 Lin Kesheng), circa 1939 (courtesy the American Bureau of Medical Aid to China Archives, Rare Book & Manuscript Library, Columbia University's Butler Library).

sonal ambitions. This patriotic appeal inspired a small but critically important number of similarly minded doctors in China to give up their successful careers and work for the lowest of salaries under the worst of circumstances in the war zones. The egalitarian vision of the Chinese Red Cross/Medical Relief Corps inspired this group of Chinese physicians much as the International Brigade medical service had inspired a group of European physicians.

However, Dr. Lin's cadre of physicians answered a nationalist appeal to serve their country against the Japanese invaders. By contrast, most of the International Medical Relief Corps' physicians had been drawn together by a global internationalist appeal to fight against the fascists who had already forced them to leave their native lands. Dr. Lin and his colleagues knew that "[t]hey would be up against the corruption, nepotism, and incompetence in the army hospitals and would have to work tactfully if they are to be allowed to enter them at all."[54] Despite these concerns, some of Dr. Lin's former students at Peking Union Medical College and other similarly motivated Chinese physicians chose to follow him to Tuyunguan, the Chinese Red Cross/Medical Relief Corps' new headquarters in southwest China. Other physicians included Drs. Peng Tah-moi (Class of 1933), Thomas Ma (Class of 1935), and Loo Chih-teh (Class of 1929). A few physicians from the University of Hong Kong, including Drs. Sze Tsung Sing (Class of 1931) and Eva Ho Tung (Class of 1927), similarly followed his lead.

This group of Chinese medical volunteers also included the radiologist Dr. Rong Dushan, the physiologist Dr. Lui Anchang, public health experts Dr. Peng Damau and Dr. Ma Jiaji, thoracic surgeon Dr. Wang Kaixi, and the internist Dr. Zhou Shoukai.[55] Dr. Shoukai became Chief of Internal Medicine of the Emergency Medical Service Training Schools and helped to train thousands of Chinese healthcare workers.

In addition to his support from the Chinese medical organizations, Dr. Lin began to obtain much assistance from the overseas Chinese communities. They could easily identify with him, an overseas Chinese physician from Singapore. Because his training had been abroad, at the University of Edinburgh, Dr. Lin could not write Chinese, and his children spoke English with a heavy Scottish accent. In this regard, it was easier for him to develop close ties with the British and American relief organizations.

However, his identity in China as an "overseas Chinese" or "foreign physician" was not without limitations. For example, when nominated for membership in the prestigious British Royal Society, prominent scientists, such as Joseph Needham argued that it would have been preferable to nominate a true Chinese physician rather than an overseas physician.[56] The fact that Dr. Lin could overcome the wary acceptance of his overseas and foreign-trained background further attests to the trust his colleagues had in his patriotic efforts to provide medical assistance to all Chinese soldiers and civilians.

Evidence for Dr. Lin's support from many different diplomatic corps members comes from the journalist Freda Utley. She wrote in 1939 that the British Ambassador thought so highly of Dr. Lin that he gave Dr. Lin the first grant he had ever had out of the Lord Mayor's Fund. Similarly, the American Consul in Hankow gave him a grant, out of American relief funds. Prior to that, Dr. Lin had even received funds from the German Red Cross in 1938.[57] His individual fundraising success quickly became unprecedented in wartime China's medical establishments.

With the support of the Chinese government, the overseas Chinese, and the British and American diplomatic and relief organizations in place, Lin turned to the task of medical care. Lin gathered the remnants of the Army Medical Corps' medical equipment, brought together medical personnel and scrapped together whatever aid he could. Much as the International Medical Relief Corps' members who chose to answer the call of Spain, this band of Chinese physicians now put their personal wellbeing aside as they chose to answer the call of China.

However, the logistics of how to best develop the Medical Relief Corps as the Chinese Army retreated west after the Rape of Nanjing in December of 1937 was daunting. In October 1937, the Chinese Red Cross built a 3,000 bed hospital in Nanjing under the direction of Dr. Pang Jingzhou (庞京周 C.C. Kohlhaus Pang).[58] When the Imperial Japanese Army took over Nanjing, the Chinese Red Cross had lost its major-medical resource. In many ways, the crisis of the Japanese invasion accelerated the push to develop decentralized, large-scale public health resources, much as Drs. Grant and Lin had advocated during their Peking Union Medical College days.

With a critical ongoing absence of trained physicians and an inability to maintain large hospitals in central China, the National Health Administration funded Dr. Lin's Medical Relief Corps to establish the first Emergency Medical Service Training Schools to serve the anti-epidemic corps, the National Health Administration, and the Army Medical Corps.[59] The Emergency Medical Service Training School provided brief courses in first aid for lay people and soldiers, thus enabling basic supplementation of biomedical services. Within two years, the Emergency Medical Service Training School went on to train more than 4,000 medical aid workers on the basics of public health and first aid.[60] The pragmatic Dr. Lin later shared with the Chinese Red Cross leadership his argument explaining why it was important to first develop as many basic medical aid personnel as possible rather than trying to fully train a cadre of physicians:

Because of China's educational backwardness, when the war began, there were less than 6,000 qualified doctors and less than 5,000 qualified nurses in the whole country. Today China's front line troops number about 3 million with several million more in training. An army medical service should constitute about 10 percent of the total strength of the army, so in China's case there should be 300,000 men in the medical service. Of these 300,000, 10 percent should be medical officers but from the figures given above it is evident that the vast majority must be unqualified.[61]

Hsia Yi-yung, a research assistant for American Bureau for Medical Aid to China, further added in 1946, "only 1,000 or 1,500 of these modern doctors might be classified as properly trained and that of these, possibly only a few hundred would be considered well qualified by American standards."[62]

Establishing Emergency Medical Service Training Schools in the face of the Japanese western advance forced numerous relocations. By February 1939, just five months before the International Medical Relief Corps' physicians would begin to join them, the Japanese assault forced the Chinese Red Cross/Medical Relief Corps and its Emergency Medical Service Training School to withdraw deep into southwest China. They relocated to the hamlet of Tuyunguan, near the city of Guiyang in Guizhou Province. This became the central headquarters of the Chinese Red Cross/Medical Relief Corps throughout the war.

From there, Dr. Lin was able to communicate the plight of the Chinese medical services to such future allies and adversaries as the Generalissimo and Mme. Chiang Kai-shek; her sister, Mme. Sun Yat-sen of the China Defence League; General Joseph Stilwell, the future chief commander of the allied forces in China; and Dr. Co-Tui of the American Bureau for Medical Aid to China.

By 1940, most medical observers and politicians in China agreed with Mme. Chiang that, after three years of warfare, the Chinese Red Cross/Medical Relief Corps "constituted the only qualified medical service caring for the sick and wounded in military hospitals and stations."[63] The Chinese Red Cross/Medical Relief Corps was to become the story of a strong-willed group of Chinese and Western physicians who had the audacity to place their vision of a more humane and egalitarian world in front of their personal interests.

International Medical Relief Corps Predecessors During the War

Before the International Medical Relief Corps' physicians arrived in China in 1939, the fledgling Chinese Red Cross/Medical Relief Corps had been bolstered by a continuum of well-intended foreign volunteer physicians and material aid, including groups of physicians—hailing far and wide, from Abyssinia to Yugoslavia—who had answered Dr. Lin's plea. The first waves of medical supplies and personnel came from overseas Chinese, particularly from the Dutch East Indies and from North America. In addition, several missionary and other physicians served in different and shorter capacities with the Chinese Red Cross/Medical Relief Corps (see Appendix C).

Dutch East Indies

The overseas Chinese from the Dutch East Indies were among the first to respond to the Chinese Red Cross/Medical Relief Corps' plea for help. Without the Dutch East Indies' early medical support, the Chinese Red Cross/Medical Relief Corps could not have functioned nearly as well. In addition to medical supplies and funding, several physicians from the Dutch East Indies reached the Chinese Red Cross/Medical Relief Corps. They included a team led by Dr. Kwa Tjwan Sioe (柯全寿 Ke Quanshou) and Dr. Go In Tjhan (吴英璨 Wu Yingcan) from Batavia, Dutch East Indies (present day Jakarta, Indonesia). However, the Japanese closely monitored and progressively limited the humanitarian efforts from the Dutch East Indies. They would later imprison Dr. Go in the Dutch East Indies for sending medical aid to China.[64]

The names of the Dutch East Indies' regions and cities attached to the Chinese Red Cross/Medical Relief Corps curative unit reports reflect the financial support that the Chinese Red Cross/Medical Relief Corps received from the Dutch East Indies. This included the 23rd Oost [East] Java Unit, the 46th Java Unit, the 26th (Menado [Sulawesi, Indonesia]) Unit, the 31st (Palembang [Sumatra, Indonesia]) Unit, the 35th (Toko de zone [Java, Indonesia]) Unit, the 5th Telok Betoeng [Sumatra, Indonesia] Unit, and the 2nd Semarang [Java, Indonesia] Unit.[65] As the war progressed, the Dutch East Indies could not sustain this level of support.

When Dr. Wu, secretary general of the Chinese Red Cross, traveled to the Dutch East Indies in 1939 to seek additional medical support, the Dutch East Indies government was already under pressure from Japan to stop supporting Java's dozen Chinese Red Cross/Medical Relief Corps units in China.[66] Such cowering under the growing menace of Japanese aggression in Asia also would result in the closure of the British-controlled Burma Road and put a stop to the transfer of medical relief supplies from the French-controlled Indo-China.

The folly of Britain and France's failed efforts to appease German and Japanese aggression would soon be all too apparent in both Europe and Asia. However, the overseas Chinese maintained a strong preference for continuing to support one of their own throughout the war. They would always regard the Singapore-born Dr. Lin's integrity and patriotism in the fight against Japan as being beyond reproach. Despite the threat and subsequent imposition of the Japanese-imposed embargo in Indo-China and the closure of the

Burma Road, some medical supplies continued to filter in from the overseas Chinese in the Dutch East Indies throughout the war.

North America

Chinese, American, and Canadian organizations were largely unsuccessful in their efforts to encourage medical volunteers from North America to go to China. The best-known exceptions were Dr. Norman Bethune (the Canadian-born Spanish Civil War veteran) and the American doctor Charles Edward Parsons. A Canadian nurse, twenty-six-year-old Jeanne Ewen, would also join them. Jeanne Ewen denounced the Canadian Communist Party that her father, Tom Ewen, founded and Dr. Bethune supported.

Dr. Bethune left Vancouver for China on January 28, 1938, on *The Empress of Asia*. Before leaving, he received a refresher course in general surgery, especially in incisions and sutures, from Dr. Louis Davidson, a professor of surgery at Columbia University.[67] Dr. Davidson also had served as a mentor and recommended Dr. Adele Cohn for service with the Chinese Red Cross. As such, Dr. Davidson was involved in the training of both North American physicians who would serve wartime China. It is not known if Dr. Bethune met Dr. Cohn during his brief period of remedial medical training in New York. Dr. Parsons faced an even greater challenge. A last-minute addition to the group, his alcoholism was not recognized when the sponsoring committee had asked him to lead the medical unit.

In 1938, Drs. Bethune and Parsons met with Dr. Lin, Agnes Smedley, and Zhou Enlai in Hankou, China. [After the fall and rape of Nanjing in December 1937, Hankou (part of the three city complex now known as Wuhan) became China's capital until October 1938.] During that meeting, Dr. Parsons told Dr. Lin that he "came to China to start a hospital so that the American people would have something to support and know is their very own."[68] Dr. Lin was probably not too impressed with Parsons' vision of trying to create a large American hospital in China.

However, Dr. Parson's ambitions became irrelevant as it soon became clear that he was suffering from a relapse of rapidly deteriorating alcoholism. An episode of delirious rage required institutionalization and Dr. Parsons had to return to America. His sponsoring organization, the China Aid Council, remained perturbed by Dr. Parsons' personal failure. As the senior physician of the group, Dr. Parsons had the responsibility for overseeing Dr. Bethune's conduct.

As it happened, Dr. Bethune had some problems of his own: "Bethune was pretty egotistic[al] and certainly driven by a demon of his own: He wanted to be a hero or a martyr of the revolution, at any cost," wrote the New Zealand journalist Jack Bertram.[69] Despite these issues, Bethune continued to badger

Dr. Lin until the latter finally permitted him to head off to the Chinese Communist Party's Eighth Route Army in Yan´an. Dr. Bethune, like most of the International Medical Relief Corps' Spanish doctors, was a staunch supporter of the communist party and he clearly wanted to serve only with the Chinese Communist Party's Eighth Route and New Fourth Armies.

Dr. Bethune's journey, however, did not go as planned. He could not find his way to Yan´an. The Canadian missionary doctor, Robert McClure, found Bethune in the Hwaiking (Huaiqing) area of Henan Province, about 600 kilometers southeast of Yan´an. Dr. McClure later recalled that Bethune had been on his way to the Chinese Communist Party's Eighth Route Army when he lost his way: "When he had gone astray, he got confused and hit the bottle.... I got him when he'd been under for about two or three weeks and we dried him out."[70]

To Dr. Bethune's credit, when he finally reached the Chinese Communist Party's Eighth Route Army in Yan´an, he was able to conquer his personal demons and provide exemplary medical service in 1938–39 under incredibly challenging medical circumstances. During the year he spent in China, he worked tirelessly for the good of the Chinese patients he served. Indeed, he reached his goal of becoming a hero of the revolution, much as Jack Bertram had predicted. Chairman Mao wrote in his *Red Book* that every Chinese communist must learn from his experience.[71]

Dr. Norman Bethune remains the most well-known Canadian in China today. The twenty-one foreign volunteer physicians and six allied healthcare providers of the International Medical Relief Corps had similar hopes of reaching their goals as they began their travel to China.

4. The Journey to the Chinese Red Cross Headquarters

Between 1938 and 1940, the International Medical Relief Corps' members traveled thousands of miles by every imaginable means. From steamship to Studebaker to sampan, they came in small groups or as individuals, with or without the support of friends, families, or relief agencies. Along the way, they were vilified, interned, and befriended. They braved an uncertain voyage to a world they knew little about. Buoyed by an unwavering faith in anti-Fascism and an international humanitarianism without ethnic, economic, or geographic borders, they did not strive to change people's faith or to seek fame or fortune. The International Medical Relief Corps' volunteers came to help.

Following the defeat of the Spanish Republican government in 1939, the China Medical Aid Committee of London succeeded in obtaining the release and temporary asylum in England of several of the refugee physicians from the French internment camps. This group now consisted of the German doctors: Herbert Baer, Rolf Becker, and Carl Coutelle; the Polish Dr. Rosa (Sussmann) Coutelle (wife of Dr. Carl Coutelle); the Austrian Drs. Fritz Jensen, Walter Freudmann, and Heinrich Kent; the Spanish nurse Maria (Rodriquez Gonzales) Kent (wife of Heinrich Kent); the Czechoslovakian Dr. Bedřich Kisch; the Romanian Dr. David Iancu; and the Bulgarian Dr. Ianto Kaneti. The married physicians, Drs. Carl Coutelle and Heinrich Kent secured longer visas in England and arrived in China a year after the others. At the same time, the Norwegian China Medical Aid Committee obtained sponsorship and succeeded in getting the direct release of ten additional physicians from the French internment camps.

Travel to the Chinese Coast

THE VOYAGE OF THE *EUMAEUS* FROM ENGLAND TO HONG KONG

"We were the scouting party of a group of sixteen doctors that were seeking a logical continuation of the Spanish Civil War that had found a temporary end,"[1] Dr. Fritz Jensen wrote about this first group of the European International Medical Relief Corps' physicians to reach the Chinese Red Cross/Medical Relief Corps' headquarters in Guiyang. This scouting party of Drs. Becker, Jensen, and Kisch left from Liverpool, England, on May 20, 1939, aboard an old, 8,000-ton cargo ship of *The Blue Funnel Lines*, the *Eumaeus*.[2] Thirty years later, Dr. Becker would reminisce on his departure:

> Farewell, beautiful, green England, vibrant and sooty London, I will see you again much changed after almost nine years. The parting is brief but cordial. Even a few members of the bourgeois press appeared; obviously, they cannot hide a slightly pitying shrug. But perhaps it is only our lack of English vocabulary. We cast off from Liverpool and slowly started on our southerly course. We three at the railing watched the shores of England and Europe slowly disappearing.[3]

The *Eumaeus* steamed south and then eastward through the Mediterranean Sea and the Suez Canal. The first three International Medical Relief Corps' physicians to reach the Chinese coast, Drs. Becker, Jensen, and Kisch crossed the Indian Ocean and entered the Haiphong port, in French Indo-China. From Haiphong, they cruised eastward past Hainan Island and on to Hong Kong.[4] The Hong Kong Port Health Office wrote that they arrived in Hong Kong on July 8, 1939.[5] It is likely that these three physicians stopped in Haiphong, traveled to Hong Kong, and then quickly returned to Haiphong to ease the clandestine transfer of medical supplies and information from the Chinese Defence League or Foreign Auxiliary-Chinese Red Cross in Hong Kong to the Chinese Red Cross in Tuyunguan. Dr. Becker chose not to describe his whereabouts in his diary during that part of his voyage in early July 1939, as he probably needed to conceal his clandestine activities.

THE VOYAGE OF THE *AENEAS* FROM ENGLAND TO FRANCE

Drs. Baer, Freudmann, Iancu, and Kaneti were the second group of International Medical Relief Corps physicians to depart from England. They had arrived in London from Spain in June 1939, and left from Liverpool for Hong Kong on August 5, 1939. The China Medical Aid Committee of London gratefully acknowledged the help of the British Fund for the Relief of Distress in China. This organization was formerly known as the Lord Mayor Fund, and was founded by Dr. Harold Balme (巴慕德 Ba Mude). He had served as a missionary physician in China and as President of Cheloo University from 1921 to 1927. The Lord Mayor Fund paid for the passage of the physicians on both the *Eumaeus* and the *Aeneas*: "Thanks to the British Fund's secretary, Gordon Thompson's good efforts, all but one of our seven and all ten of the Norwegian committee doctors would be granted free passage on the *Blue Funnel Lines*."[6]

Dr. Iancu described their hurried departure, on the *Aeneas*,[7] which embarked on its journey to Hong Kong about ten weeks after the departure of the *Eumaeus*. Their journey got off on the wrong foot when they missed a train connection to Liverpool. As the belated International Medical Relief Corps' physicians ran up the gangplank of the *Aeneas*, there was no time for farewells or fanfare.[8] But, with much relief, they were finally on their way to China.

Dr. Freudmann wrote the *Aeneas* had room for fifty first-class passengers. The extravagance of this luxury cruise made him very uncomfortable. He viewed the life of these bourgeois first-class travelers with disdain, and it was clear that he did not fit in with these folks. Fortunately, two Chinese students were heading from Scotland back to China on the *Aeneas*.[9] Dr. Freudmann added that,

> They were friendly, likeable in an Eastern sort of way and exceedingly helpful. One of them, [Hsin Ti] Wang, found pleasure in teaching us Chinese. We had been told that this language was impossible to learn. But after the first days of study we began to have the wildest hopes. From our daily progress we concluded that we would soon master the language. This optimism was actually quite useful.[10]

Like the *Eumaeus*, the *Aeneas* sailed down the foggy French coast and into the Bay of Biscay. Dr. Freudmann bunked with Dr. Iancu, and Dr. Kaneti roomed with Dr. Baer.[11] As the *Aeneas* passed through the Gibraltar Straits, they all reflected with great sadness that they were leaving Spain, a defeated democracy, in the hands of the fascists. They hoped they could achieve a better result in China.

The *Aeneas* steamed past Spain's Costa Brava and arrived in Marseille, France, on August 12, 1939. In the port of Marseille, Drs. Freudmann, Iancu, Baer, and Kaneti celebrated the reunion on the *Aeneas* with ten more China-bound medical International Brigade colleagues. These International Brigade internees had only been released a day earlier from the French internment camp at Gurs, and Dr. Freudmann noted that the connection was very tight, as the Gurs Camp was nearly 600 kilometers from Marseilles. The recently liberated arrivals on the *Aeneas* were Drs. Flato, Taubenfligel, Jungermann and his wife Edith, Drs. Kriegel, Kamieniecki and his wife Mania, and Drs. Kranzdorf, Schön, and Volokhine. They were now twelve male physicians and two women, one a medical student [Edith (Marens) Jungermann] and the other a laboratory technician [Mania Kamieniecka] on their way to China.[12]

A calm summer routine of Chinese lessons, political discussions, and planning for the unknown did not foreshadow a world that was now on the brink of global war. The *Aeneas* crossed the Gulf of Aden, steamed through the Strait of Malacca and arrived in the British port of Singapore on September 1, 1939. Upon their arrival, Dr. Iancu recalled, they learned of the start of World War II in Europe: "We found there the English fleet in alarm, a submarine in full military exercise.... I soon found out the cause of this bustle: It was the beginning of war. Hitler's armies had attacked Poland."[13]

Dr. Freudmann recalled a slightly earlier sense of outrage and unease before they arrived in Singapore:

> The news of the outbreak of the war reached us in mid-ocean.... In the Straits of Malacca we heard that German airplanes had already bombed all major cities in Poland. When we arrived in Singapore I and two of my colleagues that were German nationals [Baer and Martens] were already enemy aliens. This was not pleasant. We were not allowed to leave the ship in Singapore.[14]

Several members of the International Medical Relief Corps wanted to return to Europe as soon as possible to fight against the German fascists. They sent a telegram to Dr. Mary Gilchrist of the China Medical Aid Committee of London, asking her if they could return to Europe. However, the China Medical Aid Committee reiterated that the International Medical Relief Corps' physicians should continue as planned on their medical mission to China.[15] Dr. B.K. Basu and the other Indian physicians who had just begun to serve in China with the Chinese Communist Party's Eighth Route Army that week expressed similar sentiments about wishing to return to their home countries to fight the fascists there.

> Dr. Ma Hai-teh [马海德马海德 Dr. Ma Haide, formerly George Hatem][16] came at 11 a.m. and stunned us with the news of the European war which broke out a week ago; Hitler's Germany had attacked Poland and Great Britain had declared war against Germany; USSR remained neutral. We were thinking of many possibilities in India and were at a loss to decide our future course of action. Dr. [M.M.] Atal[17] preferred returning to India. I hesitated, thinking it was better to stay here and later go to USSR. After lunch, Dr. Atal accompanied Dr. Ma Hai-teh to Yan'an to interview Chairman Mao Zedong, for his analysis. According to Dr. Atal, Mao's opinion was that Japan and Italy would stay away from the fracas if not join with Britain.[18]

The *Aeneas* steamed into the port of Hong Kong on September 28, 1939, more than seven weeks after having left Liverpool.[19] In much less time, the German Army had blitzed into Warsaw, Poland, and the Imperial Japanese Army had marched to the outskirts of Changsha, in central China. Despite these ominous global events, Mrs. Hilda Selwyn-Clarke, the secretary of both the Chinese Defence League and the Foreign Auxiliary-Chinese Red Cross cheerfully greeted the new International Medical Relief Corps' arrivals at the port of Hong Kong. Hilda Selwyn-Clarke was both a political activist and a well-connected member of the British diplomatic community. She clearly was striving to assist these medical recruits in their goal of serving China in the war against Japan.

She informed the German and Austrian physicians, Drs. Baer and Freudmann, of the potential complications that their newly minted "enemy alien" status could cause in the British colony of Hong Kong. Since there was now a formal declaration of war between Britain and Germany, German and Austrian citizens in Hong Kong were at risk for arrest and internment. Under

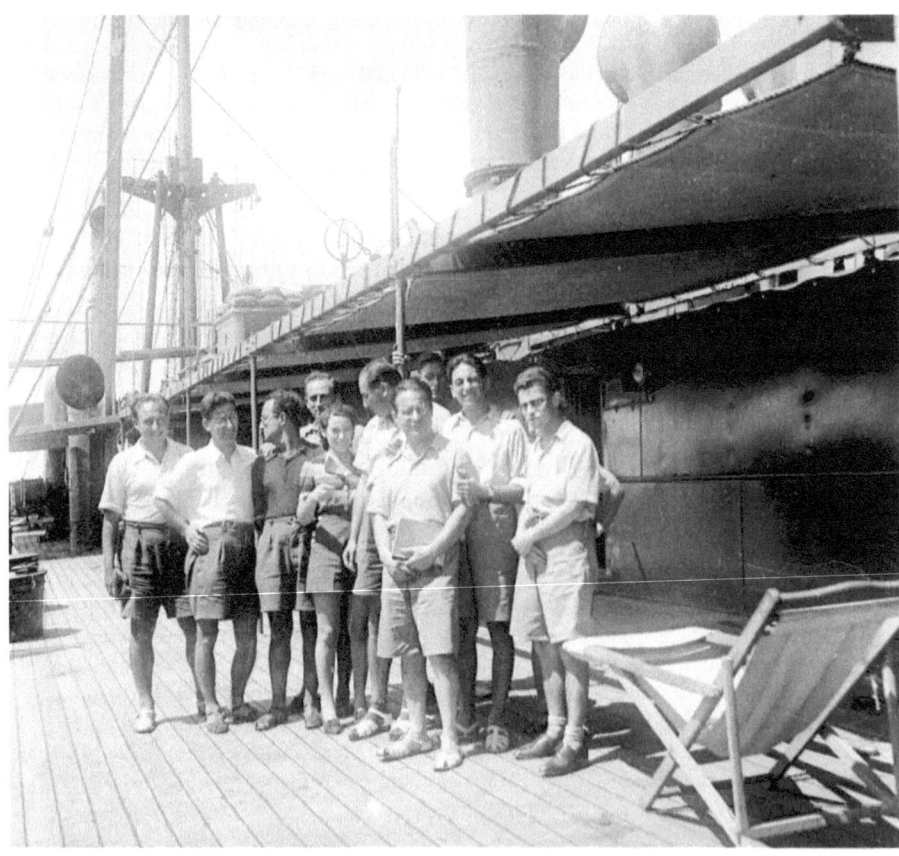

The arrival of the *Aeneas* in Hong Kong on September 28, 1939. Left to right: Drs. Frantisek Kriegel, Iacob Kranzdorf, Leon Kamieniecki, Stanislaw Flato, Mrs. Mania Kamieniecki (directing Wolf and Leon to look at the photographer), Wolf Jungermann, Herbert Baer, Alexander Volokhine, David Iancu, Ms. Edith Marens (hidden with hand on Iancu's shoulder), and Walter Freudmann (courtesy Peter and Joseph Somogyi).

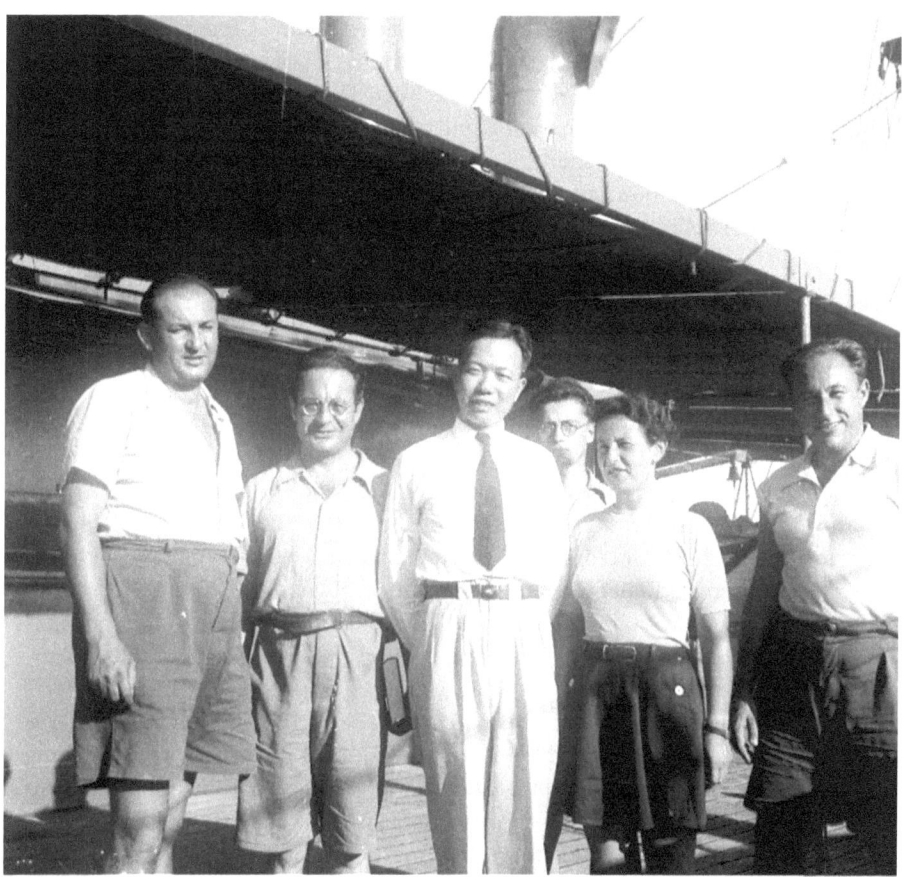

A group of Spanish Doctors disembarking on their arrival in Hong Kong in September 1939. From left to right: Drs. Wolf Jungermann, Herbert Baer, an unidentified Chinese colleague, Walter Freudmann, Edith Marens, and Frantisek Kriegel (courtesy Peter and Joseph Somogyi).

Hilda Selwyn-Clarke's patronage, and with the help of the Foreign Auxiliary of the Chinese Red Cross, the German and Austrian physicians were fortunate that they could escape immediate arrest by the British in Hong Kong.

The British and Chinese authorities spent two weeks considering how to get the International Medical Relief Corps' arrivals in Hong Kong to the Chinese Red Cross/Medical Relief Corps' headquarters in southwest China. With the help of the Chinese Defence League and the Foreign Auxiliary-Chinese Red Cross, Drs. Baer and Freudmann continued to avoid internment. As they waited to embark on their inland journey, the International Medical Relief Corps' members eagerly anticipated a visit with Mme. Sun Yat-sen, chairperson of the Central Committee of the Chinese Defence League.

Dr. Kranzdorf was not disappointed. He wrote of, "her real human greatness and was to later often recall with admiration what a lifelong treasure this meeting was."[20] Dr. Freudmann echoed Dr. Kranzdorf's sentiments of Mme. Sun Yat-sen's great human dignity. At the same time, he could not comprehend why she vehemently dictated that their deployment would be restricted to the Guomindang Nationalist Party, which controlled central and southwestern China rather than the Chinese Communist Party that controlled the northwest.[21]

Despite the intelligence and charm of Mme. Sun Yat-sen, most of the doctors were more concerned with helping the communists than the Nationalists. They envisioned the communists as able to initiate a new order that would be more representative of their values.

While the group waited in Hong Kong, they received more attention from the press than the more solitary arrivals of Drs. Cohn, Courtney, Coutelle, Kent, Mann, Mamlok, and Wantoch, and the wives, Gisela Kranzdorf and Susanne Wantoch. The front page of the *New York Times* included the brief blurb, "18 doctors who served in Spain arrive in China."[22] The International Medical Relief Corps' members did not welcome this publicity from the foreign press. Dr. Fritz Jensen later lamented that from then on, the Japanese would know all too well about their presence in China and that, if captured, they would be imprisoned or worse.[23]

Although the International Medical Relief Corps did not welcome the attention from the press, they did enjoy another warm welcome in Hong Kong, this time from Miss Joan Staniforth (唐莉华). Staniforth had come to China as a domestic assistant for the Selwyn-Clarke family in January 1938 aboard the *Naldera*.[24] In a letter to her mother in England, describing a rare moment of relaxation with the group, she exclaimed, "Mummy, I am with some of the International Brigade doctors. There are Poles, Romanians, Bulgarians, Austrians and Germans here!"[25]

However, the moments of relaxation were fleeting as the International Medical Relief Corps' members came to grips with the harsh medical realities of wartime China in the British colony of Hong Kong. They encountered epidemics of tropical diseases and severe malnutrition: things that they had only seen in textbooks. They realized that when and if they could leave Hong Kong, their medical task would be daunting.

The Voyage of the Jean Laborde from France to China

On August 4, 1939, eight days before the *Aeneas* left Marseille, Dr. Erich Mamlok sailed by himself from Marseille to Hong Kong on the French steamship the *Jean Laborde*.[26] He had just completed his medical studies at

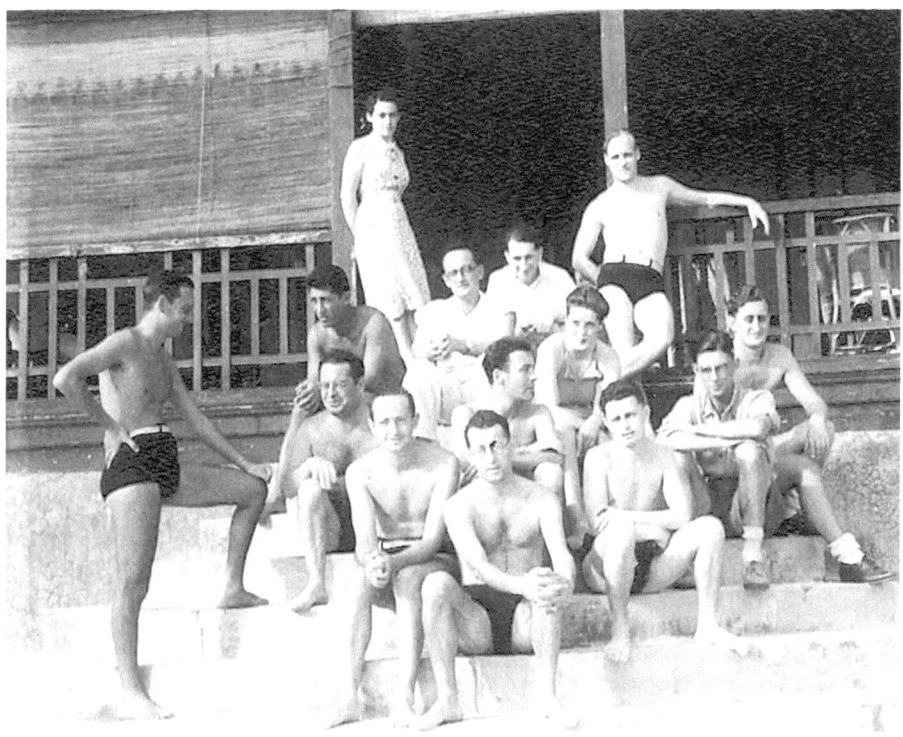

The Spanish doctors enjoying a brief seaside rest in Hong Kong before their travel to the Chinese Red Cross Headquarters in Guiyang, China, October 1939. From left to right: front row: Drs. George Schoen, Iacob Kranzdorf, and Walter Freudmann; second row: Drs. Ianto Kaneti (standing), Herbert Baer, unknown, Ms. Joan Staniforth, Alexander Volokhine, and unknown colleague; third row: Drs. Wictor Taubenfligel, Leo Kamieniecki, and unknown colleague; back row: (standing) Mrs. Mania Kamieniecki and unknown colleague (courtesy Bernard Becker).

the University of Basel, Switzerland. The Basel class of 1939 included the China-bound Dr. Hans Müller (汉斯•米勒博士 Hansi Mileboshii) and an unidentified Chinese physician returning to his homeland. Before Dr. Mamlok arrived in Hong Kong on August 30, 1939, he continued to worry about his parents. His mother and father continued to debate whether to leave Europe in the face of rising anti–Semitism in Nazi Germany. This was a common topic of discussion among many of the Jewish families of the International Medical Relief Corps:

> I see the outlook in all countries as rather gloomy, and am aware of the huge and unforeseeable difficulties as well. On the other hand, I'm convinced that by staying in Germany, our family members are in great danger of being killed. The daily events confirm the general and firm conviction that it is no longer possible for Jews to have a life in Ger-

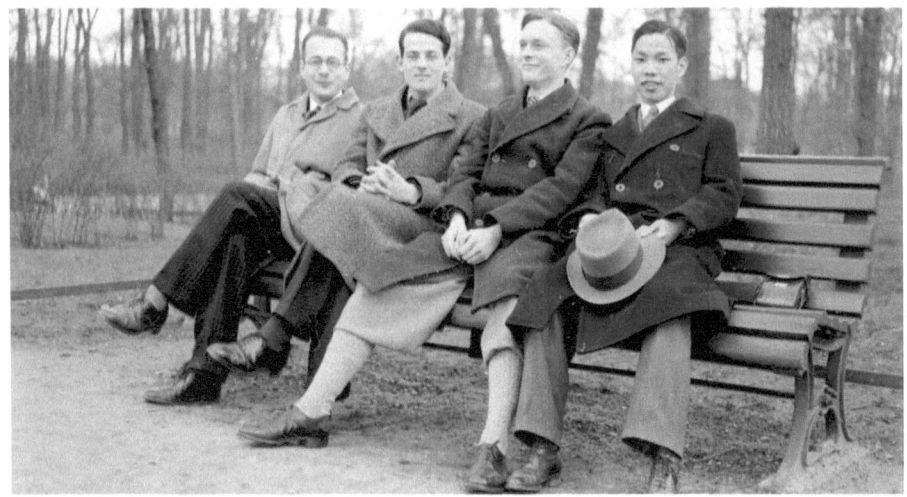

International medical students enjoying one of their last peaceful day in a park near the University of Basel, Switzerland, 1938. Left to right: Dr. Erich Mamlok, with unknown Swiss and Chinese medical students (courtesy Robert Mamlok).

many any longer. They are suspended in constant danger, and all young people are striving to get their families out of Germany. The difficulties are of course very large, but even the greatest fear for Hans [his older brother] and I would of course be easier to withstand than if the parents would stay in Germany.[27]

Dr. Mamlok's father, Dr. Alfred Mamlok, endured the forced closure of his medical practice and sale of his family's sugar beet farm. He remained in Berlin with his wife, scurrying between safe houses, trying to secure travel documents for his family to leave Germany. Strict quotas, international indifference, and the "Catch 22" logic of German Nazi bureaucrats had severely limited the immigration options for Jewish refugees by 1939. For example, proof of passage booked on a ship was required for a visa, and proof of a visa was required to book passage on a ship.[28] South America and Shanghai became popular destinations for Jewish refugees, as they did not require uncertain years of waiting for visa approval.

To Alfred's relief, his oldest son, Dr. Hans Mamlok, could immigrate to the United States in 1938. It was somewhat easier for him to obtain a U.S. visa, as he was a well-established physician, having graduated from the University of Bonn medical school in 1933. However, as an enemy alien in the United States, Hans could not join the U.S. Army in Asia until he became a U.S. citizen in 1944. The use of enemy alien physicians was restricted to essential civilian posts in 1942 by the U.S. War Department.[29]

Much like Drs. Heinrich Kent, Fritz Jensen,[30] and Teddy Wantoch, Dr. Erich Mamlok had been unable to obtain a visa to the United States. His parents wanted him to travel with them to South America.³¹ To their dismay, Erich, at twenty-six years of age, had been exploring other options. In July 1939, he wrote to his uncle Robert:

> As you know, over the past three months I have wanted to go to China. At the wish of my parents, who immediately were opposed to this idea, we tried to obtain a visa to the United States. However, this plan failed.... I believe that my parents have gradually come to terms with China, as far as I can understand their thoughts.³²

Mamlok heard from his parents just as the *Jean Laborde* disembarked to China:

> Dear Little One:
> You can understand that I am writing this letter in a wistful voice, as it will be the last one that is directed to a European address. As you know, it would be our preference to direct the course of the ship to the West, but on the other hand we cannot find the grounds to decide, what your intentions will lead you to.
> As we already have stated several times, you have our full support for your projects that have a reasonable chance of making you happy and content. Where this will be we have some ambivalence about, and we must with heavy, heavy hearts think of the probability of ever seeing you again. That is why we hope that we will have the pleasure of hearing of good news and seeing your wellbeing. Who knows today what is right and even those who believe they are prudent and wise have not succeeded. Maybe, you'll laugh at us all and also Hans yet, and you will feel happier in the east when we are all together.... Even if with each parting day you are now distancing yourself from us, you must be convinced that we are closer to you in our thoughts than ever before. Continents and oceans cannot separate us from one another.
> Please be assured that your parents accompany you in thoughts everywhere you are. We wish you all the best in all your ways; stay healthy and gladden us quite often through detailed reports, from which we can see how you are doing and how you feel...
> . If it should go so well again that we could take to China, then we would be the happiest of people, as we could embrace our youngest son again.... So, dear little one, keep your old parents in good remembrance. Enjoy, despite the sweltering heat of the Red Sea, your trip abroad and please let us hear from you soon.³³

Parental concern and conflict over decisions made during this difficult period were common among the doctors volunteering to serve in Spain. Dr. Volokhine had broken off ties with his White Russian family when he went to fight with the Republicans in the Spanish Civil War. Dr. Becker rejected fascism and joined the Communist Party; his support for the Spanish Republicans resulted in a break of all his ties with his family in Germany. When Dr. Coutelle was forced to immigrate to the Soviet Union, he too had to break off all contact with his family: "His father, who helped him to find contacts to get to the USSR, had to formally disown him. He did not like what his son was doing, but in his contribution to the Coutelle family history record, he acknowledged the consequence and honesty with which his son stuck to his beliefs as true 'Huguenot values.'"³⁴

70   Part I: The Physicians' Fight Against the Global Rise of Fascism

After the International Medical Relief Corps' members defined their political and professional preferences with their families, they considered the logistics of how to get to China. The communication of Drs. Wantoch and Mamlok with the Chinese Red Cross prior to their travel from Europe is not available. They did not have the organizational and financial support of the British and Norwegian China Medical Aid Committee or the Comintern.

Documents from the Guiyang, China, Archives show that the sponsorship for Dr. Mamlok to join the Chinese Red Cross came from his Swiss professor, Dr. Hermann Mooser. As a League of Nations' Health Organization representative in China, Dr. Mooser could easily help his Swiss alumni. Dr. Mamlok wrote to his family and told them that he finally arrived in Hong Kong on August 30, 1939, with separate visas for Hong Kong and China and that all was well in the world.[35]

However, on September 1, 1939, he, too, learned of the German invasion of Poland. Dr. Mamlok now realized that he had become an enemy alien in a British colony and sought the help of the Chinese Red Cross leadership. Dr. Changyao Wu (伍长耀), Secretary General of the Chinese Red Cross in Hong Kong, provided him with a certificate that read: "On the order of Dr. Kho-Seng Lim [Dr. Robert Lin], Dr. Mamlok is heading to Guiyang to serve for the medical relief. Please take care of Dr. Mamlok and try your best to escort him to help him out. Thank you very much. We appreciate your kind help. September 2nd, 1939."[36]

However, when Great Britain declared war on Germany the following day, the good intentions of the Chinese Red Cross did not carry as much weight as the patronage of the British Hilda Selwyn-Clarke and the China Medical Aid Committee of London in the British colony of Hong Kong. Despite his well-intended anti–Fascist efforts, Dr. Erich Mamlok was confined to his first British internment camp.

The creation of enemy aliens by Britain's declaration of war on Germany affected the Chinese Red Cross in mainland China, too. For example, on September 3, Dr. Bob McClure (then with the Friends Ambulance Unit) was out on a convoy transporting medical relief supplies. His immediate reaction was mainly one of annoyance as he sought to continue his work but some German-Jewish refugees with whom he had been working had suddenly become enemy aliens because their passports were German. As Dr. McClure had already noted, "it was a silly world."[37]

The Voyage of the *Deucalion* from England to China

In 1940, Drs. Carl Coutelle and Heinrich Kent spent a memorable period in Great Britain. Carl and Rosa Coutelle celebrated the birth of their son

4. The Journey to the Chinese Red Cross Headquarters   71

The unsuccessful effort of Dr. Robert Lin and the Chinese Red Cross to help Dr. Erich Mamlok reach the Medical Relief Corps Headquarters in Guiyang from Hong Kong in September 1939 (courtesy Robert Mamlok).

Charles in 1939, and Heinrich and Maria Kent slowly acclimated as refugees in a new land. Dr. Kent's sister, Edith, wrote that her brother, Heinrich, applauded the Spanish-speaking Maria's efforts to learn English. Although happy events punctuated their lives, the frustration of being inactive in a world at war gnawed at them. Like many of the other International Medical Relief Corps' members, this inactivity was something Dr. Kent's friends knew he could not live with:

> Through the help of Dr. [Tudor] Hart of the China Medical Aid Committee, he [Dr. Kent] got a visa to England for several months. It was anticipated that he would go with [Maria] yet to China in September 1939.... He was not allowed to work in England but his wife became a good dressmaker. He was unhappy as he was unable to work. He was not able to take his wife to China and sailed alone. They had tried to go to the United States and applied to emigrate from Paris to the United States in March 1939 but were told it would take 3–4 years.[38]

Rosa and Carl Coutelle were happy with their good fortune to have obtained temporary asylum in England. Progressive British sympathizers, particularly Dr. Mary Gilchrist, secretary of the China Medical Aid Committee of London, helped them. The Coutelles had been able to work temporarily as lodger-housekeepers for a group of Quaker men whose wives were evacuated from London.[39] Housekeeping was one of the few jobs for which asylum seekers could obtain a British work permit in 1939. However, the goal of joining their International Brigade medical colleagues in the fight against fascism remained their main objective.

On July 30, 1940, Drs. Kent and Coutelle finally departed from Liverpool on the *Blue Funnel Line* steamship the *Deucalion*. Their wives were not allowed to accompany them to China, as the *Deucalion* was an armed commercial steamer, not permitted to carry woman and children. Drs. Kent and Coutelle traveled with five Chinese students who were returning to China. Maritime records indicate that the two doctors were destined for Singapore and the Chinese students were planning travel to Hong Kong. The thirty-year-old Dr. Coutelle was listed as a German (and hence an enemy alien in the eyes of the British); the thirty-two-year-old Austrian Dr. Kent was listed as of Spanish nationality.[40] Dr. Coutelle described the *Deucalion*'s departure:

> We passed miles of mine sunk wrecks then, on the open sea. They were, like all men on board, included in the night-watch rotation, but otherwise they were strictly separated from the other passengers, even with separate meal times. In Singapore, a representative of the Chinese Red Cross invited Drs. Coutelle and Kent for dinner, but this turned out to be a very formal event without any of the cordiality they remembered from their previous reception in Spain. However, as their sea voyage ended in Rangoon in 1940; they were received by very well meaning and helpful British missionaries who understood their humanitarian aim well and helped them on their journey.[41]

Several other future International Medical Relief Corps' members embarked on solitary journeys to China under very different circumstances. This included the English Dr. Barbara Courtney; the Austrians Dr. Theodor and Susanne Wantoch; the Romanian Gisela Kranzdorf; and the American, Dr. Adele Cohn. Many of the details of their journey to China remain unknown.

However, it is known that in 1940, Dr. Courtney reached the headquarters of the Chinese Red Cross in Guiyang, China from India with the help of the Friends Ambulance Units. She previously had been working in tropical medicine at the Haffkine Institute in Mumbai, India.[42]

In September 1938, the Wantochs married, just as Teddy Wantoch finished his medical studies at the University of Vienna. They fled to England with the help of Susanne Wantoch's sister, Elisabeth Eisenberger. Having previously emigrated from Austria to England, Eisenberger could sponsor Teddy, Susanne, and Teddy's brother for their visas to England. This appeared to work out well for all: Elisabeth married Teddy's brother and they remained together in England throughout the war. Susanne and Teddy Wantoch departed from England to China in November 1938.[43]

In 1940, Gisela Kranzdorf may have had the most harrowing—but unfortunately the least documented journey to China of any of the volunteers. She took the overland route to China, from Europe through Russia, Manchuria— and, for that matter, much of the countries embroiled in World War II.[44] When the Kranzdorfs finally reunited, their Chinese colleagues described them as, "very affectionate, especially the loving Gisela. In the evening after dinner, she is often holding her husband's arm, walking in the mountains, and they are found studying medicine together."[45]

The Voyage of the *California*

Dr. Adele Cohn, the only American born and last member of the International Medical Relief Corps to reach China, traveled from San Francisco to Manila to Hong Kong in the fall of 1941 on a Java-Pacific steamship line, the *California*. After arriving in Manila, Dr. Cohn expressed great thanks to the Philippine Tuberculosis Society for sheltering her, "or else I would have been completely bankrupt long ago."[46] Dr. Cohn also recognized the help of Hilda Selwyn-Clarke of the Foreign Auxiliary-Chinese Red Cross: "She was most kind to me in Hong Kong and in facilitating my travel to Chungking [Chongqing], among all the other splendid things she did for me." At the same time, Mrs. Selwyn-Clarke wrote to Dr. Co-Tui at the American Bureau for Medical Aid to China, "Foreigners arriving in Hong Kong need some kindness and hospitality and it is advisable to send them directly to us."[47]

Ardent anti–Fascism clearly linked the two female physicians, Drs. Cohn and Courtney with the male International Medical Relief Corps' physicians.

However, they differed from their male medical colleagues by more than their sex. Drs. Cohn and Courtney's wish to serve in China did not originate from the persecution and/or internment that had displaced the other International Medical Relief Corps' physicians in exile in foreign lands. In this sense, Drs. Cohn and Courtney's volunteerism can be viewed in the purest of forms as it would have certainly been easier and safer for them to have remained in their native lands; something that the other International Medical Relief Corps' members could not easily have done in 1939.

Travel from the Chinese Coast to Guiyang

Drs. Becker and Jensen were the only German or Austrian International Medical Relief Corps' members to reach the Chinese Red Cross/Medical Relief Corps headquarters through French Indo-China. This was still possible as the French and British had not yet declared war on Germany. On July 11, 1939, while in Haiphong, Dr. Becker wrote that his Germanic sense of punctuality struggled to adapt to China time:

> The wait in the sweltering heat of that tropical port city soon became unbearable. Meanwhile we spend the days watching the scurrying lizards on the walls of our hotel room, strolling through the rain-soaked alleys and watching the hustle and bustle of the inhabitants of the city. Despite our impatience, nothing remained for us but to learn the virtue of waiting. Finally, a representative of the Chinese Red Cross, the surgeon Dr. Wang, appeared after many days. He took us in his no longer quite new Studebaker, in which the five of us squeezed in with our luggage.[48]

The crowded Studebaker truck they rode in was a staple of transportation in wartime China. The Chinese Red Cross' decision to use Studebakers reflects this automobile manufacturer's acceptance of the relatively small number of vehicles that the Chinese Red Cross could order. In addition, the Studebaker was well adapted to the limited infrastructure of wartime China. For example, Dr. McClure of the Friends Ambulance Units shared his problems with Chevrolets: "[We] went back to Rangoon and picked up some Chevy ambulances for the Friends Ambulance Units. They were six inches too wide to cross the bridges of the Burma Road and had to be traded."[49]

After their interminable wait in tropical Haiphong, Drs. Jensen, Kisch, and Becker continued north on a long and dangerous trip into the interior of wartime China:

> The journey took us through the tropical heat of the Red River delta by rice plantations and jungle forests to Hanoi and from there northward to the Chinese border, which we reached on the second day. We are on one of the few roads that have been preserved for the supply and connection of the vast subcontinent with the outside world. So we reached Lang-Son, the Chinese border town, and a frequent target of Japanese bombers.

4. The Journey to the Chinese Red Cross Headquarters

> For us, a new phase of life begins. A hurried, nervous crowd at the border crossing, lines of trucks in the dust and heat, houses and huts made of bamboo, between restaurants.... For days we are enveloped in clouds of dust on the rutted roads, here and there, bomb craters or battered trucks leaving along the way; always watching with a heavenward gaze for the Japanese planes that appeared suddenly and unhindered.
> We climbed through the south China Mountains on switchback—through numerous villages and towns on our way to our goal, the provincial capital of Guiyang. This included the picturesque, much sung about Liudschou with its conical mountains. The road passes onto rickety river ferries, before which the traffic accumulates for hours or even days as the bridges are all destroyed.[50]

They arrived on July 27, 1939, at the Chinese Red Cross/Medical Relief Corps' headquarters in the small village of Tuyunguan near the city of Guiyang. This was the beginning for some of their nine-year long medical service to China.

Two months later, the China Medical Aid Committees needed to explore different routes to get the crew of the *Aeneas* from Hong Kong to the interior of China. Before the Japanese invasion, they envisioned that it would be relatively easy to go directly by train from Canton [Guangzhou] (75 miles northwest of Hong Kong) to Hankou, deep in the heart of China. However, the Imperial Japanese Army had now halted all travel on the east–west Canton [Guangzhou]–Hankou line. At the same time, Japan was pressuring the French to stop the north–south transport of supplies and labor from Indo-China to China.

Even so, it still seemed like it would be possible for the International Medical Relief Corps' members to take the Indo-China route to Guiyang. Once Britain and France declared war on Germany in September 1939, this route was foreclosed. The German and Austrian enemy aliens, Drs. Baer and Freudmann, could no longer enter French Indo-China. In contrast to the German, Dr. Becker, and the Austrian, Dr. Jensen, before them, Drs. Baer and Freudmann needed to find an alternate route out of Hong Kong.

Fortunately, the China Medical Aid Committees secured air passage for Drs. Baer and Freudmann over the Japanese lines. They flew 690 miles from Hong Kong to Chongqing, the western wartime capital of Free China, and then traveled overland 230 miles south to Guiyang. The remainder of the group would trace the northern 610-mile journey of Drs. Becker, Jensen, and Kisch from Haiphong to Guiyang. This group was fortunate that, due to the relative unity of the Chinese Communist Party and the Guomindang Nationalist Party's Second United Front, they could still pass through both the Japanese and the Chinese Communist Party-controlled areas to reach the home of the Chinese Red Cross in the Guomindang Nationalist Party-controlled area of southwestern China.

While Drs. Baer and Freudmann had an uneventful flight into Chongqing, the rest of the group trudged slowly north by boat, train, car, and foot.

They left Hong Kong in a small coastal steamer, which was not well equipped for an intense tropical storm that left them seasick and miserable. As the International Medical Relief Corps' members passed through Indo-China and into China, crowds of enthusiastic, young people near the cities of Nan-ning and Liu-chow (Liuzhou) greeted them. Much as with their arrival in Spain, Soviet revolutionary songs were music to their ears. However, these celebrations would be short lived. As they traveled further north, Dr. Iancu wrote that the authorities took measures to prevent these welcoming gatherings.[51]

By the time the International Medical Relief Corps' members reached Guizhou province, the excitement grew much weaker and the travel became much harder. The perils of ground transportation through Yunnan and Guizhou province in China during the late 1930s are legendary. The author W.H. Auden wrote:

> The road twisted and struggled, and the car clung to it like a mongoose attacking a cobra. Pedestrians screamed, cyclists overbalanced into paddy-fields, wrecked hens lay twitching spasmodically in the dust-storm behind us. At every corner we shut our eyes, but the chauffer only laughed darkly as befitting one of the Lords of Death, and swung us round the curve with squealing brakes.[52]

After a few days of traveling over makeshift switchback roads and dodging Japanese bombers, the second group of International Medical Relief Corps' members arrived at the Chinese Red Cross headquarters.[53] It was October 16, 1939. Britain was not as fortunate that day, as the German Luftwaffe began the bombing of Britain. The whole world seemed to be zigzagging along on a very unpredictable path.

Although Dr. Mamlok arrived in Hong Kong a few days before the *Aeneas*, his German enemy-alien status forced him into taking an even more circuitous and arduous southwestern route to Guiyang. Writing from Shanghai in September 1939, he shared his travel and good fortune with his family:

> Please excuse me for not having written in such a long time. In the last months everything has been a bit up in the air, and I can now tell you things more definitively. In a few hours, I will leave today with a steamboat from here [Shanghai] to Ningpo [Ningbo] and from there deep into inner China to the south central province city of Guiyang, Guizhou. In my German atlas, this city is referred to as Kueijang. I will be hired as a physician with the Chinese Red Cross and will be sent to Guiyang where I expect that I will be working in an interesting hospital, and I am very happy to do so. In and of itself I traveled first to Hong Kong and I wanted to travel directly further with the Chinese Red Cross, as the war broke out, but because of my German passport I was interned in a highly respectable internment camp for six days, where I was treated gleamingly; but was then deported to Shanghai. I am naturally very happy that despite the war etc., things worked out with the Chinese Red Cross.[54]

4. The Journey to the Chinese Red Cross Headquarters 77

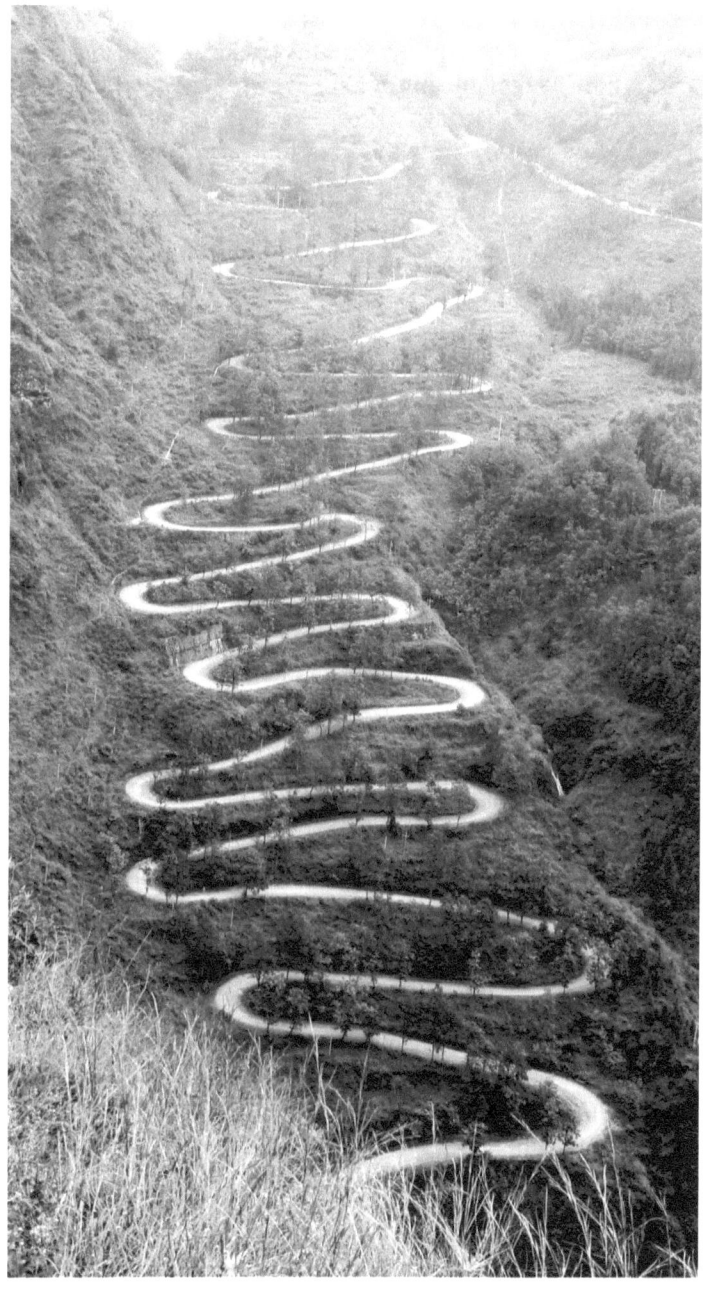

The northeast extension of the Burma road in China's Yunnan Province showing the restored remnants of the hazardous twenty-four hairpin curves segment in 2015 (courtesy Robert Mamlok).

This 959-mile trip through the Japanese lines from Shanghai to Guiyang in 1939 was more dangerous than Dr. Mamlok let on. He probably did not want to concede to his parents that it might have been a better and safer idea to go with them to South America. However, the overseas Chinese physician, Dr. Chung would have sided with Dr. Mamlok's parents. Dr. Chung wrote that travel from Shanghai and Ningbo through northeastern Kiangsi [Jiangxi] and Chekiang [Zhejiang] provinces was a remarkable journey at the best of times, but during the confusion of war-torn China under enemy occupation only the most intrepid dared set foot abroad.[55]

Even the short coastal journey from Shanghai to Ningbo was fraught with peril. Agnes Smedley wrote in *China Weekly* in May 1939, a Japanese naval officer on a destroyer stopped a medical relief boat, the *Tembien*, traveling between Shanghai and Ningbo with medical supplies and food. This ship, with ten Chinese doctors and twenty-one nurses aboard, returned to Shanghai; otherwise, the Japanese would have fired upon it. The Japanese naval officer told the physician in charge, "We do not want to help the wounded Chinese, we want them to die."[56]

Despite these warnings and having been deported from the British colony of Hong Kong to Shanghai, Dr. Mamlok was pleased to be traveling again—and striving to reach his goal: the headquarters of the Chinese Red Cross/Medical Relief Corps. He wrote to his family about the beauty of China, though he again sheltered them from the more precarious aspects of his new life.

> The Chinese landscape is wonderful. In some mountainous areas in this province, which have been developed only after the war began, highways have been built with a certain resemblance to the Dolomites road. [The Dolomites are a mountain range in northeast Italy listed as a World Heritage site by UNESCO. They feature vertical walls, sheer cliffs, and numerous narrow, deep, and long valleys.] It looks just like the Dolomites with rice fields; they look wonderful. I hope that I will again be able to travel a few thousand kilometers here again. It will take a few weeks but in China time and distance play a small role.[57]

Therefore, we can see that time and distance played a major role in wartime China. In fall of 1939, wave after wave of refugees and soldiers headed thousands of miles to the west. They ported the remnants of China's institutions and industry, piece by piece, from the occupied coastal cities to the freedom of the western provinces.

Many historians view the good fortune of this exodus, probably the largest migration in human history, much like the miracle of the British evacuation from Dunkirk, France to Dover, England in spring 1940. These Chinese refugees had the difficult choice of following the main roads and canals and be strafed by Japanese aircraft or following rural paths where gangs of bandits were almost as feared. Either way, the hazard of travel in central

China in 1939 were far more perilous than Dr. Mamlok and the other International Medical Relief Corps' members chose to share with their anxious friends and families who awaited their fate abroad.

On December 20, 1938, Dr. Wilhelm Mann had departed on the fully booked *Victoria* from the port of Genoa, Italy, to Shanghai. He noted that Shanghai had become a last-resort refugee destination after 1936, as England and other European countries, North America, South America, New Zealand, and Australia became closed to immigrants fleeing the Nazi regime. At the age of twenty-three, Dr. Mann had settled into the wartime Shanghai ghetto of Hongkou. This restricted sector for stateless exiles became, during World War II, a haven for more than 20,000 Jewish refugees, including more than 408 foreign refugee doctors and dentists.[58] Hongkou was liberated on September 3, 1945. Almost all the Shanghai Jews left by 1949. Although wartime conditions were austere and unpredictable, the Jewish population in Hongkou found relative safety and tolerance.

However, Dr. Mann's main frustration was not being able to continue his work in biochemistry. With the help of Dr. Erich Landauer, who had served together with Dr. Mooser in the League of Nations' Health Organization, Dr. Mann also embarked on the long and perilous journey from Shanghai to Guiyang. Under the cover of darkness, he left the stifling tropical humidity of Shanghai with Dr. Landauer. They traveled overnight to the port of Ningbo, and headed south, through occupied Chekiang [Zhejiang] Province toward the headquarters of the Chinese Red Cross/Medical Relief Corps. Dr. Mann wrote of the mayhem and crush of humanity as the Chinese fled to the west in every conceivable form of transport.[59]

Coincidentally, and probably unknown to each other, Drs. Mamlok and Mann trekked separately through wartime China from Shanghai to Guiyang in September 1939. Taking the path less traveled was to be a common characteristic of both the Chinese Red Cross/Medical Relief Corps and the Western International Medical Relief Corps' members.

The clear majority of Jewish refugee physicians chose to stay in Shanghai throughout the war. Dr. Mamlok, however, chose to leave Shanghai after three weeks. Dr. Mann left after eight months to join the Chinese Red Cross. Although there were more than 400 Jewish doctors and dentists in Shanghai, relatively few of the others joined the Chinese resistance against the Japanese invasion. Notable exceptions were Dr. Jacob Rosenfeld (羅生特 / 罗生特 General Luo, or Luo Shengte) and Richard (Stein) Frey (Fu Lai). The Jewish-Austrian physician Dr. Jacob Rosenfeld joined the Chinese Communist Party New Fourth and Eighth Route Army in 1941. He was a Urologist who graduated from the University of Vienna Medical School. It does not appear that he had any contact in China with his Austrian International Medical Relief Corps classmates, Drs. Freudmann, Jensen and Wantoch. Richard (Stein)

Frey was another member of the Austrian Communist Party and immigrated in 1939 to Shanghai at the age of nineteen. He became self-trained in acupuncture and medicine and served the Chinese Communist Party's Eighth Route Army in 1941.

After living in Shanghai for two years, Dr. Jacob Rosenfeld and Richard Fry joined the Chinese Communist Party Army's Medical Corps. Much like Drs. Bethune, Jensen, Kisch, and Becker before them, the physicians who found the conviction to serve China during the war were exceptional and did not have passive personalities. Decisions to oppose the Nazis, to go to Spain and/or the interior of China, and to reject the relative comfort of remaining in or immigrating to Shanghai, Hong Kong, Prague, Montevideo, Paris, or New York required considerable courage and determination. For the International Medical Relief Corps' members, doing nothing was an option that they would never willingly accept.

When the German Dr. Coutelle and the Austrian Dr. Kent's ship, the *Deucalion*, docked in Rangoon, Burma in 1940, they already knew that they could no longer reach the headquarters of the Chinese Red Cross in central China through either Hong Kong or Indo-China. Much like the German Dr. Baer and, the Austrian Dr. Freudmann before them, Drs. Coutelle and Kent flew directly to Chongqing over the beautiful terraced rice fields and karsts of southwest China to the terrible ruins of the now heavily bombed Chongqing. The spectacular and iconic South China Karst terrain extends through Guizhou, Guangxi, and Yunnan province and is a UNESCO World Heritage Site. Drs. Coutelle and Kent tempered their admiration for the natural beauty of China with their worries about a world at war.

Dr. Adele Cohn also shared these worries as she completed her long, transpacific voyage to China. Dr. Cohn wrote that she was fortunate to have had the opportunity to acclimatize to her new world with stops in Manila and Hong Kong. This was important, as the shock of the grim horrors of death, starvation, and human misery in wartime China was everywhere: "How common corpses were on the streets. Young and old had large ulcers on their legs, bodies emaciated and legs that were swollen three to four times their normal size."[60]

Although travel had already enriched Dr. Cohn's understanding of China, she arrived in Chongqing with only forty dollars in her pocket. Her clothing and personal possessions would arrive several months later. Much as Drs. Becker, Coutelle and Mamlok had already learned, time and distance had different meanings in wartime China than in the urban West. By good luck, Dr. Robert Lin arrived in Chongqing at the same time, and they rode together for two days through the province of Guizhou to her new home at the Chinese Red Cross headquarters, where she was now more than 7,600 miles from her home in Rochester, New York. Dr. Cohn welcomed the opportunity to get to know Dr. Lin on the drive from Chongqing to the Chinese Red Cross' headquarters in Tuyunguan "He is a source of inspiration to me and his fellow workers and they all feel as I that we are fortunate to work with a man who can and will do so much for China."[61] However, not all of the International Medical Relief Corps' members had such a cordial initial impression on reaching the Chinese Red Cross' headquarters.

Getting to China was one major thing but surviving there was another, as subsequent chapters reveal. Certainly, the minority of Jewish physicians who did serve with the Chinese Red Cross Medical Relief Corps appear to have been quite different from those who remained in Shanghai. They were adventurous, had a great sense of commitment to humanity, and were socially and politically idealistic internationalists. Perhaps they also were more stubborn and willing to sacrifice themselves for their deepest beliefs. These traits tightly linked the Jewish and non–Jewish physicians of the International Medical Relief Corps as they began their service in wartime China.

II. THE INTERNATIONAL MEDICAL
RELIEF CORPS IN WARTIME CHINA

5. Political and Cultural Conditions at the Chinese Red Cross Medical Relief Corps Headquarters

Political Conditions

From the north, west, and south of China, the International Medical Relief Corps' members were finally approaching a mixed reception at the headquarters of the Chinese Red Cross. Dr. Mann, now more than 5,000 miles from home, described Guiyang on October 7, 1939, as an ancient fortified city on an elevated plateau surrounded by mountains. Its gray skies remained hot and humid in the summer, dry, and cold in the winter. More striking than the topography was the abject poverty. "The population lived in thatched mud and bamboo huts and wore long coats stuffed with any available material in the winter."[1] The poverty that they witnessed had recently been exacerbated by the burden of caring for thousands of refugees fleeing the war zones. However, long before the war began, economic development in Guizhou lagged significantly behind China's east coast provinces.

The final four miles of the International Medical Relief Corps' members' journey took them from Guiyang to the Chinese Red Cross/Medical Relief Corps' headquarters in the village of Tuyunguan.[2] This short stretch was fittingly straight uphill. The New Zealand journalist, James Munro Bertram (贝特兰 Bei Telan), described his arrival to the Chinese Red Cross headquarters in 1939:

> The buildings at Tuyunguan are primitive affairs of plaster and logs with mushroom thatched roofs. They sink into the landscape as unobtrusively as a native village. In one sheltered valley are the long wards that house the 1,000 bed 167th base hospital, which was attached to the school of the training hospital.... On the opposite hill are the dor-

83

mitories of the students–long barn-like buildings where students sleep in three tier wooden bunks under a straw roof. Scattered around is an ambulance park, a repair shop and several units where students still sleep in tents.[3]

When the Spanish doctors from the *Aeneas* arrived in Tuyunguan, Dr. Freudmann shared his initial disappointment. In contrast to Spain, he did not receive a hero's welcome among thousands of united raised fists.

> We were taken to a shack that served as a storeroom and was filled to the roof with old boxes. At last some workers were found who stacked the boxes so that enough space for ten people was made. The two wives [Mania Kamieniecki and Edith Marens] were accommodated in another shack. The comrades expressed their surprise that in the vast buildings of the Red Cross headquarters no better accommodation could be found for them than this half open warehouse where the wind blew through the gaps between the wooden planks and where there was not even a table or a chair available. "Nice welcome!" Dr. Canti [Kaneti] said to me.[4]

When Dr. Adele Cohn arrived later at the Chinese Red Cross/Medical Relief Corps headquarters, not much had improved:

> I found there was no place for me to live. The dormitory where foreign doctors lived resembled a pig pen more than living quarters and was overcrowded, eleven people living in three small stalls. I was finally put up with one of the staff, in a room that was originally intended to be a bathroom of the house. My room has a dirt floor, no ceiling, and a tile roof that leaks when it rains. The only light in the room comes from the doorway, and when I leave the door open, I must entertain about two dozen chickens, a rather flea besieged and lousy dog, and occasionally a cat. The rats are a more serious problem and at times rather filthy.... The house has no electricity, so there are candles and charcoal for heating the room when it is unbearably cold.[5]

While this degree of austerity was unanticipated, most of the International Medical Relief Corps' members eagerly awaited the opportunity to visit with Dr. Lin and the leadership of the Chinese Red Cross/Medical Relief Corps before they would make any conclusions about their new medical home.

As a journalist, James Bertram felt very fortunate to have been present during the first meeting between Dr. Lin and the International Medical Relief Corps' physicians in Tuyunguan. He described the abrupt informality and revolutionary medical ideas that Drs. Kisch, Becker, Jensen, and Lin shared as thoughts that would have pleased Dr. A.J. Cronin, the medical ethicist and author of *The Citadel*.[6] James Bertram recalled that their mutual admiration included the following back and forth consensus:

> "Most modern drugs are nonsense ... we try to cut down our supplies to a dozen essentials, and those we need in bulk." ... "Front line surgery is a romantic legend. You do a marvelous job and the patient dies. Immobilization is the thing and a decent transport system to get the patient back. Everything is a matter of organization and courage" ... "The sanitation job we are doing is worth a dozen divisions to the Army, if we can only

get the commanders to take it up." "You found that in Spain? Now in China." "Lin is a realist and his measures are eminently practical."[7]

Dr. Jensen credited Dr. Lin for his willingness to use the Spanish Civil War medical experiences on the Chinese front. Dr. Freudmann quoted Dr. Lin as saying that the decision to push the Medical Relief Corps units to the frontlines was a new experiment of great significance for the Chinese Red Cross.[8] However, prior to the arrival of the International Medical Relief Corps, some of the Spanish Civil War medical military innovations may already have been implemented. These strategic advances may have occurred because of Dr. Lin's meeting with Dr. Bethune in 1938. Whether Drs. Lin, Bethune, or the International Medical Relief Corps' physicians had initiated the policy of using frontline medical units in China, the International Medical Relief Corps' physicians clearly supported their personal deployment to the front lines. The medical service of the International Brigades had learned that morbidity and mortality could be limited by increasing timely access to blood components, surgical intervention, and immobilization of fractures. However, the term "mobile army surgical hospital" (MASH) was not popularized until twenty years later by the U.S. military in Korea. The Chinese Red Cross adapted this strategy, by dividing small, mobile medical units drawn close to the front into different functions: curative, preventative, and ambulance. Although Dr. Lin clearly embraced the concept of front line medical military care, some members of the Chinese Red Cross/Medical Relief

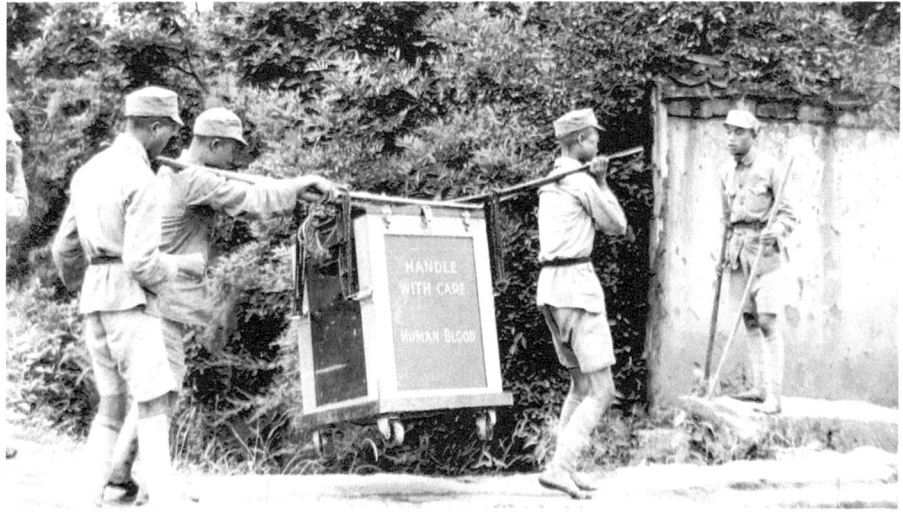

Mobile units often worked in areas inaccessible by trucks. These Chinese soldiers are carrying heavy, refrigerated blood bank bottles to the Chinese Headquarters (National Archives: 208-FO-OWI-3395).

Corps resisted this idea. For example, Dr. Coutelle would later write that convoys of ambulances departed with much fanfare to the "front" long after hostilities had ceased.[9]

All of the International Medical Relief Corps' members initially admired the charisma and inspiration of Dr. Lin. Dr. Mann, for instance, wrote about Dr. Lin's wide ranging influence to recruit and motivate volunteer medical personnel from China and abroad.[10] Dr. Jensen recognized that Dr. Lin was, a lively, eloquent, artistically and scientifically very talented man whose motives were scientific, humane and, gentlemanly.[11] Dr. Cohn added that "Dr. Lin is a source of inspiration to me and his fellow workers and they all feel as I that we are fortunate to work with a man who can and will do so much for China."[12] Writing later for *Asia Magazine*, Freda Utley concluded that Dr. Lin

> combines the best of China with the best of the West. He has the patience, the good humor and the tolerance of a Chinese, combined with a western determination and indifference to face saving, a western scientific training and absolute personal integrity. He understands and loves his own people without having any illusions about them.[13]

China had clearly found the right man to lead the Chinese Red Cross/Medical Relief Corps. Dr. Lin reciprocated the International Medical Relief Corps' members' accolades with his clear admiration for this highly motivated group of foreign trauma surgeons and physicians. He shared the common vision of their solidarity and selflessness, in his August 1939 report to the President of the Chinese Red Cross, Dr. Wang Zhengting (王正廷; Wáng Zhèngtíng) :

> Three foreign surgeons from Spain [Jensen, Becker, and Kisch] have arrived in Kweiyang [Guiyang]. All appear to be excellent individually and we are now testing their technical ability in our hospital here. We found them well qualified, and expect them to be very helpful to our services. All have seen service for about two years in Spain and will have salaries paid for by the London medical aid committee. Dr. Kisch, an experienced surgeon, has already been sent to the Northwest to our Group I, to work with our front units. Drs. Jensen and Becker will soon go into the field in central China. I would like to stress that we would be glad to have as many doctors of this type as can be sent to us. They want to help China, make no complaints, are experienced in war, and are competent and technically experienced.[14]

In summary, Dr. Lin had a very positive initial experience with the highly motivated International Medical Relief Corps anti-fascist, refugee physicians. In 1939, he clearly wanted to recruit more foreign refugee physicians to China. Dr. Lin forwarded his preferences to Hilda Selwyn-Clarke of the Foreign Auxiliary-Chinese Red Cross who shared Dr. Lin's thoughts with the China Aid Council:

> Through experience we have discovered that doctors who come to China for political reasons rather than humanitarian reasons or because they are refugees and cannot

make a satisfactory living in their own countries are very much more satisfactory. Their political understanding of China's struggle against aggression, their international approach to the anti-fascist study makes them prepared to adapt to Chinese conditions and gives them the stability and the courage to endure the very hard conditions of China that is rarely possible for doctors without this background.[15]

A couple of months later, on October 24, 1939, Dr. Lin acknowledged the subsequent arrival of fourteen more foreign volunteer doctors from the London and Norwegian China Medical Aid Committees. He noted that two had arrived on October 11, Drs. Freudmann and Baer, the enemy aliens who had to fly in to Chongqing. The rest of the group arrived through Indo-China on October 16.[16] Dr. Lin wrote on November 5 that they were working at the 167th Base hospital and would soon be sent to the field. He acknowledged that he appointed as reserve doctors the other two foreign doctors (probably Drs. Mamlok and Wantoch) who had also arrived.[17]

Dr. Lin informed Dr. Wang at the Chinese Red Cross headquarters that this second group of International Medical Relief Corps' physicians was off to the front in December 1939: "The 14 Spanish doctors who had been assigned to Groups IV and V in Hunan and Kiangsu [Jiangsu] left Kweiyang [Guiyang] on December 8th. They were accompanied by five Chinese doctors and a number of other personnel. All of them will go to the various divisions to push our new program of Front Line Medical Service."[18]

While there remained an undeniable need for more physicians to head to the front lines in China, it soon became clear that the International Medical Relief Corps member's honeymoon period with Dr. Lim's Chinese Red Cross/Medical Relief Corps would be short lived. Many Chinese Red Cross/Medical Relief Corps' members simply did not want them there. Dr. Jensen tried to explain:

> Our welcome in Chiang Kai-shek's China, the China of the Kuomintang, was cold and heartless. Our colleagues from the Faculty of Medicine wasted no time in making it clear to themselves and to the patients of the Red Cross Hospital where we began working that we, a group of politically and racially persecuted people who had come to their country, were very questionable volunteers. Some of us, they said, were released from concentration camps and others emigrated because of an impending internment. And just what kind of doctors could they be who had to run away from their own country?! In their eyes, we had "lost face." Such a reception felt like a sudden crash. From the heart-warming solidarity and the flaming-hot internationalism with which the Spanish people had taken us in, we came suddenly into the frostiness of Chinese bureaucracy.[19]

Dr. Coutelle similarly wrote that the Chinese could not understand how or why a German would leave his country as a traitor or be forced to leave as a criminal; both associated with loss of honor or "losing face." As the International Medical Relief Corps' members would learn, "losing face" by being openly criticized or not fitting into perceived standards was one of the worst things that can happen to you in relation to social acceptability in Nationalist China in the 1930s. However, in the Chinese Communist Party-controlled Chinese Eighth Route and New Fourth Armies, the two best known Jewish refugee physicians, Drs. Jacob Rosenfeld from Austria and Dr. Hans Müller from Germany, did not report any prejudice due to either their foreign refugee or subsequent enemy alien status. Dr. Coutelle would later suggest that part of the mixed tolerance for the Jewish refugee physicians might well have originated from the fact that many members of the Guomindang Nationalist Party were sympathetic toward Hitler.[20]

However, the malicious anti–Semitism imported into China by Europeans did not take root. Jewish journalists in wartime China noted that China did not have a history of anti–Semitism.[21] It has been argued that the anti-Semitic image of the wealthy, business focused, politically influential Jew was admired rather than detested by the Chinese as both Jews and Chinese celebrated success and wellbeing and identified with a common history of persecution.[22]

Dr. Becker pointed to political differences as a more probable cause of the International Medical Relief Corps' very mixed initial reception:

> Dr. Lin built a well-organized medical aid center. He and his staff had come from the Japanese occupied territories of the eastern coast and the capital Beijing. Among them one finds next to the few doctors, many students and pupils who have left their families in order to join the anti–Japanese struggle.... We sensed very soon that the majority of them sympathized with the progressive forces of the Left and looked hopefully to the northwest of the country. They are careful and cautious in their political statements, because in the province of Guizhou there is a reactionary regime that, despite the "truce" with the Communists, cruelly persecuted their sympathizers.[23]

The dichotomy between the desperate need for more physicians in the Chinese Red Cross and Army Medical Corps and the Chinese Red Cross/Medical Relief Corps' mixed tolerance for the left-leaning International Medical Relief Corps' refugee physicians slowly became more evident. Both Drs. Iancu and Freudmann ominously described episodes of espionage. They wrote that some of the International Medical Relief Corps members' clothes and wallets were stolen shortly after they joined the Medical Relief Corps. The police located their missing belongings the next day and none of their valuables was missing though some of their personal documents disappeared.[24] It was clear to Drs. Iancu and Freudmann that this was the work of intelligence agents rather than thieves.

The alleged Chinese Red Cross/Medical Relief Corps' spying and wary regard for the International Medical Relief Corps' members can be best attributed to the Spanish doctors' communist party membership and their well-known wish to serve with the Chinese Communist Party's New Fourth and Eighth Route Armies. The Guomindang Nationalist Party–controlled Chinese

Red Cross certainly knew about the Spanish doctors' political convictions. At the same time, the International Medical Relief Corps' members were eager to understand how the covert Chinese civil war between the Chinese Communist Party and the Guomindang Nationalist Party could limit their medical role in China. Through their link with the Comintern, the Spanish doctors sought clarification from Zhou Enlai, the Chinese Communist Party's representative to the Guomindang Nationalist Party in Chongqing. Dr. Iancu wrote that Zhou Enlai recommended that for the time being "we should go wherever the Chinese Red Cross/Medical Relief Corps decides to send us."[25] Dr. Mann wrote that Dr. Flato, who was now the official communist party representative of the Spanish doctors, was similarly told by Zhou Enlai that, "You shall continue to treat your soldiers ... we are all Chinese!"[26]

Despite these pleas to continue their service with the Guomindang-Nationalist-Party–controlled Chinese Red Cross/Medical Relief Corps, a sense of cautious political and social segregation remained in Tuyunguan. The International Medical Relief Corps physicians wrote that they felt quarantined, as they were not allowed to have social relationships with their colleagues.[27] Dr. Freudmann added that, in spite of their social quarantine some of the bilingual female Chinese physicians in Tuyunguan warned him of the potential danger of the ongoing political intrigue:

> They do not trust you! ... Your good intentions are not being recognized here, nor are your talents or your wish to fight the Japanese with your own means. They might not even want to use you.... At any rate, they will be gathering detailed information about you. There is something that does not suit them, of this I am sure.[28]

The clandestine support for these International Medical Relief Corps' members points to the political heterogeneity that was already present in the Chinese Red Cross/Medical Relief Corps in 1939. The Guomindang Nationalist Party would subsequently send observers to Tuyunguan to counter Chinese Communist Party objectives in the Chinese Red Cross/Medical Relief Corps. Some of the Chinese Red Cross/Medical Relief Corps' Chinese Communist Party members, such as D.C. Zhang, would leave Guiyang due to the perilous political situation.[29] Although the degree and timing of Chinese Communist Party infiltration of the Medical Relief Corps has been debated, the International Medical Relief Corps' experience clearly supports its existence in 1939.

It is probable that another group of Chinese Red Cross/Medical Relief Corps' members did not choose to embrace or reject the International Medical Relief Corps, but simply did not know what to make out of them. When the English writer Robert Payne visited Tuyunguan, he spoke of one of the Chinese physician's difficulty in comprehending the motivations of the International Medical Relief Corps' members:

> He liked the Europeans, who had come to serve the Chinese Red Cross with a kind of paternal affection, but they were such queer animals, they behaved in such extraordinary ways and he could not understand the complex and sometimes contradictory reasons which impelled young medical graduates to come out to China: "I had never met people like them before I came here. There were Jews, of course, extraordinarily skillful Jews, who could easily have obtained appointments in England or America, but they preferred to live and work and die in this wilderness. Yes, they died."[30]

Finally, there was a third cadre of physicians in Tuyunguan, who shared the International Medical Relief Corps' united vision of anti-Fascism. Dr. Arthur Chung spoke of the International Brigade like internationalism of working with Poles, Germans, and Austrians from Spain, overseas Chinese from the United States and Southeast Asia, and compatriots from most of China's provinces. Both their humanitarian medical interests and the fight against Japan linked this predominantly Asian yet truly international brigade.[31] They believed the need for a united defense would remain stronger than China's domestic conflict and the International Medical Relief Corps' physicians still hoped that the Chinese Red Cross/Medical Relief Corps would not discriminate against the Chinese Communist Party's Armies.

While different groups in the Chinese Red Cross/Medical Relief Corps shared their like and dislike for the presence of the International Medical Relief Corps, the International Medical Relief Corps shared their initial impressions of rural China. They wrote extensively and concurrently about their admiration for the hard-working Chinese people and their contempt for the corruption they witnessed in the medical institutions that they served. As we have seen, the low military pay and status of the military in China in the 1930s resulted in an understaffed and economically challenged cadre or medical providers. It is not surprising that under these circumstances, corruption was pervasive and destructive. The overseas Chinese physician, Dr. Chung, shared his experiences with black marketeering:

> The division headquarters overlooked the border checkpoint where often I would see officers doff their uniforms, put on civilian garb, and saunter across the border to barter for goods. The brothels must have been doing a roaring business as well. At my initial encounter with an army doctor I innocently accepted two cans of condensed milk made in France. A week later the doctor took me aside and asked if I would like to "exchange" a bottle of our quinine tablets for something I desired. I circumvented the subject with some difficulty for the fellow was quite persistent. He did not understand why government issued goods could not be surreptitiously sold for personal profit. "Who would miss them?" he asked.[32]

Anna Wang, (王安娜; Anneliese Martens) a German born journalist, wrote that when the International Medical Relief Corps physicians returned from the front, they often poured out their hearts to her in Chongqing. She wrote that it was not the primitive conditions of their lives and their work that shocked them so bitterly, but rather the ever-worsening corruption that permeated all spheres of public life.³³

Dr. Lin was aware and obviously shaken by the allegations of institutional corruption. He tried his best to shelter his organization from these charges. As early as September 1938, he wrote to the American Bureau for Medical Aid to China: "We welcome anytime a liaison officer from America, if only to refute the many lying rumors about graft, etc. We may be incompetent (I doubt so) but we are honestly doing our best and working without any rest."³⁴

The International Medical Relief Corps' members continued to write about the institutional corruption that surrounded them. However, this dishonesty was in stark contrast to the strength, good spirits, and integrity of the broad Chinese population they served:

> Sometimes we met peasants with their tools on their backs. When they suddenly saw a strange, European face wearing the well-known uniform of the Red Cross, they always displayed a priceless surprise on their faces, that never changed into an unfriendly stare or a hostile gesture. That their nature was kind and free of malevolence was always a pleasant revelation.³⁵

Dr. Becker agreed with Dr. Freudmann:

> They [the Chinese] are always up for a joke, completely reliable and honest, even [in case where] there once was a small dispute over the payment. During the long years in the interior of China nothing has ever been stolen from me, even if I left my suitcase at any bus stop. I am always amazed about the open cooperation of the rural population, so in contrast to what we have heard from the Chinese. Of course, war and looting by the army and civil service have led individual peasants and runaway soldiers to go to the mountains and join together in bands that attack the traveling merchants, as a means to escape poverty that is unimaginable for us.³⁶

Dr. Schön clearly voiced his support for the hardworking, underpaid carriers. These peasants were given the manual tasks of stretcher-bearers and supply transporters in the mobile Chinese Red Cross/Medical Relief Corps units that they served. Dr. Schön defiantly told the Chinese Red Cross Medical Relief Corps headquarters, "I cannot ask the carriers to spend half their salary to obtain the requested photographs and the unit does not have a fund to do so."³⁷

Dr. Coutelle wrote:

> [W]hen you visit a Chinese village, they come out to look at the "foreigners," the "foreign ghosts," the "big-nosed" and ask questions like do you have chickens and how many children. When a farmer showed us his hut, you had the feeling that he is giving you a privilege, and not the other way around. The "Middle Kingdom" was for good reason regarded as the navel of the world of the Far East, and some of this spirit was still alive in its people.³⁸

Dr. Becker added:

Everywhere we meet working farmers who hospitably invite strangers to their meal, with rice, peppers and vegetables. Whereupon [with] even the most hungry beggar there is a commandment of courtesy and consideration, with the question "Have you eaten?," which is respectfully answered, "Thanks, I've already eaten." In a country where the satisfaction of food is a priority, the ceremonial salutation appears natural.[39]

The humble kindness and acceptance of the International Medical Relief Corps' physicians' efforts by the Chinese people remained a universal and uplifting experience for them through the war years.

Despite their palpable empathy for the Chinese people, the limitations imposed by the harsh political and cultural realities of wartime China had quickly become apparent to the International Medical Relief Corps' physicians. Although the first meetings between Dr. Lin and the International Medical Relief Corps physicians showed their mutual admiration, it soon became clear that not all in the Guomindang-Nationalist-Party-controlled Chinese Red Cross/Medical Relief Corps' shared this view. There were factions that embraced them, others that denounced them, and yet others that did not know what to make out of them. Drs. Jensen and Coutelle pointed to their refugee status and the loss of face of having to leave their native lands as an impediment to their acceptance.

Drs. Becker, Freudmann, and Iancu wrote more ominously about the political danger of their support for communism in the Guomindang-Nationalist-Party–controlled Chinese Red Cross. Yet others pointed to xenophobia and jealousy of a preference by some Chinese for western physicians. In addition, the International Medical Relief Corps members' outspoken condemnation of institutional corruption was not welcomed by those profiting from wartime misery. As we will see, the left-leaning political convictions of many of the International Medical Relief Corps' members would ultimately prove to be untenable in the Guomindang- Nationalist-Party-controlled Chinese Red Cross/Medical Relief Corps.

Cultural Conditions

Although buoyed by the acceptance and support of the Chinese population, the International Medical Relief Corps' physicians continued to confront soul-searching dichotomies. The Chinese Red Cross/Medical Relief Corps were admired by some and rejected by others. The rural Chinese population appreciated their personal efforts; however, they often discounted their views on the merits of biomedicine versus cheap, widely available, herbal remedies they had used for centuries. The International Medical Relief Corps' physicians had come to China to fight fascism and improve public health; yet, they did not anticipate being thrust into the broader and longer standing political conflict between the Chinese Communist Party and Guomindang Nationalist Party and the cultural conflict between biomedicine and Chinese medicine.

Indeed, the conflicting views of biomedicine and Chinese medicine would remain a barrier between much of the rural Chinese population and the bioscientists of the Chinese Red Cross/Medical Relief Corps. The term biomedicine is used to depict the "Western medicine" or "scientific medicine" that the western trained physicians practiced. To understand the different approaches, Dr. Jensen wrote of China's tenuous belief in modern biomedicine in rural China in the 1930s:

> The traditional system based on Ben Tsao, herbal medicine or acupuncture, and even on Taoist magic is still very vigorous. Partly because they are much cheaper, and partially because they use a genuine core of empirical knowledge that has not yet been investigated. There is a movement by the Minister of Education, Mr. Chen Li-Fu [陈立夫], and his powerful brother Mr. Chen Kuo-Fu [陈果夫 Chen Guofu], to favor the traditional herbal medicine at the expense of modern medicine for nationalistic and reactionary reasons.... The value of modern medicine is not yet a foregone conclusion in modern China and doctors and instructors will need to be careful not to antagonize the half believers in Chinese traditional medicine.[40]

The Ben Cao Gang Mu (Compendium of Materia Medica) is a comprehensive study of the principles and species of roots and herbs. It was compiled in the late sixteenth century by the physician Lee Shi-zhen (東璧 Dongbi) and has been referred to by UNESCO as the most comprehensive medical book ever written in the history of Chinese medicine.

Although some bioscientists summarily dismissed Chinese medicine, Dr. Jensen knew that Chen Lifu and Chen Guofu, the "CC Clique," were a potent political force with whom they needed to coexist. After the war, the CC Clique continued to argue that the Peking Union Medical College biomedical elite's efforts amounted to an American colonization of medicine in China.[41] However, Dr. Jensen recognized that the politicizing of medicine between the Anglo-American and German-Japanese trained medical factions in China was already long underway and fraught with professional danger.

The Chief of Surgery at Stanford University and former International Brigade physician, Dr. Leo Eloesser, shared Dr. Jensen's observations on the lack of acceptance of biomedicine after having spent a year in China:

> China has the oldest existing civilization, but scientific medicine is still in its swaddling clothes, and the mass of people have had little or no contact with it. The average Chinese, not only the peasant, but the more educated, regard the doctor's visit with a mixture of mistrust, abhorrence, and a little veneration as one might with a man who has sold his soul to the devil.[42]

However, eminent bioscientists, such as the pragmatic Dr. Lin also saw the limitations of biomedicine in rural wartime China. For example, he would not allocate precious public health resources to the establishment of cardiovascular and neurosurgery services in wartime China. As such, Dr. Eloesser's request to join the Chinese Red Cross did not come to fruition until after the war.[43] It appears that Dr. Eloesser ultimately shared Dr. Lin's view on state medicine as Dr. Eloesser later devised basic medical programs to help the rural poor in underdeveloped countries and published a textbook for rural midwives.

The obstacles to the rural population's acceptance of biomedicine in wartime China were large as the understanding of the value of public health had not yet been well established.[44] It is also clear that the International Medical Relief Corps and Western-trained Chinese biomedical leadership displayed little faith and patience for the superstitions and Chinese medicine they encountered in the interior of China in the 1930s. They had been trained to rely on evidence- based biomedicine practices that established causative relationships between microbes and diseases. This had revolutionized the prevention, pathogenesis, and management of such infectious diseases as smallpox, malaria, diphtheria, typhoid fever, cholera, and tuberculosis. It is not surprising that the International Medical Relief Corps' physicians would show contempt for such practices as managing cholera epidemics with rituals to exorcise demons rather than receiving lifesaving vaccinations.

However, the biomedical leadership did not have the resources to scientifically validate or refute the efficacy and safety of Chinese medicine that often coexisted with scientific medicine in the 1930s. In addition, they often did not recognize the political and cultural contentions that underpinned the tensions between biomedicine and Chinese medicine in rural China in the 1930s. This topic has continued to interest historians and has been extensively reviewed.[45]

What is clear is that the Nationalist government viewed bioscience as an important component of modernization of the Ministry of Health and the National Health Administration. To the Chinese Red Cross/Medical Relief Corps, Army Medical Administration, and the National Health Administration biomedical practitioners, Chinese medicine represented the past. However, Chinese medicine practitioners countered that Chinese medicine was the essence of Chinese culture and called for the promotion of Chinese medicine to counter foreign cultural and economic invasion.[46] They argued that the denial of the merits of Chinese medicine was a tool of cultural superiority grounded in racial prejudice rather than fact.

Many of the International Medical Relief Corps physicians had witnessed this argument in a different context. In the 1930s, the German National Socialists forbade Jewish medical practitioners from treating Aryan patients. The Nazis exclusion of non–Aryan bioscientists into isolated enclaves in the 1940s, such as the Jewish Hospital of Berlin, would deprive the world of many of their medical breakthroughs. For example, in the field of gastroenterology, this resulted in a generational delay of such advances as flexible fiber-optic endoscopy and fecal occult blood testing.[47] In addition to the direct effect of Nazism on patient care, the delay in adaptation of these medical advances contributed to an incalculable amount of human misery and loss of life.

In contrast to the universal and ongoing acceptance of these diagnostic medical advances, many of the potential merits of Chinese medicine remain areas of evolving study and more temporal use. For example, in the 1920s, K.K. Chen and Carl F. Schmidt's isolation of the asthma medication ephedrine from the Chinese herb ma huang heralded hundreds of international studies and wide use of this novel Chinese medicine compound.[48] Over time, ephedrine was replaced by far more effective and safer asthma medications. It subsequently became popularized as a weight-reduction supplement until it was ultimately banned by the U.S. Food and Drug Administration due to its cardiovascular risks.

More recently, scientists such as the 2015 Nobel Prize in Physiology and Medicine laureate, Youyou Tu (屠呦呦 Tu Youyou) have been able to combine their knowledge of Chinese medicine with prospective evidence-based data with great success. The rigor of randomized, double-blinded, placebo-controlled animal and clinical trials resulted in the repudiation of some practices and the validation of such compounds as Qinghao (Artemisinin) in the treatment of malignant malaria. However, most practitioners of biomedicine and Chinese medicine continue to emphasize the need for more rigorous, randomized prospective studies.[49] These studies are complicated by the recognition that hundreds of thousands of compounds have been used over the ages, and most remedies are combinations of many herbs, each of which may contain dozens of potentially bioactive compounds.

What remains clear is that in the 1930s, the paucity of biomedical healthcare providers serving with the Army Medical Corps and Chinese Red Cross/Medical Relief Corps in rural China created a public health and biomedical vacuum that perpetuated a reliance on superstition and Chinese medicine. Dr. Lin recognized that it was not economically feasible for Chinese biomedical practitioners to adequately serve the rural healthcare needs. He maintained that "[t]he few doctors and nurses, who are trained by the handful of good medical and nursing schools, are now only sufficient for the cities to which they nearly all go for the reason that they are unable to make a living."[50] The coexistence and merits of biomedical practitioners and the far more numerous Chinese medical practitioners in rural China in the late 1930s was something that not only Drs. Jensen and Becker had to weigh.

A Chinese military officer wrote that "many of the 600,000 Chinese 'herb doctors' put themselves and their ancient recipes at the service of the troops and, despite the scoffing of the Western medical men at their traditional remedies, they proved psychologically helpful and valuable. "In surgery, of course, they could be of little assistance."[51]

The International Medical Relief Corps' physicians learned that they needed to work diplomatically to coexist with what they referred to as the "herb doctors." For example, Dr. Becker lamented that on the one hand some Army Medical Corps division surgeons had essentially no formal medical training. On the other hand, if the herb doctors felt that they were losing face to the foreigners, they could easily undermine all the division's medical activities.[52]

The concurrent delivery of Chinese medicine and biomedicine and the population's varied perception of the relative value of ethnic Chinese and Western healthcare providers continued to evolve. However, there is no question that there were eminently trained ethnic Chinese biomedical practitioners who served selflessly with the Chinese Red Cross/Medical Relief Corps in rural China. They had graduated from elite medical schools in Europe and North America as well as from such excellent Chinese medical schools as the Peking Union Medical College, Hong Kong University, Tongji and St. John's (in Shanghai), Xiangya (in Changsha), and Jilu (in Jinan, Shandong).

Dr. Cohn noted, from the Chinese Red Cross' headquarters in November 1941 "The Peking University Medical College surgeons, Drs. Chang Hsien-Lin[53] and Wang Kai Hsi are excellent. They compare favorably to some of the best surgeons I have seen at home…. Dr. Wang gave up a promising career at Peking University Medical College to come and work with Dr. Lin."[54]

Paradoxically, some of the Chinese only wanted to receive medical care from the Western International Medical Relief Corps' physicians. For example, when Dr. Jensen was working in Kiangsi [Jiangxi] Province, he became the personal physician of Chiang Kai-shek's son, Chiang Ching-Kuo (蔣經國 Jiànfēng).[55] In October 1941, Dr. Kent assisted his Chinese medical colleagues by advising some high officials, who, he notes, "are more likely to hear [sic] to the word of a foreigner, than of a Chinese."[56]

Even if the Western physicians were preferred in some settings, they remained accountable for the death of their patients. Dr. Becker noted that when a "patient died, two [of our International Medical Relief Corps] doctors were arrested without trial for several weeks and only released by the intervention of the Red Cross' efforts through the government."[57] The English missionary physician and former Dean of Medicine at the Cheloo Medical School, Dr. Harold Balme (巴慕德 Ba Mude) wrote in 1939 that the tradition of holding caregivers accountable for all bad outcomes had its origin in the Rituals of the Chow (Zhou) Dynasty (1122 BCE), when physicians were classified by their percentage of cures over a given time.[58]

However, Dr. Lin's intervention on behalf of the arrested International

Medical Relief Corps' physicians speaks against the Chinese Red Cross/Medical Relief Corps' tolerance of the ancient traditions that Balme described. In addition, Dr. Lin's actions are further evidence of his ongoing support for the International Medical Relief Corps' physicians he had previously praised. Fortunately, no other International Medical Relief Corps' physicians are known to have been arrested or punished for poor medical outcomes. Allegations of political wrongdoing rather than medical malpractice became the main concern.

Dr. Cohn wrote that she was not surprised that the perceived preference for foreign-trained physicians, whether justified or not, would result in some resentment: "I come to China and there is still a minority feeling—sometimes latent, other times quite obvious—that of the resented foreigner. It is a cloud on the horizon of my work and while I feel little interference now by my colleagues in the things I want to do, I am worried that it will come."[59] Dr. Schön wrote, similarly, of how much the Chinese physicians disliked being shown up in the field.[60]

The interpersonal, cultural, and political battle lines that appeared in the Chinese Red Cross/Medical Relief Corps were not as well demarcated as the no man's land of the Hunan front of central China but arguably just as treacherous. Some selfless Chinese physicians, such as Dr. Lin, clearly had the vision to focus on opposing Japan, providing medical assistance based on need, and downplaying the political, cultural, and interpersonal divisiveness of medicine in wartime China. Others placed their political convictions, personal ambitions, and distrust of the Chinese Red Cross/Medical Relief Corps' motives far in front of these goals. The International Medical Relief Corps' support of Dr. Lin's vision of biomedicine, public health and egalitarian medical care added an important voice to this discourse.

6. Medical Conditions in Wartime China

While the political and cultural complexities that confronted the young International Medical Relief Corps' physicians on their arrival in China would remain for them inexplicable, the medical problems that they encountered were more predictable, but certainly no less overwhelming. Over the next five years, nutritional disorders and infectious diseases quickly became a pervasive and inescapable duality of their professional lives.

Nutritional Disorders

The medical mission of the Chinese Red Cross/Medical Relief Corps largely focused on fighting against the consequences of widespread chronic malnutrition and susceptibility to infection. Not only did malnutrition contribute to the prevalence of infectious diseases, but infectious diseases also contributed to malnutrition in an ongoing vicious cycle.

For example, the malabsorption associated with dysentery and parasitic infections was a common effect that often contributed to lethal outcomes. Dr. Gordon Seagrave,[1] the "Burma Surgeon" graphically described the relationship between parasitic infections and poor outcome in an intraoperative report:

> The intestine had been badly torn [by a bullet] and, as in the case of so many Chinese, roundworms were escaping from the various rents and exploring the abdomen on their own. One was actually lying in the abdominal wound, its body cut in two by the bullet.... A respectable number of my abdominal cases have been known to live, but not one where roundworms filled the abdominal cavity.[2]

Many other factors contributed to the progression of malnutrition in wartime China. At this time, China was, compared to the West, a relatively impoverished agrarian economy that struggled to meet the basic dietary needs of its more than five-hundred-million citizens. The production and delivery of food became increasingly precarious as the Japanese invasion pushed one of the largest human migrations in history ever further westward and into misery. The dire nutritional status of the Chinese was exacerbated by an ever-tightening embargo of imported relief goods and by the destruction unleashed by modern warfare, manmade floods, and devastating droughts. Widespread malnutrition and near-starvation became core challenges that confounded the delivery of basic medical care. Of course, these problems were compounded by questions of politics and the devastation of war.

Evidence for the severity of malnutrition in wartime China comes from several International Medical Relief Corps' physicians. Dr. Erich Mamlok reported in 1939 from Chinese Red Cross/Medical Relief Corps Unit 32 on the Hunan front:

> Medical work is made much more difficult because of the chronic malnutrition from which most of the patients are suffering. Autopsies made by Dr. Wu with special permission of the military authorities, disclosed in almost every case, signs of chronic underfeeding, disappearance of subcutaneous fat and of the fat of the omentum, anemia, and atrophy of the intestine, soft bones etc. In some cases of enteritis the inflammation of the intestine was so slight that the patients must have died of malnutrition and not a result of enteritis at all. The deficiency is a qualitative one, lack of albumin and vitamins.[3]

Under normal circumstances, it was extremely difficult to obtain permission for an autopsy. It was a common attitude to presume that the patient had suffered enough and should not have to undergo an autopsy. In addition, many Chinese believed that if a patient were not buried whole, their ghost would return to haunt people until it found its lost parts.

At the same time, Dr. Hans Müller, Dr. Mamlok's classmate at the University of Basel, Switzerland, had similar observations in northwest China: "At least a third of the deaths are due to lack of medicines and nourishment."[4] Dr. Landauer added in October 1940 that "[m]alnutrition in the New 4th Army soldiers invariably contributed to hemoglobin rarely above 80 percent [predicted] and usually around 60 percent."[5] This degree of anemia further contributed to the mortality and morbidity from concurrent chronic medical conditions from which most of these patients suffered.

John Rich, the Quaker representative in China, wrote in his diary that malnutrition and starvation among the civilian population often created grim and despairing medical and morale decisions:

> At the hostel gate, I was distressed to find a small girl crouched in a corner—a poor forlorn little waif. I urged Bob [Dr. McClure] to bring her in and feed her but Bob insisted that she was bound to be lousy and couldn't be touched. At least, I argued, tell

her we would feed her in the morning. By then he said a hundred starving people would be at the gate and two hundred before the day was over. It is hard to pass by such tragic little creatures and I reproach myself for not acting on my original impulse.[6]

The common use of the term "lousy" to refer to "bad or poor" has its origin in the concept of being lice-ridden.

The severity of malnutrition and nutritional disorders similarly hampered the combat readiness of the Chinese Army. Their officers acknowledged "[p]rolonged malnutrition rendered the soldiers acutely susceptible to xerophthalmia [severe dry eyes], trachoma, skin infections and all sorts of parasitic infections and anemia."[7] The inadequate Chinese military diet and civilian malnutrition became topics of continuous debate among the military, the Chinese Red Cross, the International Medical Relief Corps, the National Health Administration, and the supporting relief organizations.

Among those debates was talk of vitamins. In the 1930s, the diagnosis and treatment of vitamin deficiencies were already well known. For example, the neuropathy and nutritional edema of beriberi resulted from the low vitamin B1 (thiamine) intake caused by using polished or stale rice. Dr. William Wu of the 1st Chinese Red Cross Unit wrote that "[a] special ward with 50 beds in Guiyang was kept constantly filled with such patients. Special diet and vitamin B tablets were prescribed ... and over 90 percent were cured and discharged."[8] Night blindness was a common and easily recognized early sign of Vitamin A deficiency, though it could advance to blindness if left untreated.[9] According to the International Medical Relief Corps' Dr. Wilhelm Mann, the laboratory of the Chinese Red Cross in Guiyang became responsible for producing Vitamin B1 preparations for patients with beriberi and Vitamin A preparations for patients with xerophthalmia and night blindness.[10]

It appears probable that the official Chinese Red Cross' reports did not accurately reflect the amount of food that the Chinese soldiers ate. The Chinese Red Cross estimated that the daily diet provided by the Guomindang Nationalist Party to the Chinese Army in 1940 included, "953 grams of rice, 273 grams of vegetables, 10 grams of lard and 13 grams of salt."[11] From a practical standpoint, this meant that the soldiers tried to survive on two meals a day consisting of a dish of vegetables with some meat or, more commonly, just soup, rice, and congee (a rice-water porridge).[12]

While the caloric load was marginally adequate, the diet was essentially void of protein and vitamin supplementation. The Chinese Red Cross wrote that "[t]he basis of the low nutrition is the economic status of the country."[13] However, widespread corruption and misappropriation of the limited supplies on hand reduced the soldiers' daily food intake to near starvation levels.

Several organizations questioned the adequacy of the dietary allowances for the Chinese Army. In 1941, the Chinese National Institute of Health wrote that the diet was far less than minimum requirements.[14] The Chinese National Health Administration added that only 40 percent of the 4.5 million new conscripts were physically fit. They estimated that more than 50 percent became sick with nutritional or infectious illnesses before they could enroll in the army.[15] Simply put, this army could not march on its stomach.

The International Medical Relief Corps' members did a remarkably good job of adapting to the Chinese Red Cross/Medical Relief Corps diet. This was no small task. Several foreign volunteer physicians had previously failed to last more than a few months with the Chinese Red Cross/Medical Relief Corps because of the poor diet and living standards. For example, Dr. Bob McClure wrote, "A foreigner, even born out here cannot stick it on the food they get there [at the Chinese Red Cross/Medical Relief Corps] and there is no money to get anything better. [Dr. Arthur F.] Bryson tried it and others just as good, no Westerner can live like the Chinese Red Cross doctors."[16] Dr. Arthur Bryson was a Chinese-born and English-trained orthopedic surgeon who returned to China in 1939 with the Council for World Mission. He worked intermittently with the Chinese Red Cross until he was captured by the Japanese in 1941 and interned in Camp Lungha. After the war, he served as an orthopedic surgeon in Nigeria.

Agnes Smedley begged to differ with Dr. McClure. She wrote that the sixteen International Medical Relief Corps' members she met in Tuyunguan were able to adapt to the diet and lifestyle of their Chinese colleagues:

> These men were entirely different from any other foreigners I had met in China. Despite definite political differences, they were united as anti-fascists. Unlike several other foreign doctors whom I had known, moreover, they dressed, ate, and lived like the Chinese.[17]

It was not that their dedication to anti–Fascism strengthened these volunteers' physiology; rather the International Medical Relief Corps' members who were stationed at the base hospitals often had adequate supplementary resources to avoid overt malnutrition. However, Drs. Schön and Kamieniecki self-reported signs of hunger edema when they served on the I'Chang front.

International Medical Relief Corps' physicians did what they could to stay properly nourished. As inflation mounted, however, several, such as Dr. Cohn could no longer afford the supplementary diet they needed to maintain their health on their Chinese Red Cross salary. Dr. Lin acknowledged this fact in a report to the American Bureau for Medical Aid to China: "We are paying Dr. Cohn NC $409/month. This is not enough as she has to buy her own food etc. She is doing good work and does not complain."[18]

Despite their personal nutritional needs, the International Medical Relief Corps' physicians continued to write about the discrepancies between the official reports of nutrition and diet and their observations in the Chinese

Army. Much as Drs. Müller and Mamlok indicated in their earlier reports, Drs. Kamieniecki and Schön wrote of the loss of life due to malnutrition and disease that they observed on the I'Chang [Yichang] front in Hupeh [Hubei] province on the Yangtze [Changjiang] River.

> The 18th Division is the only one receiving the full rations of 24 ounces [680 grams] of rice, which every commander receives for each registered soldier. In all other divisions, they are not getting more than 20 ounces [567 grams]. Only in hospitals is the squeeze [the corrupt practices of kickbacks and bribes] allowed to be reduced to 16 ounces [454 grams] of rice due to the fear of over weakening the troops.... Even quantitatively this is insufficient, but qualitatively this is appalling. The vegetable protein and vitamins in the rice is completely destroyed by the time the two to three year old rice gets to the soldiers.[19]

These frontline medical observations were at considerable odds with the Chinese Red Cross' and National Institute of Health's official estimates (953 grams and 773 grams, respectively) of daily rice consumption. Although chronic malnutrition was obvious to the International Medical Relief Corps' physicians, not all of the international relief organization's leadership shared their view.

For example, the American Bureau for Medical Aid to China director, Arthur Kohlberg, a staunch anti-communist and future ally of Senator Joseph McCarthy and the John Birch Society, aggressively defended the Guomindang against all charges of corruption and misappropriation of medical and military supplies.[20] He argued that the observations of Drs. Kamieniecki and Schön were unique to their area of service on the I-chang front and not representative of what he saw 200 miles to the south around the Tungting lake area in northeast Hunan Province.[21] Father Patrick Scanlon,[22] an Australian Trappist Monk, disagreed with Kohlberg. He believed that undernourishment was common, in 1942, among the troops in the Tungting Lake area.[23] The head of the British Red Cross, Dr. Wilfred S. Flowers, similarly took offense at Kohlberg's views:

> I see troops that are semi starved falling by the wayside. I see them sick and wounded from malnutrition and disease. There is a great need for better food, vitamins, fats and salt so lacking in their diet. Kohlberg is deriding the views of more experienced men such as Dr. Bachman [of the American Bureau for Medical Aid to China] and Mr. [Dwight] Edwards [of the United China Relief]. There is widespread semi starvation among civilians and the soldiers and I have wired the International Red Cross Committee about this.... Kohlberg's assessment is based on a very selected guided tour in Hunan.[24]

Kohlberg complained to American Bureau for Medical Aid to China's parent organization, the United China Relief, about Drs. Edwards[25] and Bachmann's support of Drs. Kamieniecki and Schön's assessment of chronic malnutrition. Kohlberg was convinced that the United China Relief's concerns of corruption and malnutrition in the Guomindang Nationalist Party army "smelled like treason" and that their misrepresentation was evidence of Communist infiltration in the United China Relief.[26] The board of directors of the United China Relief ultimately intervened with a vote of confidence and thanks for Dr. Edwards in the face of Kohlberg's accusations.[27] Their decision helped to vindicate the observations of the International Medical Relief Corps physicians, British Red Cross, and United China Relief that malnutrition was indeed pervasive and widespread.

In contrast to the eventual inability of the Chinese Red Cross/Medical Relief Corps to defend itself from the Guomindang Nationalist Party's charges of communist infiltration in its ranks, the United China Relief was able to survive a similar assertion from the Arthur Kohlberg led American Bureau for Medical Aid to China.

When the Chinese military command was confronted with the prevailing conditions of chronic malnutrition they often argued, "Never mind, the one thing we have plenty of in China is men."[28] However, this would prove to be a pervasive myth. There would never be enough men to serve both the insatiable manpower needs of the army and the labor needed to feed it.[29] As forced and barbaric conscription maintained the ranks of the military, a vicious cycle of increasing military demand and decreasing agricultural supply unfolded. As less food became available, malnutrition and disease killed more and more troops. As more soldiers died, more men were taken from the farms and into the war, reducing the labor needed to plant, sow, and harvest the food so desperately needed by the troops.

While debate continued over the extent to which Chinese civilians and troops were suffering from chronic malnutrition, acute famine remained an indisputable cause of great horror. For example, more than 3 million people died during the famine of 1942 in Henan Province on the North China Plain. The American journalist, Theodore White described the Henan Province famine as the worst disaster of the war in China, and one of the greatest famines the world has known. Weather-related crop failures coupled with hoarding and speculation had catastrophic results. White wrote that

> [T]he people were slicing bark from elm trees, grinding it to eat food. Some were tearing up the roots of the new wheat; in other villages people were living on pounded peanut husks or refuse. Refugees on the roads had been madly cramming soil into their mouths to fill their bellies, and the mission hospitals were stuffed with people suffering from terrible intestinal obstructions.[30]

Famine spread beyond Henan and continued after 1942. Dr. Jensen noted that in the Swatow area, on the eastern coast of Guangdong province,

> [t]he greatest killer was the famine of 1943, which was to some extent manmade by hoarding and the forcing up of prices by speculators. In Swatow coffins were lined up

by a charitable Buddhist organization and patients staggered into them waiting to die in order to ensure some form of burial.[31]

A lack of government control over the distribution, transport, and pricing of agricultural resources and the all too familiar curse of institutional corruption clearly contributed to the severity of acute famine in wartime China. However, the International Medical Relief Corps' experience supports the historian, Hans Van De Ven's contention that even under the best of circumstances; China remained an agrarian society that simply could not cope with the heightened nutritional and medical demands imposed by modern warfare.[32] The inability of the Guomindang Nationalist Party to provide the Chinese population with adequate food and public health became a key factor in its ultimate demise.

Infectious Diseases

In 1937, Dr. Lin wrote that "[t]he Chinese people are predominantly (80 percent) rural, supporting a culture which may still be described as medieval, and existing on a pittance varyingly estimated at $30–50 per capita per annum."[33] In this disadvantaged setting, infectious diseases and epidemics were, throughout the war years, feared and frequent events. Reducing the medical impact of these pervasive public health problems became the main medical priority for the Chinese Red Cross/Medical Relief Corps.

In wartime China, epidemics of cholera, plague, smallpox, typhoid fever, and dysentery were taking an enormous toll on life. In June 1938, Dr. Wu, Secretary General of the Chinese Red Cross, noted that several organizations, including the League of Nations, had been working with the Chinese to help prevent and diagnose these disorders:

> Mass vaccination, with the help of League of Nations Anti-Epidemic Commission Unit No. 2 is under way. This is currently directed against typhus in the northwest. Typhoid fever is everywhere, but plague remains rare.... We are using anti-meningococcal and anti-dysenteric sera widely.... Malaria is worse in the southwest; cholera is epidemic in central China, especially Hunan [province]. We currently have 50 [medical relief] units in the field.[34]

Despite these combined efforts, epidemics of infectious diseases remained rampant in 1938:

> An epidemic broke out in Guangdong, Hunan, and Henan. Around 20 percent of those sick at the Yangtze River front suffered from dysentery and another 10 percent from other enteric diseases. In August whole regiments were infected with malaria and an entire division stopped in its tracks.[35]

In 1939, as the Japanese invasion thrust further westward, the refugee crisis continued to mount. The risk of epidemics in crowded refugee camps grew as the paltry Chinese public health resources were stretched well beyond their means. Dr. McClure and others argued that terrorizing the population by spreading disease was a deliberate objective of the Japanese assault. He wrote that, "breakdown of civilian morale is the goal of modern war and military technique has been altered to deal with it. Medical work naturally suffers in this new attack, for a satisfactory medical service is an essential part of civilian morale."[36]

Among the many diseases to plague China was malaria. Malaria had been a well-recognized scourge throughout southwest China since the Han dynasty (206 BCE–220 CE). In the southern Chinese provinces of Yunnan and Guizhou, malaria was endemic and pervasive. This disease contributed to the historic lack of growth and development of this region.[37] Most new migrants to the area during the war were completely lacking in immunity to malaria, and many died because of ensuing epidemics. Guizhou Province, where the International Medical Relief Corps' members were based, suffered from approximately 800,000 malaria cases in 1938 and saw 80,000 malaria-related deaths per year during this period.[38]

As the war progressed, malaria in China became a national rather than a regional curse. This shift resulted from the large migration of troops from malaria-endemic areas in the southwest to mid- and northern China. The migration of refugees from the flooded Yellow River area further helped to spread the disease westward. It affected almost all medical providers in the Chinese Red Cross, from the lowest soldier on up to the organization's leader. In July 1940, Dr. Lin apologized to his American Bureau for Medical Aid to China supporters: "I have had a bout of malaria and am just beginning to attend to correspondence.... Please excuse [the] short note. This explains why some of your letters are not as yet answered."[39] The scope of the problem of malaria, and the relative absence of effective medical prophylaxis to combat it, was a persistent problem throughout the war.

A review of the Chinese Army estimated that malaria's prevalence in some districts was up to 95 percent of the population. Although the Chinese Army prepared considerable quantities of an indigenous compound, fraxine, to combat the disease, there was no reliable data on its efficacy.[40] The Chinese Red Cross noted that the modern pharmacotherapy for malaria remained very limited in 1938: "General prophylaxis with quinine is cost prohibitive, hence the main focus is on prevention through mosquito netting and prompt diagnosis and treatment."[41]

The direct effect of malaria on Chinese troops was devastating. In 1938, the Chinese Red Cross noted:

> [a]n entire division was paralyzed by what turned out to be malaria.... A notice put up by the postmaster said "Business suspended during malarial attacks!" It was a common

sight to see soldiers with towels around their heads stumbling and all possible clothing and blankets wrapped around their shoulders, shivering and stumbling along to the rear.[42]

Next to malaria, the most devastating disease was bacterial dysentery. The Chinese Red Cross wrote:

> Along the Yangtze front, approximately 20 percent of the population suffered from this though, another 10 percent had various other forms of diarrhea. The Chinese Red Cross produced large amounts of sodium sulfate and some emetine for the Army hospitals in the Wuhan area. However, drugs were largely ineffective without proper diet and nursing care. For the troops at the front, the Chinese Red Cross prepared bamboo tubes filled with bleaching powder with a small spoon fitted to the stopper to ladle out sufficient chlorine for a water bottle. Chloramine tablets would be better but are far too expensive. For others, it was better to rely on boiled water than to trust any chlorination.[43]

Drs. Jensen and Chung shared the horror of the primitive care for patients suffering from dysentery. The military hospital's dysentery ward was crammed with soldiers lying in misery and excrement on the earthen floor. The patients lay squeezed tightly together, side-by-side, unable to escape the horrible stench as their excrement flowed together into a pool. The death of a patient was diagnosed by his neighbors from the cold of his body. Hospital attendants would eventually respond to the weak cries of the neighboring patients and drag the corpses out of the ward.[44] Dr. Chung wrote that, "the image of those gaunt, skeleton-like shadows of men haunted me to no end. I seemed to feel their groping hands touching me, imploring me for help, and I shuddered involuntarily."[45]

Malaria and dysentery were not the only illnesses to plague China. Lice were everywhere. It was not an exaggeration to say that the Chinese Red Cross/Medical Relief Corps had to start from scratch as the entire army was infected with lice.[46] By the 1930s, physicians knew that both typhus and relapsing fever were caused by the prevalence of fleas carried by rats.[47] Yet, in 1938, few army facilities were available for delousing or bathing, even in the base hospitals.

The disease typhus is transmitted by the human body louse, which becomes infected by feeding on the blood of patients with acute typhus fever. Infected lice excrete rickettsia onto the skin while feeding on a second host, who becomes infected by rubbing louse fecal matter into the bite wound. Relapsing fever also is transmitted by the human body louse. These infected lice excrete bacteria of the genus *Borrelia*, which are similarly transmitted.

"No typhus has yet appeared," the Chinese Red Cross reported,

> but relapsing fever is present at several sites. Its prevalence was estimated at 10 percent of the sick, but the absence of microscopes and the coexistence of malaria makes this difficult to estimate. Treatment with neoarsphenamine [an arsenic derivative] and san-

itary measures are needed to keep things in check. We hope to extend delousing to all base hospitals and make this a prerequisite to admission.[48]

Although local infections were present on all fronts, the base hospitals were at greater risk for outbreaks of relapsing fever; these included an outbreak in two hundred patients in Ichuan. Although less fatal than typhus, relapsing fever appeared to be more widespread.[49] Despite the widespread illnesses, the commanders largely ignored measures to prevent lice-transmitted relapsing fever and typhus because they involved "increased" costs.[50]

In 1939, other units of the Chinese Red Cross/Medical Relief Corps, outside of Ichuan, wrote that typhus was less common (and occurred principally in the northwest), but they also recognized that many cases went undiagnosed. Prophylaxis by delousing was the only effective measure as typhus vaccine was usually not available.

Lice and fleas did not only afflict the Chinese. The rat-infested sleeping quarters of the International Medical Relief Corps' members in Tuyunguan added to these physicians' worries of flea-transmitted typhus and relapsing fever. Dr. Mann wrote that there were an awful lot of rats, big as cats. When the rats ran along the ceiling of their barracks, they called it "The Wild Chase."[51] Among the International Medical Relief Corps' members, recurrent febrile illnesses were common, though it remained difficult to distinguish among malaria, recurrent fever, typhus, and typhoid fever. Dr. Coutelle was reported to have suffered from bouts of relapsing fever. Dr. Becker survived the scourges of malaria and typhus, and Drs. Schön and Kisch had unidentified febrile illnesses.[52]

In addition to typhus, dysentery, and malaria, China was afflicted with cholera (霍乱 Huoluan). A highly contagious and dreaded infectious disease, cholera results from the spread of bacteria—in this case, *Vibrio cholera*—in contaminated food and water supplies. Dr. Lin recognized the danger that cholera epidemics could pose and placed a high priority on obtaining funding for cholera vaccine from relief agencies for the Chinese Red Cross and Chinese National Health Administration.[53] Initially, the cholera vaccine was purchased at low cost from The Hanoi Institute in French Indo-China.[54]

Despite such anti-epidemic efforts, several International Medical Relief Corps' physicians, such as Dr. Becker witnessed a large outbreak of cholera shortly after their arrival in Guiyang in 1939. He wrote that the hospital system in Guiyang could not cope with the number of cases that quickly spread in this overcrowded city. Countless dehydrated corpses quickly lined the roads, waiting for a burial when the epidemic would wane.[55]

The threat of cholera epidemics in crowded cities and refugee camps brought together all the available public health resources in China. To highlight the scale of these combined efforts, Dr. McClure estimated that 6 million people received vaccinations for cholera during one three-week anti-epidemic effort. He credited Dr. Pollitzer of the League of Nations, "for having saved the lives of millions in a dedicated, low profile life of great scientific but humble service."⁵⁶

As the Japanese embargo from Indo-China tightened, the Chinese Red Cross developed its own vaccine production facility in Guiyang. Dr. Wilhelm Mann noted that all Chinese Red Cross/Medical Relief Corps' employees were inoculated against cholera and typhoid.⁵⁷ In addition, the institution of large-scale vaccination of millions of civilians ensued and a dab of dye was put on one finger to act as a certificate of vaccination and avoid dodging or overlapping.⁵⁸ By 1943, the American Friends Service Committee estimated that "6,000,000 doses are made annually of cholera, typhoid, diphtheria, tetanus, and typhus biologicals. The equipment is limited but surprisingly good and the technical skill excellent."⁵⁹

Although vaccination reduced the severity and occurrence of cholera epidemics, other infectious diseases took hold. Diphtheria, for example, is another contagious bacterial disease caused by the person-to-person spread of bacteria—in this case, *Corynebacterium diphtheria*. Since routine immunization with diphtheria toxoid was not widely available in China until after the war, epidemic outbreaks of diphtheria occurred in wartime China.⁶⁰ Those outbreaks were also not limited to Chinese troops and civilians. Jensen recounted the misery and good fortune of his personal experience:

> For three days I lay in bed with fever and chills, thinking that it was only an ordinary flu until I could find a mirror and two candles and noted suspicious white stains noted on the back of my pharynx. This was the dreaded pseudomembranous stigmata of diphtheria. I was carried in a sedan chair for two days until I came to a larger village from where I telegraphed a dignitary, who knew how to get a car and gasoline. This brought me back to Kanhsien where I used my Zeiss microscope to diagnose diphtheria. The Catholic sisters in their hospital nursed me back to health. From time to time one came into my room and asked me if I did not repent for my sins. Since I refrained, they assured me, that God will forgive me; because I am so good to the poor. I was lucky and soon recovered.⁶¹

Dr. Jensen and others like him recovered from the disease, but other illnesses sparked fear in physicians, civilians, and the troops. Among those was plague (鼠疫 Shuyi). The bacterium responsible for plague, *Yersinia pestis*, was already well known in China. The Swiss microbiologist Dr. Alexandre Yersin first isolated the plague bacillus during the Hong Kong Plague outbreak of 1894. At that time, plague resulted in the death of more than sixty thousand people in Canton [Guangzhou] in just a few weeks.⁶²

The Chinese Red Cross voiced fears of plague outbreaks in endemic areas and of the use of plague as a biological weapon by the Japanese forces throughout the war. Evidence for Japan's use of plague as a biological weapon came from both Drs. Jin Baoshan and Robert Lin of the Chinese Red Cross.[63] Extensive reviews of the probable use of plague as a biological weapon in China also were described by the Allied command during the war.[64] Other reports of plague, probably of an endemic nature, came from Yunnan, Fukien [Fujian], and Chekiang [Zhejiang] Province.[65] Although *The International Medical Team in Guiyang* reported Dr. Barbara Courtney as having died of plague, her International Medical Relief Corps colleagues' observations do not support this. However, Drs. Heinrich Kent and Tan Xuehua isolated *Yersinia pestis* from a girl who died of plague in Changde (Hunan province).[66] In November 1941, Dr. Kent reported the difficulties of their epidemiological efforts to the Chinese Red Cross headquarters:

> Many sudden deaths and dead rats in a village 45 Chinese Li from Changteh. An acute epidemic of bubonic plague was found which had already lasted for one month. Rats and humans showed the signs of acute plague. Dr. Pollitzer and I have gone on to focus on the plan for fighting this outbreak. By this time, 23 people had died out of a village of 800 persons and many others had run away in the country and so made the control very difficult.[67]

Scabies, caused by the *Sarcoptes scabiei* mite, was another highly contagious disease. While not as lethal as plague and cholera, it was incredibly prevalent and the cause of much misery. In 1940, Dr. Lin described scabies on the battlefield:

> I have seen during my recent trip that the soldiers and civilians up at the front are practically all inflicted with lice and scabies. The latter leads to gross impetigo and really huge ulcerations of the skin, especially of the leg. We would probably have to go back to the Middle Ages in Europe to define such conditions! Sulfur is required by the time for treatment, and we are using the lime water method as Vaseline is now unobtainable and lard, which might be used as a substitute, is too good of a food![68]

The presence of lice and scabies was not limited to the battlefront areas of central China. Lice was prevalent in the Chinese Communist Party New Fourth and Eighth Route Armies. Even Chairman Mao was described as "earthy enough to startle a visitor by reaching into his baggy trousers to deal with lice."[69]

Just as scabies, plague, and malaria were long associated with China, so too was tuberculosis (结核 Jiehe). In fact, tuberculosis was known in China 2,600 years before the Christian era and was widely spread throughout the population.[70] During the war, the disease resumed its spread. Dr. Jin Baoshan at the National Health Administration wrote that China's wartime tuberculosis mortality was

> 3–4 times higher than it should be owing to the lack of preventative and therapeutic facilities. Recent reports from the U.S. indicate that less than 30 percent of U.S. college students are tuberculin positive while in China close to 100 percent of students are

tuberculin positive.... Due to the war crisis we do not envision the building of sanatoria; patients will be cared for in the organizations where they are currently treated.[71]

International Medical Relief Corps' physician, Dr. Adele Cohn, established one of the first tuberculosis-inpatient units in 1942. The pressing need for earlier intervention was apparent: "twenty-five beds were allocated in the training hospital for TB under the charge of Dr. Cohn. Approximately 50 percent died within one month, as they had advance[d] disease and little treatment options. Earlier diagnosis of recruits is needed."[72] Despite efforts to contain the disease, tuberculosis remained an insidious and chronic condition that would contribute to the death of many, including some of the foreign volunteer physicians.

Although not usually fatal, trachoma was another disease the International Medical Relief Corps' physicians had to battle with. Trachoma is a contagious, potentially epidemic eye infection caused by the bacteria *Chlamydia trachoma*. The ocular secretions from infected patients account for its rapid spread and trachoma continues to be a leading cause of preventable blindness. It is not surprising that the International Medical Relief Corps' physicians repeatedly reported cases of trachoma, given the conditions of war: "Trachoma is also a scourge. I have seen in Kansu [Gansu] whole troops of blind men, the blind leading the blind."[73] In 1941, "[o]ver 70 percent of the population of the North West [of China] suffer from trachoma and this means thousands of blind."[74]

In Guiyang, Dr. Heinrich Kent noted that "[w]ashing faces with dirty rags in ramshackle highway inns after meals is probably a cause of the spread of trachoma."[75] The German-speaking International Medical Relief Corps' physicians referred to these ubiquitous guesthouse washcloths that were dipped in hot water, wrung out, and often thrown across the room to a guest to wipe his face as trachoma *Tücher* (towels).

Unlike the chronicity of scabies and trachoma, typhoid fever, was an acute, often fatal illness in wartime China. The responsible bacterium, *Salmonella typhi* is spread in sewage-contaminated water supplies and by infected food handlers. Several of the International Medical Relief Corps' members developed symptoms of typhoid fever. One died in Yunnan Province, and others barely survived their encounter with this dreaded disease.

The medical conditions that these young physicians confronted in China provided a unique professional challenge that would shape many of their lives. Although the Spanish doctors were already familiar with malaria, dysentery, and scabies, the breadth of tropical disease and the severity of infections and malnutrition were things that none of them had ever seen before. They began their medical mission with the intellectual excitement of managing

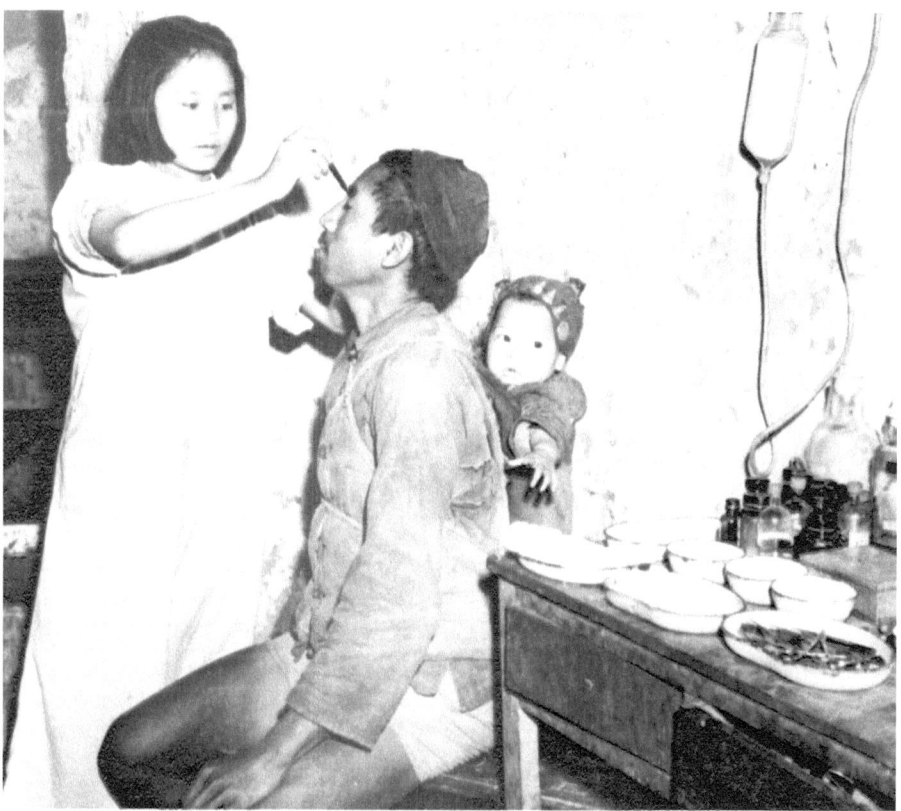

A Chinese Red Cross nurse treating a countryman with an eye infection (undated) (National Archives: 208-FO-OWI-5791).

exotic tropical diseases and ended with the discouraging reality of the insurmountable nature of many of the dilemmas their patients faced.

However, the process of trying to solve some of wartime China's medical problems provided them with a profound professional experience. The International Medical Relief Corps' physicians would learn that the medical impact of public health measures far exceeded the impact of individual medical and surgical interventions. It is not surprising that many of the International Medical Relief Corps' physicians who survived the politics and battlefields of China would later be drawn to careers in public health.

7. Travel to and from China's Battlefields: 1939–1940

The reasons for the movement (and, subsequently, lack of movement) of the International Medical Relief Corps' physicians onto the battlefields in China were complex. They included the waxing and waning of the animosity between the Guomindang Nationalist Party and the Chinese Communist Party, the military strategies devised to impede the advance of the Imperial Japanese Army, and the eventual involvement of the Allied forces in Asia. The International Medical Relief Corps' members continued to speak out and fight against what they saw as the main impediments to improving the health of the Chinese people they served: malnutrition, rampant infectious disease, and an understaffed, overwhelmed, and often corrupt military healthcare delivery system.

Prior to the International Medical Relief Corps' members' arrival in 1939, movement of medical supplies and physicians between the Guomindang Nationalist Party and the Chinese Communist Party controlled areas was relatively easy. This united effort was consistent with Dr. Lin's vision of using the Chinese Red Cross/Medical Relief Corps to aid all the Chinese. Recognition of the Chinese Red Cross/Medical Relief Corps aid to the Chinese Communist Party's Armies comes from several sources. For example, Dr. C.C. Shen (沈其震 Shen Qizhen), a chief medical officer of the Chinese Communist Party's New Fourth Army shared his appreciation of Dr. Lin in January 1938: "Dr. Robert K.S. Lin has earned our gratitude ... the supplies contributed by the medical relief commission were brought back to Nanchang… . Dr. K.S. Lin then came to inspect our hospital and said that it was the best hospital in the third war zone."[1] Dr. Norman Bethune similarly thanked Dr. Lin for the medical care that was extended to the Chinese Communist Party's Eighth Route Army:

Dr. Robert Lin has a supreme control over all medical relief work under the Chinese Red Cross. We have had the privilege of many conversations with this remarkable man and have been tremendously impressed with his organizational ability, vision and drive.... I regard the work of his commission to be of the greatest importance and recommend its support to the entire world as I see the commission has the vision and organization to render the greatest assistance to the heroic Chinese people.[2]

Although Dr. Lin could provide medical assistance for the Chinese Communist Party's Armies in 1938, by the time Drs. Becker, Kisch, and Jensen joined the Chinese Red Cross/Medical Relief Corps in 1939, much had changed. These International Medical Relief Corps physicians hoped to serve with the Chinese Communist Party's Eighth Route Army, in the northern province of Shensi [Shaanxi]. After all, the five Indian physicians (see Appendix C), Dr. Müller, and Dr. Bethune's group (Dr. Richard Brown and Jean Ewen, RN) had recently succeeded in doing so. But their aspirations ran contrary to Mme. Sun Yat-sen's and Mrs. Hilda Selwyn-Clarke's forewarnings in Hong Kong that travel to the Chinese Communist Party-controlled regions in the north would no longer be possible.

In summer 1939, Drs. Becker, Kisch, and Jensen sought the council of Zhou Enlai, the Chinese Communist Party representative to the Guomindang Nationalist Party. They hoped that he could facilitate their transfer to the Chinese Communist Party's Eighth Route Army. Zhou Enlai met with these International Medical Relief Corps physicians in Chongqing, the capital of Free China. He told them that the situation was not simple on the front, and he directed these Spanish doctors to stay with the Guomindang Nationalist Party and use their medical skills to help the wounded Chinese on the Guomindang Nationalist Party-controlled front. Wherever they worked in China, he added, they would be supporting the war against Japanese aggression.[3]

While Drs. Becker and Jensen heeded Zhou Enlai's advice, Dr. Kisch, the senior surgeon of the group, tried to reach Yan´an with a small group of Chinese Red Cross/Medical Relief Corps' workers. He had been appointed to relieve Dr. Bethune, who had been operating continuously during the past year with the Eighth Route Army. Dr. Bethune probably did not know that Dr. Kisch, his former medical commander in Spain, was on his way to help him. On November 12, 1939, Dr. Bethune died from septicemia due to an intra-operative scalpel wound on his finger. Concurrent tuberculosis, poor nutrition, and the absence of antibiotics and basic medical care undoubtedly contributed to his demise.

Dr. Kisch was urgently reappointed to replace Dr. Bethune; however, continued obstruction from the Guomindang Nationalist Party Army again thwarted Dr. Kisch's efforts to reach the Chinese Communist Party's Eighth Route Army. "Dr. Kisch was twice forced back across the Yellow [R]iver," journalist James Bertram wrote; "he is now working in a military hospital in

Shensi [Shaanxi]. Only one foreign volunteer doctor, a young German anti-Fascist [Dr. Hans Müller], is attached to the Eighth Route Army Headquarters in Shensi [Shaanxi, 陝西] province."[4]

Crossing the Yellow River a few times was, in fact, a major undertaking. Several Chinese Red Cross units did not want to go to Shensi [Shaanxi], precisely because they did not want to cross the Yellow River. Yu Tao-Chen, a member of Chinese Red Cross/Medical Relief Corps Unit 61, explained why: "Everyone has a burning desire to cross the Yellow River, but once crossed; then tears will flow, for one realizes the dangers which have to be surmounted on returning." If the treacherous currents of the Yellow River were not enough of a deterrent, Yu added that the risk of being killed by the invading Japanese Army and the physical hardships of travel to the Chinese Communist Party's Eighth Route Army were.[5]

Why Dr. Müller could reach the Eighth Route Army in 1939 and Drs. Jensen, Becker, and Kisch could not is unclear. Dr. Müller later reminisced on his good fortune:

> I was impatient, and I wanted to go to the front and that was that. I had met some German doctors who had been in Spain when I visited the Chinese Red Cross (in which I did not participate) in Guiyang. The people I met during my two weeks in Guiyang were Becker and Jensen. They said that they were eager to go to Yen'an [sic] and did not want anything to do with the Chinese Red Cross any more. They asked that I should do all I can to get them to Yen'an. In a sense, they envied me, because I was on my way to Yen'an.[6]

Dr. Kisch's inability to reach the Eighth Route Army was a serious blow both to the medical team of the Eighth Route Army and to the aspirations of the Spanish doctors. The Eighth Route Army would not be able to find a trauma surgeon with the wartime medical experience and skill of Dr. Kisch to replace Dr. Bethune. The failure of the International Medical Relief Corps physicians to reach the Chinese Communist Party's Eighth Route Army was not due to lack of effort. Despite this initial disappointment, the Spanish doctors pleaded persistently to the China Medical Aid Committee of London about the need and preference to serve in the Chinese Communist Party-controlled areas:

> The Chinese people have carried on their just war against the barbarian invasion of the Japanese militarists for three and a half years. For three and a half years, they have shed their blood and their sweat in a fight waged under the most terrible conditions human beings have ever faced. In many places in which the struggle goes on, there is a lack of the most elementary necessities, which human beings need to live and a soldier needs to carry on a war. And the medical provisions are especially poor as regards both the army and the civilian population. Fifteen million civilians die in China every year. Of the number, at least half could be saved by the simplest sanitary measures. In this sacred struggle, China does not stand alone. In recognition of this fact, the peoples of the entire world and especially of England and America have organized great campaigns

of support for China, and contributed gifts of all kinds to her cause.... The area behind the enemy lines is very vast. While the occupied zone has a few thousand doctors the guerilla region has only a few score. Free China has opportunities to receive supplies from the coast and from abroad, the guerilla areas seldom have these opportunities.[7]

At this point, Dr. Lin and the International Medical Relief Corps' physicians' shared vision of providing medical care for all the Chinese placed them squarely in the crosshairs of competing political interests. Mme. Sun Yat-sen, the head of the Chinese Defence League, disliked Dr. Lin because of his close ties with her sister and archrival, Mme. Chiang Kai-shek. In Mme. Sun Yat-sen's view, accepting the United Front to the point of working mainly through Dr. Lin meant handing over medical supplies and money to the hopelessly corrupt Nationalist government of Generalissimo Chiang Kai-shek.[8] In contrast, others seeking relief aid for China, such as the overseas Chinese in the Dutch East Indies, the American Bureau for Medical Aid to China, Agnes Smedley, and Hilda Selwyn-Clarke, still firmly believed that Dr. Lin was the best person to lead China's wartime healthcare system.

With the gateway—and safe passage—to the guerrilla areas of the Chinese Communist Party in the north closed, and the admonitions of Zhou Enlai and Mme. Sun Yat-sen to remain with the Guomindang Nationalist Party controlled armies, the International Medical Relief Corps' physicians turned to the medical tasks at hand in 1939. Drs. Kisch, Jensen, and Becker left Guiyang for the Hunan and Kiangsi [Jiangxi] front on September 6, 1939.

As this would be more than 500 miles, the International Medical Relief Corps' physicians needed to learn how to march over long distances in wartime China. Their extended travel over difficult terrain required several adaptations to maintain survival, if not exactly comfort. For example, Dr. Becker marveled at the value of the bedroll known in China as the *pugai*. He described how the Chinese could compact mats, pillows, bedsheets, and the indispensable mosquito nets into a tight package hung from bamboo rods. Although there were no pack animals available, he was amazed that the peasants assigned to their unit could easily haul forty-five kilograms, up to thirty kilometers a day.[9] Dr. Mamlok wrote to his family, "traveling in China is the best of all. One travels with bed linen or even better, as in Goethe's time, with one's own private bed roll often going through completely medieval areas, hardly occupied by civilization."[10] Further assimilation of the International Medical Relief Corps' physicians into the Chinese Red Cross/Medical Relief Corps on the Changsha front in 1939 included their choice of footwear. Dr. Freudmann wrote that after a few days of marching, the soles of their feet became one large blister.[11] They had to abandon the high leather boots that many favored in Spain and adopted the cloth slippers that the Chinese used.

As they marched along, the International Medical Relief Corps' physicians described the horror of modern warfare, in stark contrast to the beauty of ancient China. Dr. Becker spoke of ascending over hills on scarlet and gold paths lined with azaleas and enormous bushes of wild roses. They descended into valleys with clear rushing rivers and rice patties that were greener than anything they had seen. However, the continuous flow of downtrodden refugees tempered this beauty. It included, "a father with a boy on his back, blind from hunger and the starving girl on the roadside."[12]

Similar flows of refugees also appeared in Poland in September 1939 as World War II began in Europe. In China, it had already been eight years since the first Japanese invasion of Manchuria and more than two years since the start of the second Sino-Japanese war. The ardent anti–Fascists, Drs. Becker and Jensen, were eager for any information from Europe, as they marched toward the Changsha front. During a short stay in a German missionary house, they learned that some of the German missionary members did not share their anti–Fascist views: "There the missionaries were sitting around the radio and enthusiastically commenting about the march of Hitler's troops in Poland!"[13]

At the base hospital in Tuyunguan, other Europeans in China similarly tested the unequivocal anti–Fascist sentiments of the International Medical Relief Corps' members. Dr. Mann described a member of the French Foreign Legion of the pro–Vichy French Petain Mission in Guiyang who was seeking medical care:

> Since we were in a military hospital in Tuyunguan, they sent him to us.... He had heard that the Red Cross up there were all Jews and Communists! So, he asked if that was true. And as the Polish doctor, stood up and introduced himself, he said emphatically: "My name is Moishe Shmuel [Stanislaw] Flatow!" And, of course, the Frenchman was then gone.[14]

In contrast, to these encounters with fellow Europeans, the International Medical Relief Corps' members did not report episodes of Chinese anti-Semitism throughout their travels.

Drs. Becker, Jensen, and Kisch continued to move by motorcade and foot toward the Changsha front. When they arrived on September 15, the continuous Japanese bombardment forced them to retreat with the 49th Brigade.[15] Dr. Kisch headed north again to Xi'an in the unrealized hope of eventually reaching the Eighth Route Army. Meanwhile, the outbreak of war in Europe weighed heavily on a restless and already disillusioned Dr. Jensen. The following day, September 16, he pleaded to Dr. Len Crome in England to help him return to Europe:

> I am very anxious to get back to Europe and to take my place anywhere in the fighting line near Germany. I feel that nothing is actually as important as that the right people should be at the right time on the right spot. The efficiency rate of my work here is not at all so satisfying that I could take the risk not to be there when we are going to smash Hitler and to provide him with a good successor.... I ask you therefore as my friend

and comrade to do all in your power to provide a place for me anywhere where men are fighting for our common sake; be it that there are existing units of volunteers of Spaniards, Czechs, Austrians or Germans or be it that the English or French Army would take a man like me with the Spanish Nationality and valid Spanish papers born in Prague (Czechoslovakia).[16]

The Polish members of the International Medical Relief Corps also wished to return and fight for the liberation of German-occupied Poland. However, Dr. Kamieniecki, the 57th medical team captain, and Dr. Flato continued to serve near the front lines in Xiangxi with the 3rd Squadron teams.[17] Pushing small mobile units of medical providers to the front remained the focus of the Chinese Red Cross/Medical Relief Corps' efforts throughout fall 1939.

Dr. Freudmann wrote that "Dr. Lin wants to send us to Changsha to build up some sort of model sanitary service that could be organized in a similar way for other front units."[18] However, the International Medical Relief Corps' physicians' advance to the front lines resulted in as mixed a reception as did their initial arrival at the Chinese Red Cross' headquarters in Tuyunguan. Dr. Becker wrote to the China Medical Aid Committee of London from the northwestern Kiangsi [Jiangxi] front: "We are received here by the military like rain in a very dry summer."[19]

However, Dr. Freudmann wrote that Dr. Kaneti received several anonymous letters in bad English requesting him to leave his post and to withdraw the International Medical Relief Corps' foreigners from their units. If he refused to "obey," the lives of none of the foreigners would be spared. Dr. Kaneti, who was responsible for the whole section of the frontline, had made enemies by sending Chinese Red Cross/Medical Relief Corps units of Chinese doctors to some front divisions who had urgently asked for medical help. Dr. Freudmann added that the Chinese doctors protested vehemently against such a degrading imposition. Having to leave their comfortable life far from the frontlines affected them deeply, and they refused to obey orders.[20] It appears that the experiences of the International Medical Relief Corps' physicians were varied and often determined by the leadership of the different divisions with whom they served.

The International Medical Relief Corps' physicians were learning that after the fall of Hankou in 1938, the military strategy of the Chinese became "defense in depth." With this strategy, the Chinese tried to stop the advance of the Imperial Japanese Army by creating a buffer zone free of all roads and supplies. While this defense hindered the invaders' advance into central China, it also resulted in an absence of frontline medical care. Under these circumstances, there was no way to bring physicians to the front. Now, there was only a perilous journey for the wounded soldiers to the distant division and base hospitals. Dr. Jensen described the horror of such a wounded soldier's plight:

Under the impression that any loss of body fluid, either blood or saliva, means a loss of living force never again to be recovered, his anxiety increases with every drop. He covers his wound with his hands and cries like every soldier in every army in the world would do: for help; for his mother; and his friends. He will be carried out of the zone of danger by his comrades. The stretcher, two long bamboo poles and a cotton cloth will sway with every step. Any broken bone fragments will rub against each other with the pace of the bearer's steps. The man keeps groaning until shock and weakness overtake his pain. There is no morphine. It is strange that this should be so in a land associated with opium use.[21]

The 100-mile buffer between the Japanese and Chinese forces became a true no man's land. Deep ditches alternating with mud walls prevented the passage of the Japanese motorized troops. Becker wrote that much like a biblical *"via dolorosa"* (way of sorrows), long sad progressions of wounded limped from the front through the scorched earth of this no man's land.[22] Dr. Jensen went on to explain that they almost never saw abdominal, chest, and head wounds in the base hospitals. He marveled that whenever any soldier arrived at the base hospitals it was an amazing feat. Most of the base hospitals remained at low capacity because of this absence of access to front-line injuries.[23] In this setting, it is not surprising that Dr. Lin had not attached much priority to the neurosurgical and cardiovascular services that Dr. Eloesser had volunteered to bring to China.

When Dr. Baer asked a division hospital leader why they had so many beds but no patients, the director reiterated the logistics. Dr. Baer pressed the question of what the purpose of an empty hospital could possibly be, and the best that the embarrassed director could reply was that Mme. Chiang had visited his hospital and spoke highly of it. Dr. Baer sarcastically whispered to Dr. Freudmann, "In that case, it has served its purpose."[24]

Through the fall of 1939, Dr. Kisch continued to work far north of his colleagues, in Shensi [Shaanxi] province in the city of Xi'an. He kept in contact with both the Chinese Red Cross and representatives of the Chinese Communist Party's Eighth Route Army. However, he was still unable to reach the Chinese Communist Party's Eighth Route Army in Yan'an, 200 miles to the north.

An Indian physician who was already with the Chinese Communist Party's Eighth Route Army, Dr. Basu, traveled to Xi'an to visit with Dr. Kisch. He wrote that they dined together with Dr. Wang, the head of the Chinese Red Cross, and Theodore White, the American journalist. Dr. Basu described Dr. Wang and White as being rude and pompous to him because of his intimacy with the Chinese Communist Party's Eighth Route Army. Dr. Basu complained of Dr. Wang's behavior to Dr. Lin at the Chinese Red Cross/Medical Relief Corps' headquarters and Dr. Lin subsequently apologized. At the same time, Dr. Basu spoke with admiration of the internationalism of the

Czech Dr. Kisch and the service of Dr. Müller to General Chu Teh and the Eighth Route Army.[25]

The polarizing ideological battle lines between the Guomindang Nationalist Party and the Chinese Communist Party were closing in on healthcare delivery. These battle lines would soon trap the International Medical Relief Corps' members in a political no man's land.

Both the wary Second United Front between the Guomindang Nationalist Party and the Chinese Communist Party, and the Imperial Japanese Army's advance into China, ground to a halt in 1940. A stalemate with the Japanese forces lasted until the start of the Japanese *Operation Ichigo* offensive in 1944. With this reduced external military threat, the Guomindang Nationalist Party and Chinese Communist Party had time to realize how unholy their union was, and strife soon reemerged. The reduction in combat with the Japanese also changed the healthcare needs for both civilians and the military.

The Emergency Medical Service Training School reported that the number of wounded in 1940 decreased to 17 percent of the 1937 total while the number of sick in 1940 increased to 283 percent of the 1937 total.[26] Dr. Lin similarly noted that "[o]ur wound casualties are only one third of the beginning of the war though our sick injuries are up 300–400 percent."[27] By spring 1940, Dr. Landauer, wrote, "the front is really more of a combat zone with raiding. Malaria and other diseases have changed the epidemiology."[28] The medical needs in wartime China were clearly shifting from battlefield casualties to anti-epidemic work.

In July 1940, Drs. Iancu, Flato, and Schön, like Drs. Jensen, Becker, and Kisch before them, met with Zhou Enlai, the Chinese Communist Party representative to the Guomindang Nationalist Party in Chongqing. Dr. Iancu continued to share his dissatisfaction, as he felt forced to work with the Guomindang Nationalist Party rather than the Chinese Communist Party at that time:

> It will be almost impossible for me to continue to work with the Kuomintang reactionaries and I asked my party [the Communist Party of Romania] leadership for advice. I immediately wrote a letter to Moscow ... where I expressed the opinion that it would be preferable to return to my country, than to work with reactionaries. Meanwhile, expecting, along with the others, that our problems would be solved, we returned to the units that we had been assigned to by the [Chinese] Red Cross.[29]

When Drs. Coutelle and Kent joined with the International Medical Relief Corps' members in Tuyunguan in 1940, Dr. Flato informed them that the Communist north of China was practically sealed off by the Guomindang Nationalist Party. Thus, neither doctors nor medical material were allowed to pass through, and that the opportunities to work with the Army units would be quite limited.[30] The prospects for many of the International Medical

Relief Corps' members to serve where they wished in China continued to diminish.

The Chinese Ministry of Foreign Affairs, which allocated the International Medical Relief Corps' members' travel permits, tightened the restriction of travel in wartime China. Beginning in the fall of 1940, Dr. Mamlok's travel permit, for example, was limited to Hunan, Hupeh [Hubei], Kwangsi [Guangxi], and Kiangsi [Jiangxi] provinces. Writing from Lukou [Lukou Zhen] in Hunan province in 1940, he chose again not to share with his family the worries of war, politics, and malnutrition that he had previously published in his unit reports. Instead, he painted a picture that one might expect a son to share with his widely dispersed and worried family. Dr. Mamlok wrote in 1940 to his family:

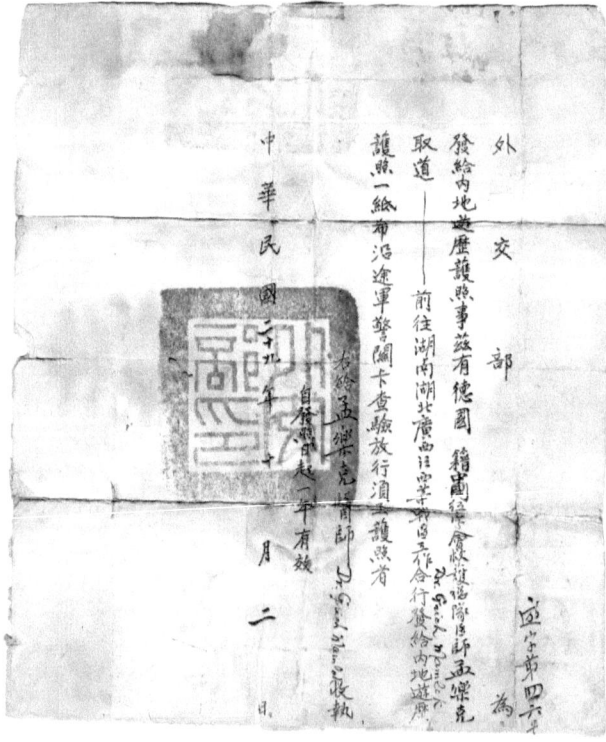

The Ministry of Foreign Affairs (Republic of China) issues the passport to the German doctor Leke Meng (Dr. Erich Mamlok), who is serving with the Medical Relief Corps, Red Cross Society of the Republic of China, to travel through mainland China. This passport is to honor that Dr. Mamlok is going to serve on the battle fields of Hunan, Hubei, Guangxi, and Jiangxi. All the checkpoints of police and army along the trip should let the passport holder pass through. The Ministry of Foreign Affairs (Republic of China), October 2, 1940 (courtesy Robert Mamlok).

Now I am working at one of the Chinese Red Cross supported military hospitals together with an exceptionally nice and perfectly English and German speaking Chinese physician. The work is very interesting. I am learning about a bunch of new diseases that I previously only knew about by name. Life in China is in general very pleasant. Great politeness and friendliness and interesting impressions.[31]

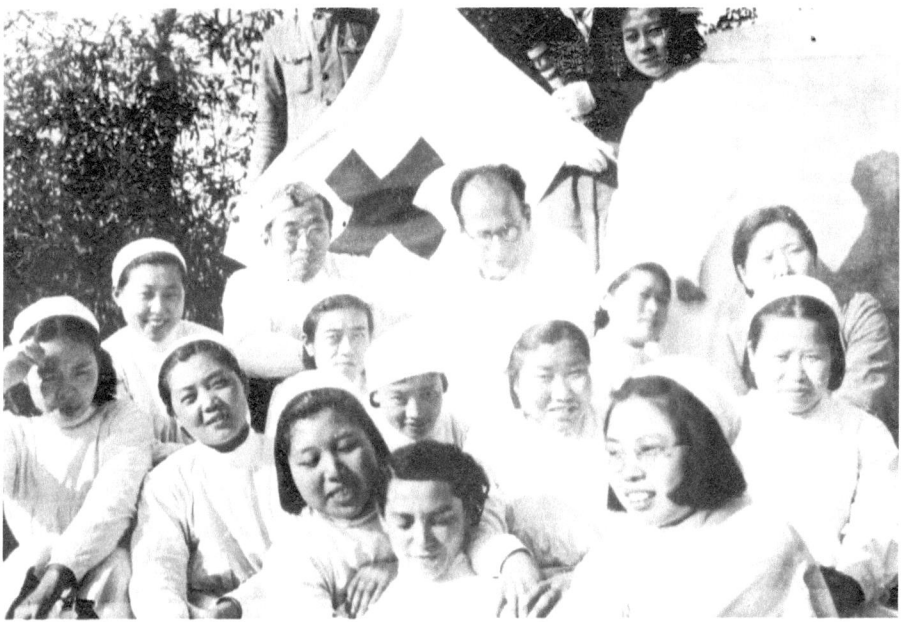

The International Medical Relief Corps Unit 32 in Lukou (Hunan Province), China on August 4, 1940. Unidentified Chinese medical volunteers with Mrs. Mania Kamieniecki (front center) and Dr. Erich Mamlok (back center) (courtesy Robert Mamlok).

A restless and underutilized Dr. Jensen continued to ask his family to seek a means for his return to Europe. In addition, he asked them to share some of his recent work with his Spanish Civil War friend, the English nurse, Patience Darton. Dr. Jensen anticipated that his duties in China would expire the next June and asked again if his family could help him return to Europe or America.[32]

The day-to-day misery that Dr. Jensen witnessed probably contributed to his wish to return to the Western world as soon as possible. For example, conscription of peasants into the Chinese Army continued to be widely and cruelly in place. The inhumane conditions of the maltreated, conscripted peasants weighed heavily on the conscience of the International Medical Relief Corps' members. In their view, the Chinese peasant's plight was not far removed from the plight of the persecuted European minorities who were forced to support the German war effort. The conscripts' ubiquitous presence was a constant reminder to the International Medical Relief Corps that they were not in a setting where their goals of humanitarian relief and egalitarian medical aid could be readily realized.

Dr. Freudmann also wrote of the political fallacy and plight of China's system of forced conscription. He spoke of endless rows of men chained together, beaten, and cursed like cattle. Dragged hundreds of miles from their rural homes, less than half would survive the maltreatment, hunger, cold, and epidemics that they endured. This constant reminder of the absence of basic humanitarian standards was one of Dr. Freudmann's most difficult trials in China.[33]

It is not surprising that Dr. Jensen observed, "the inhabitants of whole villages scatter to the hills for fear of conscription when I approached with a troop of soldiers."[34] Their flight would appear to have been warranted as the rate of loss or death of all conscripts in one year was 44 percent, (750,000 out of 1.67 million)—"a terrible indictment of Chinese leaders," in historian Barbara Tuchman's words.[35]

Travel to Hong Kong

Although the International Medical Relief Corps' medical efforts remained largely restricted to their small Chinese Red Cross/Medical Relief Corps units in central and southwestern China, Drs. Becker and Jensen managed to travel east to Hong Kong in the summer of 1940. The China Medical Aid Committee of London commissioned them to transport critically needed medical supplies from Hong Kong to Guiyang along the coastal waterway and through the Japanese lines. Dr. Becker wrote that they left Guiyang on June 16, 1940, and headed by truck to Luichow in Guangxi province:

> We arrived there two days later. They were building a new railway line. There were masses of workers. Water buffalo dragging timber beams. It reminded me of the building of the Pyramids or something like that. We took the train to the airfield in Guilin. We saw our plane leaving before us as it was overcrowded. Guilin is the most advanced city I have seen in inner China, with lots of electric lights and a quite acceptable hotel. It is too hot to write. Too hot to do anything. On June 20th, we were surprised to find another plane so soon. Soon we were climbing out of the stifling afternoon heat higher and higher to 3,000 meters, below us were the mountains, rice paddies and villages. The air gets cooler and cooler and by and by all the passengers put on their coats. Wonderful air after so many days full of dust and heat. Through the clouds beside us appears another plane. The dreaded Japanese! No, it follows its own course peacefully in a similar direction as ours. The night comes and with it, suddenly appearing out of complete darkness, the sparkling sea of light that is Hong Kong. Really like a fairytale city, like something never seen before, after such a long time in darkness and life in earth houses. The light of the city hits us like a flame.[36]

It turned out that medical supplies were not the only things that Drs. Becker and Jensen would bring back to Guiyang. Joan Staniforth, who had been working as a nanny for Hilda Selwyn-Clarke in Hong Kong, decided to join them on their trip back to Guiyang. The author Graham Peck[37] joined Staniforth along with Drs. Jensen and Becker. They sailed along the coast, past Macao and through the Japanese-held sections of the West River delta. Their harrowing journey required dodging Japanese patrol boats during the day and guerrillas, pirates, police, and smugglers during the night.[38] They completed their journey, getting past the Japanese lines into the interior of China until at last they reached the relative safety of the Guomindang Nationalist Party Army.[39] Drs. Becker and Jensen had succeeded in crossing in and out of Japanese-controlled China but had failed in their attempts to cross into the Chinese Communist Party Army controlled areas.

Travel around China had become increasingly difficult for everyone at

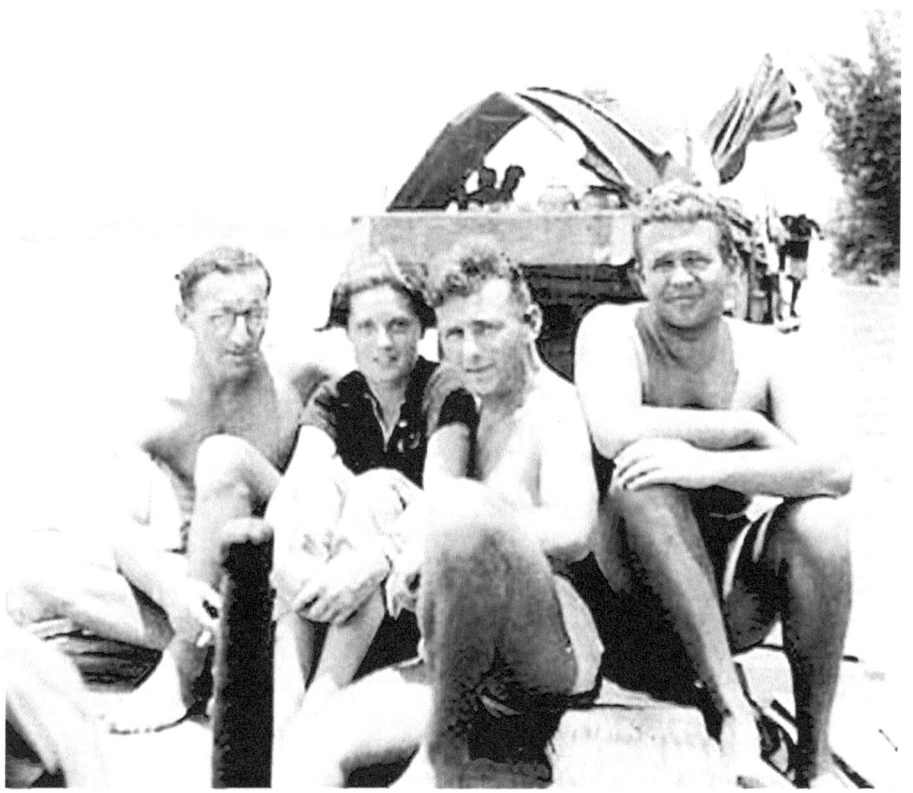

Traveling behind Japanese lines on a sampan from Hong Kong to Guiyang, June 1940. From left to right: Dr. Fritz Jensen, Ms. Joan Staniforth, Dr. Rolf Becker, and the American author Graham Peck (courtesy Bernard Becker).

this stage of the war. With France's surrender to Germany on June 25, 1940, Japanese forces increasingly threatened the British and French colonies in Southeast Asia. On July 18, 1940, the British tried to thwart the Japanese threats to Hong Kong and Singapore by closing the Burma Road for three months. When the Japanese then entered French Indo-China, the United States responded with an embargo of all steel and iron exports to Japan. Japan, in turn, signed the Tripartite Agreement with Germany and Italy on September 24, and the British responded by reopening the Burma Road on October 18. To most observers, a Pacific War now appeared certain.

Medical Relief Corps Public Health Efforts

While the International Medical Relief Corps' members remained separated from world events in small Chinese Red Cross/Medical Relief Corps' units dispatched throughout central and southwestern China in 1940, they were linked by the medical conditions that they were confronted with. Although their travel remained restricted, the need for anti-epidemic efforts was unbounded. One public health focus was the creation of delousing and bathing stations to reduce the spread of scabies, typhus and relapsing fever.

In September 1938, the Chinese Red Cross/Medical Relief Corps had only seven delousing and bathing stations in operation but by June 1940, this had grown to more than two hundred units.[40] The Chinese Red Cross/Medical Relief Corps Unit 49 shared their procedure for ridding patients of the scabies mite:

> It was found that a temperature of 70 degrees centigrade for about 15 minutes was sufficient to kill the lice and nits, and the maximum amount of clothing that could be placed in one barrel without over packing was about 4 to 5 persons' clothing. Under these conditions, delousing and bathing stations' treatment was started and within 16 days a total of 1,606 were deloused and bathed at a cost of $0.17 per person ... all other patients from other base hospitals in the district were deloused here before being transferred for further treatment.[41]

Dr. Iancu wrote of the initial difficulty in enlisting some Chinese healthcare providers in the battle against scabies. This involved the laborious task of boiling sulfuric acid and rubbing it onto countless cutaneous lesions with cotton gauze. At first, Dr. Iancu did this alone as some Chinese medical officers felt that it was demeaning to anoint a common soldier. However, he wrote that the example he set and the good results he obtained gradually changed the Chinese officers' perceptions. They learned that the International Medical Relief Corps' physicians clearly did not belong to the uncaring colonial Western stereotypes that many Chinese officers had known.[42]

The International Medical Relief Corps' physicians' efforts to promote

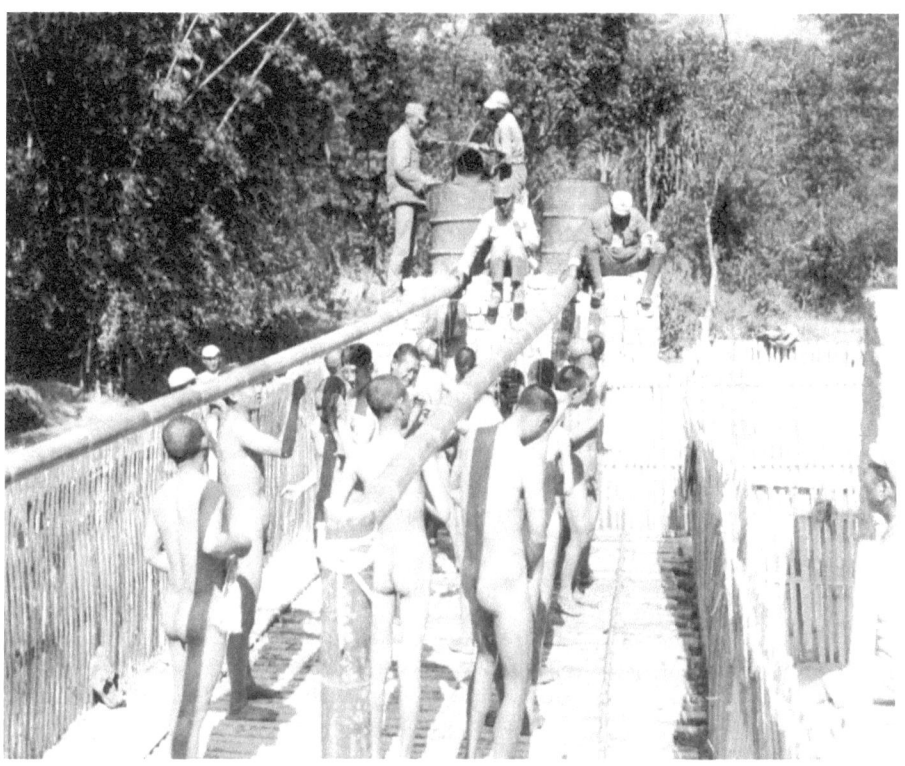

Chinese troops in the communal shower section of a delousing, bathing and scabies (D.B.S.) station receive a warm shower. Bamboo pipes deliver water and disinfectants from recycled oil drums. December 25, 1944 (National Archives: 111- SC-1276).

public health, while not as contagious as scabies, were slowly catching on. Reporter Agnes Smedley commented on this change:

> When a delousing and bathing station was erected on one front, a commander announced to his troops "Now you've got no right to have scabies!" … The Medical Corps was changing from an old boat to a new one in midstream. Henceforth, they were to re-train every Army medical worker, lecture to the troops on hygiene and first aid, build delousing and bathing stations out of whatever material was at hand, purify wells, and do other anti-epidemic work. Education and more education was the cry.[43]

Dr. Kent's innovations in the delousing and bathing stations "bathing bucket" design received much acclaim. Both General Feng Yuxiang (馮玉祥 Feng Yu-hsiang) and the commander of the 53rd Military Corps, Zhou Fucheng (周福成 Chou Fu Cheng), praised Dr. Kent's anti-epidemic work in 1940.[44] Much as with typhus and relapsing fever, the use of delousing and bathing stations proved to be the best plan to combat scabies. Reducing the prevalence of scabies, typhus, and relapsing fever through the promotion of public health measures such as delousing and bathing stations would be one of the main accomplishments of the Chinese Red Cross/Medical Relief Corps.

In 1940, the ability of the China Medical Aid Committees to continue to support the International Medical Relief Corps became more imperiled. German tanks blitzed across Europe and U-boats and airplanes decimated shipping lanes as the Battle of Britain began. The German occupation of much of Scandinavia further limited Norwegian support for the Spanish doctors' mission with the Chinese Red Cross/Medical Relief Corps. Norwegian correspondent Tor Kjesdal wrote to the American Bureau for Medical Aid to China:

> The Norwegian relief committee for Spain under Dr. Haslund agreed to support a number of surgeons and send them to Dr. Robert K. Lim. With the help of Norway's Director of Public Health, Dr. Karl Evang, a number were chosen and have given valuable support to Dr. Lim. We managed to shield these funds from the invading Nazis. When war on Norwegian soil was suspended, we went to America. Can you consider transferring funds from the National Red Cross of China to this special account [set up for the] salaries from abroad to the Norwegian group of surgeons in Free China?[45]

In November 1940, Hilda Selwyn-Clarke forwarded the Norwegian's appeal to the American Bureau for Medical Aid to China:

> Regarding the foreign doctors, 10 were sent from Norway and 9 from the London committee. They were paid 7 pound nine pence/month. Each doctor asked that only 3 pounds be given per month in national currency and that the balance be kept in Hong Kong for their return to Europe. As we could not expect that the Norwegian and London committees could pay their second year of salary, I appealed to the British Relief Funds in Hong Kong and we raised H.K. $8,000. Dr. Lin did not wish to use this money. He made each doctor a head of a curative unit and paid them NC $200/month. As he had accepted these doctors under the promise that their salary would be paid for, I feel this is unfair to him. Perhaps some of the groups that worked for Spain would help. Dr. Lin has found their services invaluable—their experience in Spain in front line work and in evacuation of wounded has enabled him to put through a new scheme for the wounded. Their political experience enables them to understand the development stage of China and they have excellent cooperation with their Chinese colleagues without criticism and misunderstanding. They are very sincere anti-fascist fighters. Drs. Becker and Jensen speak good English and will be sending reports.[46]

As 1940 ended, and the Battle of Britain intensified, Drs. Coutelle and Kent did not understand why their wives, a physician and a nurse, had not yet been able to join them in the Chinese Red Cross/Medical Relief Corps. Dr. Coutelle wrote to the China Medical Aid Committee in London that it would be better for their wives to be in China than in Britain:

> If you still have some uncertainty about the general conditions [in China] being suitable for Europeans, we can now inform you from our own experience that they are probably much better than at present in England. We hope that this letter will disperse all doubts the committee may have and that it will do everything to help our wives to depart with the first available ship.[47]

A few months later, Dr. Rosa Coutelle and Maria Gonzales Rodriquez, RN, received permission from the Chinese Red Cross to begin travel from England to China. Against all odds, they had survived the battles of the Spanish Civil War, internment in the French concentration camps, and exile in a foreign land. When they finally departed from Liverpool, England, in March 1941, they traveled northward for three days through the Irish Sea and North Channel to the Atlantic Ocean. A German Luftwaffe bomber off the northwest coast of Scotland attacked their steamship, the *Staffordshire*. Dr. Rosa Coutelle wrote that she and her son were on deck when the plane started strafing the ship. More than forty lives were lost in the attack. After about six hours in a lifeboat, a Norwegian trawler rescued Gonzales Rodriquez, Coutelle, and her two-year-old son, Charles. They were brought to the Isle of Lewis (Outer Hebrides) where the recovered dead were buried. Gonzales Rodriquez, Coutelle, and her son spent the rest of the war in the United Kingdom.[48]

In summary, from 1939 to 1940, military confrontations would escalate in Europe and decline in China. The International Medical Relief Corps' members could not return to Europe, nor travel north thru the Guomindang Nationalist Party lines or south through the Japanese sealed Indo-China and Burma Road. For the most part, they remained carefully watched by the Guomindang Nationalist Part-controlled Chinese Red Cross as they spread out in small Medical Relief Corps units throughout central and southern China.

Their travel permits confined their movement as did the no man's lands that separated the Japanese and Chinese forces. These buffer zones also separated wounded soldiers from access to the Guomindang Nationalist Party division hospitals. The International Medical Relief Corps witnessed a profound shift to preventative medicine in rural China as the management of battlefield casualties waned.

Public health efforts surged at this time as the burden of infectious disease management continued to increase and the Nationalist government adopted the state medicine system in 1940. Preventative measures such as the Chinese Red Cross/Medical Relief Corps and Army Medical Corps' increased use of delousing and bathing stations, the National Health Administration's support for mass vaccination programs, and the educational efforts of Dr. Lin's Emergency Medical Service Training School helped to protect the health of the soldiers and the civilian population in rural China.

However, the Medical Relief Corps' public health efforts and the rural county health initiatives of the National Health Administration would continue to have difficulty in obtaining political support, funding, and adequate medical staffing. Most historians agree that this clearly limited the longer-term legacy of these public health initiatives. Watt notes that by 1943, the public health service in Sichuan was struggling for its existence and approaching collapse.[49] Bu added that by the end of the war, the efforts probably did not do much to improve the limited landscape of rural health services.[50]

At the same time as these efforts were playing out in China, travel and politics had become as perilous in Europe as in China. The China Medical Aid Committee in Norway ceased to function as Norway was overrun by the German Army and the Battle of Britain began. The sinking of the *Staffordshire* would confine Dr. Rosa Coutelle and Maria Gonzales Rodriquez in England while dozens of the International Medical Relief Corps' member's Jewish relatives became trapped in central Europe by the politics of the National Socialist Party.

8. The Forced Restriction of Healthcare Delivery: 1941–1942

The continuing collapse of the Second United Front and the Guomindang Nationalist Party's restructuring of the Chinese Red Cross/Medical Relief Corps and National Health Administration brought on added challenges for Dr. Lin. Dr. Liu Ruiheng, one of Dr. Lin's strongest supporters at the National Health Administration, had been forced out of office. Dr. Wang was reappointed to direct the Chinese Red Cross.

Mr. Du Yuesheng (杜月笙 Y.S. Doo) remained as a vice president of the Chinese Red Cross. Du Yuesheng's business interests placed him in the uncommon position of supporting both the bioscientists of the Chinese Red Cross and the Chinese medicine practitioners of the Shanghai Academy of Chinese Medicine.[1] "Big Eared Du" Yuesheng was—at best—an opium-smuggling leader of Shanghai's notorious Green Gang with enormous wealth and influence. Swiss journalist Ilona Ralf Sues recalled her first impression of him in Shanghai in 1938:

> He had a long, egg shaped head, no chin, huge bat like ears, cold cruel lips uncovering big yellow decayed teeth, the sickly complexion of an addict.... He shuffled along, turning his head left and right to see if anyone was following him.... His eyes were dead and impenetrable.... I shuddered. He gave me his limp cold hand. A huge bony hand with two inch long, brown opium stained claws.[2]

Du Yuesheng's Chinese Red Cross' new medical leadership was more presentable but no less ruthless in placing an unwanted level of bureaucratic control over Dr. Lin's Medical Relief Corps' activities. Drs. Wang and Pan Ji (潘骥 C. Pan), who was appointed as the secretary general of the Chinese Red Cross in 1940, led the Guomindang Nationalist Party's mission to reestablish political and economic control over Dr. Lin's Medical Relief Corps. Pan Ji accused Dr. Lin of left-leaning politics and corruption. Specifically, this included Dr. Lin's support for the International Medical Relief Corps' Spanish doctors, his prior aid to the Chinese Communist Party's New Fourth and Eighth Route Armies, and his friendship with Agnes Smedley. These were used to label him a Communist. Chiang Kai-shek summoned Dr. Lin to Chongqing in August 1940 to defend himself against these serious allegations.[3] It would not be the last of his tribunals.

By 1941, the plan to provide health care to all in wartime China was failing on many fronts. For example, two volunteers with the British Relief Unit, Evert Barger (埃弗特·巴格) and Philip Wright (菲利普·莱特)vehemently protested when Guomindang Nationalist Party troops prevented them from transporting six tons of medical supplies to Yan'an. Although they assumed that the Generalissimo had approved this transport, the Guomindang Nationalist Party seized their medical supplies in Sanyuan, Shensi [Shaanxi]. Shaanxi is a province in Northwest China that includes the middle reaches of the Yellow River and the Loess Plateau. Its capital city is Xi'an.

To Barger and Wright's dismay, the private pharmacies in Xi'an eventually sold the confiscated medications and medical devices at black market prices. This was the last known effort to send drugs in large quantity to the guerrilla fronts until the end of 1944.

Journalists estimated that tens of thousands perished due to the lack of basic medical care during this period. This loss of life probably included Dr. Bethune, whose death from septicemia can be attributed to the absence of antibiotics.[4] However, the International Medical Relief Corps' protests against this medical supply blockade continued. Eighteen of the International Medical Relief Corps' physicians pleaded again to Dr. Mary Gilchrist of the China Medical Aid Committee of London to seek help from the British Foreign Office:

> This is an impossible situation in which we consider it the duty of all who have the victory of China at heart to see that aid reaches the heroic people and armies in the rear of the enemy. International aid to China should not be given to any single group, but to all. We seek to remedy a situation where it is not permissible to go to the area of the 8th and the New 4th armies to continue our work for the Chinese people whom we have learned to honor and to love.[5]

The British Government viewed this restriction in the transport of medical aid and personnel as a domestic Chinese issue. Anthony Eden,[6] of the British Foreign Office, wrote that the "movement of supplies in China would appear to be a matter of Chinese internal affairs and it would not be appropriate for him to intervene. It would be more appropriate for the group to take up the matter with the Chinese Ambassador to Britain."[7]

Mme. Sun Yat-sen's Chinese Defence League had previously been able to send supplies from Hong Kong to the International Peace Hospitals in Chinese Communist Party-controlled areas through Dr. Lin's Chinese Red Cross/Medical Relief Corps. But, it was now no longer possible for Dr. Lin

8. The Forced Restriction of Healthcare Delivery: 1941–1942

to handle these medical shipments. Drs. Pan Ji and Wang firmly controlled and limited the transport of supplies in and out of Lin's Chinese Red Cross/Medical Relief Corps.

The Chinese Defence League and the British Relief Unit were not the only relief organizations to feel the brunt of the division between the Guomindang Nationalist Party and the Chinese Communist Party regarding the transport of medical supplies. Dr. Bob McClure of the Friends Ambulance Units wrote to Hilda Selwyn-Clarke on September 23, 1941, about the Barger and Wright incident:

> I saw Madame Chiang, and I complained about the delay in transport and was spoken to as I have seldom been spoken to before. They referred to drugs moving in that direction that did not have papers from Guiyang. With my former International Relief Committee connections, they held me responsible. I did let them know that I had not altered my opinion one little bit and that I considered that they were making a large tactical error in trying to keep drugs from people in order to bring suffering as a form of political pressure. We closed on that note—not a very nice one.[8]

It was clear to the relief organizations in China that restricted access to medical care had become a political weapon of the Guomindang Nationalist Party. However, the British Foreign Office remained reluctant to support humanitarian needs in what they saw as a Chinese domestic issue.

Despite the reassurances given by Zhou Enlai in Chongqing of the importance of their mission in the Guomindang Nationalist Party controlled areas of central China, the International Medical Relief Corps' members' medical role and survival was threatened. The Spanish doctors in the International Medical Relief Corps maintained a clear preference for serving with the Chinese Communist Party's New Fourth and Eighth Route Armies. However, the International Medical Relief Corps' physicians had now become a restricted and endangered medical commodity as the Second United Front between the Guomindang Nationalist Party and Chinese Communist Party dissolved.

Dr. Lin's Chinese Red Cross/Medical Relief Corps could not rise above the rift between the Guomindang Nationalist Party and the Chinese Communist Party. This chasm widened when the animosity between the Guomindang Nationalist Party and the Chinese Communist Party burst into open conflict, in January 1941. The events that resulted in the New Fourth Army Wannan Incident (新四軍事件) remains an area of controversy between the People's Republic of China and the Republic of China (Taiwan).[9] However, the net result of the Guomindang Nationalist Party's attack and destruction of the headquarters of the Chinese Communist Party's New Fourth Army was the loss of thousands of lives and a *de facto* end of the Second United Front.

In the aftermath of this battle, efforts to extend medical aid to the

Chinese Communist Party armies were blocked. Mme. Sun Yat-sen wrote of the inhumanity of this outcome:

> In most countries at war, even enemy wounded are given the benefit of medical service. But the Kuomintang has drawn an imaginary line across China, on one side of which Chinese soldiers fighting Japan were entitled to care when wounded, and on the other not. Volunteer personnel, like drugs, were prevented from going north.[10]

The observations and letters from the International Medical Relief Corps' physicians clearly supported this new reality.

The Chinese Red Cross/Medical Relief Corps came under increasing pressure from the Guomindang Nationalist Party to prevent the International Medical Relief Corps' members and international aid organizations from extending assistance to the Chinese Communist Party-affiliated soldiers and civilians. At the same time, the Guomindang Nationalist Party and the Chinese Communist Party wanted international aid to continue for their mutual cause against Japan. This core conflict placed Dr. Lin's Chinese Red Cross/Medical Relief Corps' vision in an increasingly untenable position. It was not long before Chiang Kai-shek again summoned Dr. Lin to Chongqing to defend himself against accusations of being a Chinese Communist Party sympathizer.

The International Medical Relief Corps' physicians knew that their position with the Chinese Red Cross/Medical Relief Corps was now fraught with peril. Though unanimously united in their anti–Fascist belief, some International Medical Relief Corps' members differed in their political ideology. All the Spanish doctors were members of the Communist Party. In 1941, Drs. Mamlok and Lurje were the only International Medical Relief Corps' physicians in Guiyang who were not members of a national Communist Party. Drs. Cohn and Courtney were also not members of a national Communist Party, but would only reach the Chinese Red Cross/Medical Relief Corps later in 1941.

Dr. Mamlok would write to his family that one of the allegations now used by the Guomindang Nationalist Party against Dr. Lin was

> that he committed a dozen physicians [to the Chinese Red Cross/Medical Relief Corps] from the International Brigade in Spain, thus "very left leaning people," which due to several reasons here are not wanted. Outside of the "Spanish doctors," I am the only foreign physician in the Red Cross. I expect that in a short time I will be thrown out together with the Spanish doctors.[11]

In early 1941, Dr. Lin realized that the presence of International Medical Relief Corps' Communist Party members could be used by some Guomindang Nationalist Party officials to remove him from the Chinese Red Cross/Medical Relief Corps' leadership. He tried to defend the International Medical Relief Corps' members and the Chinese Red Cross/Medical Relief Corps. Hilda

Selwyn-Clarke of the Foreign Auxiliary-Chinese Red Cross forwarded Dr. Lin's political strategy to Sir Archibald Kerr, the British Ambassador to China in 1941:

> Dr. Lin would like his foreign personnel, about 23 in all, 20 of which were sent out by the China Medical Aid Committee, London, to be transferred to your committee to make things easier for him politically.... Dr. Lin is anxious to retain the services of all the foreign doctors but it has occurred to us that we should make enquiries as to whether they should return to Great Britain if necessary.[12]

Dr. Lin's fear for the survival of the Chinese Red Cross/Medical Relief Corps was well founded. He continued to insist on the neutrality of the Chinese Red Cross/Medical Relief Corps and downplayed the Guomindang Nationalist Party's fear of Chinese Communist Party infiltration. Nevertheless, in 1940, the Guomindang Nationalist Party had already sent observers to Tuyunguan to counter Chinese Communist Party objectives in the Chinese Red Cross/Medical Relief Corps. As previously mentioned, some of the Chinese Red Cross/Medical Relief Corps' Chinese Communist Party members, such as D.C. Zhang, had been pressured to leave Guiyang.[13] D.C. Zhang was a Quinghua graduate who joined Dr. Lin in 1939. He spent the rest of the war in Chongqing working for Zhou Enlai.

In February 1941, because of the charges raised by the Guomindang Nationalist Party against him, Dr. Lin resigned from the Chinese Red Cross/Medical Relief Corps' leadership. However, the Generalissimo ordered the Chinese Red Cross not to release him.[14] Chiang Kai-shek knew that Dr. Lin was still the best physician to accrue international funding and lead the Chinese Red Cross Medical Relief Corps. Agnes Smedley attended the Chinese Red Cross' board meetings in Hong Kong. She decried the Chinese Red Cross' board members' wish to force Dr. Lin from his position merely to advance their own power and prestige: "Unable to stop herself, she provoked a confrontation so offensive it ruined her arrangement for getting back into China under the auspices of the Chinese Red Cross."[15]

In 1941, the International Medical Relief Corps' physicians felt growing distrust and frustration with the Chinese Red Cross, as may be sensed in the letters of Dr. Carl Coutelle to his wife, Rosa:

> We proposed to be put for the time being under the command and the disposition of the military authorities, so that we, as highly movable units, could go any place where we were required and necessary. Naturally—the offer has been "accepted." Immediately propaganda among the Chinese for volunteers has been started and yesterday some units left for Changsha—none of us. And these units go—so far I know—not directly to the front but are deployed to a town about 45 km. away from Changsha and not at the disposal of the military authorities, but rather as regular units for the regional head of the Chinese Red Cross. So the essence of our plan has not been realized. Our plan would cost too much money!! And it is not probable, that we will be sent. But now I

got already asked—when are you going to the front? The Chinese have already left!! You see, the whole thing is treated not as a matter of necessity and duty, but as a matter of "losing face".... Finally, on October 10th—a great Chinese holiday—Kriegel, Kaneti and two Chinese doctors were sent without units as advisors;—and a most impressive, but entirely useless convoy of ambulances left for the south. At this time the action was already finished and the sense of all—to bring first aid and to organize proper and rapid evacuation could not be realized.[16]

These token efforts were clearly in contrast to the true meaning of October 10 ("Double Ten Day"), the National Day of the Republic of China (ROC). This Chinese holiday commemorates the start of the Wuchang uprising of October 10, 1911, which led to the collapse of the Qing Dynasty and the establishment of the Republic of China on January 1, 1912.

Dr. Coutelle told his family that this period of forced inactivity was one of the most frustrating and unhappy experiences in his life. It was in stark contrast to the camaraderie in Spain, which many of the Spanish doctors had referred to as the best experience of their lives. Indeed, as political intrigue mounted and military confrontations waned in 1941, discontent and inactivity increased throughout the Chinese Red Cross/Medical Relief Corps. A young overseas Chinese physician wrote, in Tuyunguan "All we see are chronic illnesses, and they are all treated according to the [Medical Relief] Corps' manual. Any nurse can do the job. We came here for an internship. What kind of training do you call this?"[17]

Less is known about the politics that may have resulted in the restriction of the International Medical Relief Corps' nursing services. On June 18, 1941, Dr. Kaneti requested permission for Gisela Kranzdorf to serve as a dresser [surgical assistants who helped with patient's wound dressings and bed sores] with her husband, the leader of Chinese Red Cross/Medical Relief Corps' Unit 383 in Kwantung.[18] However, the Chinese Red Cross/Medical Relief Corps' nursing supervisor wrote that, based on a practical nursing exam, she was not qualified for that role.[19]

Even though physicians remained desperately needed in China, the growing animosity between the Guomindang Nationalist Party and the Chinese Communist Party contributed to the Chinese Red Cross' concern that Chinese Communist Party-sympathizing physicians could jeopardize their mission. However, the Chinese Red Cross/Medical Relief Corps continued its public promotion of the need for more physicians in China. Dr. Lin told the Central News Agency in Hong Kong on February 28, 1941, that "[i]nsufficiency in doctors and nurses remains the greatest problem in medical relief in Free China despite the fact that Red Cross work has been placed on an organized and systematic basis."[20] At the same time, the existing International Medical Relief Corps' physicians' medical activities became more and more restricted.

8. The Forced Restriction of Healthcare Delivery: 1941–1942

By the end of 1941, the Chinese Red Cross/Medical Relief Corps had only 181 doctors among its more than 2,700 employees. Between June 1938 and March 1941, the medical staff of the Chinese Red Cross/Medical Relief Corps increased by only thirty physicians.[21] More than two-thirds of this increase came from the addition of the foreign physician volunteers of the International Medical Relief Corps. These few foreign doctors now constituted 12 percent of the entire Chinese Red Cross/Medical Relief Corps' medical staff in China.

Dr. McClure marveled at how such a small medical group accomplished so much:

> The fact that Dr. Lin did as well as he did in quickly putting a medical relief corps into service can be attributed to the astounding fortitude and courage of his handful of doctors and nurses. In the past year, he has [also] established Emergency Medical Service Training Schools to assist in teaching young Chinese girls and housewives the elements of nursing and preventive medicine.[22]

In fact, the Emergency Medical Service Training School probably deserves more credit than the fortitude and courage of the physicians. The historian, John Watt effectively argued that Dr. Lin's vision to use the Emergency Medical Service Training School to create brief training courses for thousands of modern medical aides was a key component in the rise of biomedicine in wartime China.[23] Had the Emergency Medical Service Training School failed, there would not have been many public health alternatives to traditional Chinese medicine in many rural areas.

The need for more physicians in China continued to be publicly promoted in the media and privately dismissed by the Chinese Red Cross. In July 1941, Dr. Co-Tui, speaking for the China Defense Supplies,[24] told Dr. Lin of a plan suggested by Henry Luce, founder of *Time Magazine*:

> [He] said that you should write a letter to JAMA [Journal of the American Medical Association] through the American Bureau for Medical Aid to China regarding the need for American doctors. If you could draft this letter, I am sure Henry would be pleased. PS: The idea of sending physicians to China is a pet idea of Mr. Luce. Let's try to make something out of this.[25]

At the same time, Freda Utley wrote in *Asia* magazine:

> Although there were many Chinese doctors in Hong Kong and the treaty ports, few of them thought of volunteering for war service.... The strength [of the Chinese Red Cross/Medical Relief Corps] was that it was a distinctly Chinese patriotic organization that persons of varying political views and affiliations could work within.... Its weakness was its lack of initial support and Lin's refusal to appease the self-seeking or moral extortionists and his insistence to send supplies to all armies fighting the Japanese.... Will not a few doctors answer Dr. Lin's call and go to China? There is nowhere in the world where they are so badly needed, and today it is being recognized that the Chinese are fighting for us as well as for themselves.[26]

The remaining missionaries in China shared the realities of a woefully understaffed medical infrastructure and the need to resurrect their efforts. Writing to Dr. Edward Hume,[27] chair of the Christian Medical Council for Overseas Work in China, Dr. McClure observed, "There is a need for more doctors to come to West China. They will be future allies for China, there is a huge influx of refugees out here, and there will be a need for missions here after the war.... Chinese docs tend to come and go, and some of the missionary docs in southern China could really help."[28]

John Rich, public relations director of the American Friends Service Committee, later shared with Dr. Lin his proposal to include the Quakers in the Chinese Red Cross' efforts to provide rehabilitation for crippled soldiers:

> To this he [Dr. Lin] was most enthusiastic. I was told that he was quoted as saying no more foreign workers, but he vigorously denied that. He said that he did not want any high specialists unable to adapt to the limitations of Chinese medicine on the field nor did he want untrained people. I pointed out that we did not have enough doctors to fulfill our agreement with the Chinese Red Cross and asked if he approved of our asking for more. He did so and agreed to exchange letters on the subject.[29]

The journalists and missionaries' pleas for the Allied command in Europe and the United States to send many more international physicians to China remained largely unanswered. The only two foreign physicians that succeeded in reaching the Chinese Red Cross in 1941 were the two women doctors: Dr. Adele Cohn from the United States and Dr. Barbara Courtney from England.

Dr. Courtney arrived in Guiyang in May 1941. She traveled from Calcutta to Hong Kong, where Mrs. Selwyn-Clarke offered her a position in a missionary hospital. However, Dr. Courtney made it clear that she wanted to join the Chinese Red Cross/Medical Relief Corps. The Friends Ambulance Units and British Relief Unit also helped her to reach Guiyang from India though records of her travel are incomplete. She worked with the three other British citizens associated with the Chinese Red Cross at that time: Michael Sullivan, Evert Barger, and Philip Wright. They petitioned the British Secretary of State for Foreign Affairs from Guiyang on February 17, 1942, for grants to support the work of Dr. Lin and the Chinese Red Cross/Medical Relief Corps.[30]

Michael Sullivan (苏立文) was an English pacifist who joined the International Red Cross Committee and then the Chinese Red Cross/Medical Relief Corps in Guiyang in 1939. He worked as a truck driver and draftsman and lived in China for six years. However, it was his appreciation of Chinese art rather than healthcare that would later make him the most famous of the international volunteers at the Chinese Red Cross Medical Relief Corps' headquarters. After the war, he became a Professor of Asian Art at Stanford and Oxford University. Upon his death in 2013, he donated what has been hailed as the largest collection of private Chinese art in the West to the Ashmolean Museum of Art and Archeology at Oxford University.[31]

Despite the addition of Drs. Courtney and Cohn, Dr. Lin continued to express his ambivalence about receiving more foreign physicians in China in 1941: "They are needed very badly, but experience with foreign doctors proves that selection must be carefully made; otherwise, good men find themselves unable to work."[32] It seems probable that Dr. Lin was alluding to the political realities of the concurrent forced inactivity of the International Medical Relief Corps' physicians in Tuyunguan at that time. He reiterated to American Bureau for Medical Aid to China, "If you cannot find a really enthusiastic foreign doctor, do not send them out here.... We are certainly disappointed that no Chinese doctors have volunteered.... The Spanish doctors have on the whole done splendidly."[33]

The International Medical Relief Corps' physicians were trying to come to grips with the reality that they were both needed by China and appreciated by Dr. Lin yet not permitted to carry on their medical work. In 1941, Dr. Iancu continued to write of his, Drs. Baer and Freudmann's detainment in Tuyunguan and Dr. Kisch's detainment in the area near Sian [Xi´an].[34] Dr. Freudmann expressed his frustration with Dr. Lin's inactivation of most of the International Medical Relief Corps:

> Dr. Lin did not react to my complaints. He did not give an opinion, he did not reply— obviously what I had told him was neither new nor interesting. Maybe it was humiliating for him to hear such complaints coming out of my mouth, the mouth of a foreigner.... When Dr. Lin said goodbye to me after the banquet, he said: "I have been thinking for some time of withdrawing all the Spanish doctors. You will soon come to Guiyang." ... For all practical purposes, this completed the first stage of my Chinese experiences.[35]

Dr. Fritz Jensen remained active in the field and had not yet been ordered back to Tuyunguan. By the fall of 1941, he began working for the industrial cooperatives in Kanhsien[36] in southern Kiangsi [Jiangxi] that the New Zealand–born writer and political activist, Rewi Alley (路易•艾黎, Lùyì Àilí) had initiated. At that time, Dr. Jensen became the personal physician of Chiang Kai-shek's son, Chiang Ching-kuo.[37]

While Dr. Jensen was heading south, Dr. Coutelle wrote, on September 6, 1941, from Guiyang that he hoped to be heading north to the Yellow River with Drs. Kaneti, Flato, and, probably, Baer. This trip did not come to fruition, however, and Dr. Coutelle was still in Tuyunguan six months later.[38] In 1942, the other International Medical Relief Corps' members trapped in Tuyunguan were inactivated. This group included:

> Dr. Kaneti in group 23 of the OPC hospital in Tuyungyan, Dr. Cohn in the x-ray department, Dr. Kamieniecki in the laboratory and Dr. Flato in environmental sanitation. They were all officially relegated to the reserve division in Guiyang, Guichou [Guizhou].[39]

As they sat dejected and medically inactive, they pondered the political irony of a world at war. In the Nazi-controlled areas of Europe, no Jewish or communist physicians were permitted to render aid to Aryan patients, while in the Guomindang Nationalist Party-controlled areas of China, no Aryan or Jewish physicians were permitted to render aid to Communist patients. The International Medical Relief Corps' hope to fight against fascism were foiled again. They remained temporarily trapped in a political no man's land, as impenetrable as the trenches and walls on the Japanese front.

The Pacific War and the Enemy Alien Medical Allies: 1942

Suddenly, on December 7, 1941, the prospects for International Medical Relief Corps' members rose, even as the battleship *USS Arizona* sank into Pearl Harbor. The Chinese were delighted to be aligned with American and British forces in what was to be called the Pacific War. But, the military campaigns started poorly for the new allies. The battle of Hong Kong ended with a Japanese victory on December 25, 1941.

The Hong Kong–based headquarters of the Chinese Red Cross and Mme. Sun Yat-sen's Chinese Defence League barely escaped to Chongqing in central China. The Chinese Defence League's treasurer, Norman French, was killed in action on December 19, 1941, as a gunner in the No. 2 Battery of the Hong Kong Volunteer Defence Corps,[40] and its secretary, Hilda Selwyn-Clarke, was interned by the Japanese soon after. The outposts of the British colonial empire in Southeast Asia continued to fall like dominos: Singapore surrendered to the Japanese on February 15, 1942, and Rangoon, Burma, [Yangon, Myanmar] on March 7, 1942.

China's declaration of war against the united Axis powers on December 9, 1941, further complicated the lives of the German and Austrian born members of the International Medical Relief Corps, since the Chinese now also viewed these doctors as enemy aliens. Being enemy aliens was nothing new: they had been enemy aliens of the British and French since September 1939 when those allies declared war on Germany. Their political convictions, ethnicity, and aid to China had made them enemy aliens of Germany and Italy even before that. And when Germany invaded the Soviet Union in 1941, they became enemy aliens of the Soviet Union.

Although Japan had invaded China in 1937, China's formal declaration of war against Japan and the Axis powers did not occur until the attack on Pearl Harbor in December 1941. At that point, the German and Austrian-born International Medical Relief Corps' physicians had obtained the dubious distinction of becoming enemy aliens of all the combatants in World War II.

8. The Forced Restriction of Healthcare Delivery: 1941–1942   139

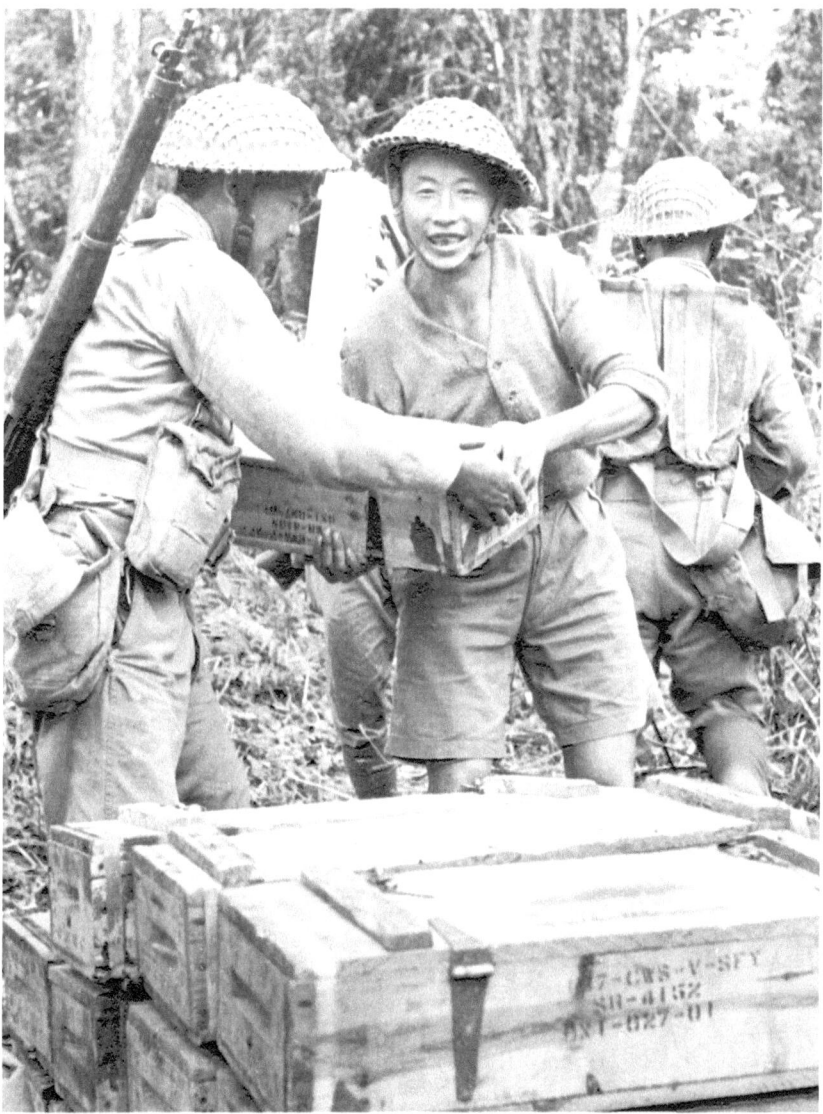

Chinese soldiers stacking United States Army ammunition in the Mogaung Valley of Northern Burma, July 13, 1944 (National Archives: 208-FA-30121).

As the Spanish doctors pondered this improbability, they shared the practical impact of their new status with the China Medical Aid Committee in London:

> There are some restrictions introduced after the declaration of war by China to the Axis countries, against the enemy aliens, Germans and Austrians, who have considerable

difficulties getting certificates, issued by the Foreign Ministry for free travel in the interior of China. This greatly affects our present work and the possibility of those who are here to do any active work in the field as they are officially not allowed to work at the front. This concerns Drs. Baer, Coutelle, Freudmann and Kent. Drs. Coutelle and Kent have certificates issued by the British Home Office. It would be very helpful for them if the home office renewed these certificates which have expired. The visas must be sent to the British Consul General in Chungking [Chongqing] from where they could get them. All the other nationals have nearly the same difficulties.[41]

The fact that Drs. Mamlok, Lurje, the Wantochs, and the German and Austrian physicians sent by the China Medical Aid Committees were anti–Fascist refugees would cause considerable confusion as they fought together with the Allied command. They would be required to report regularly to the police and struggled to obtain the travel and visa documents needed to serve with the Chinese Red Cross/Medical Relief Corps.

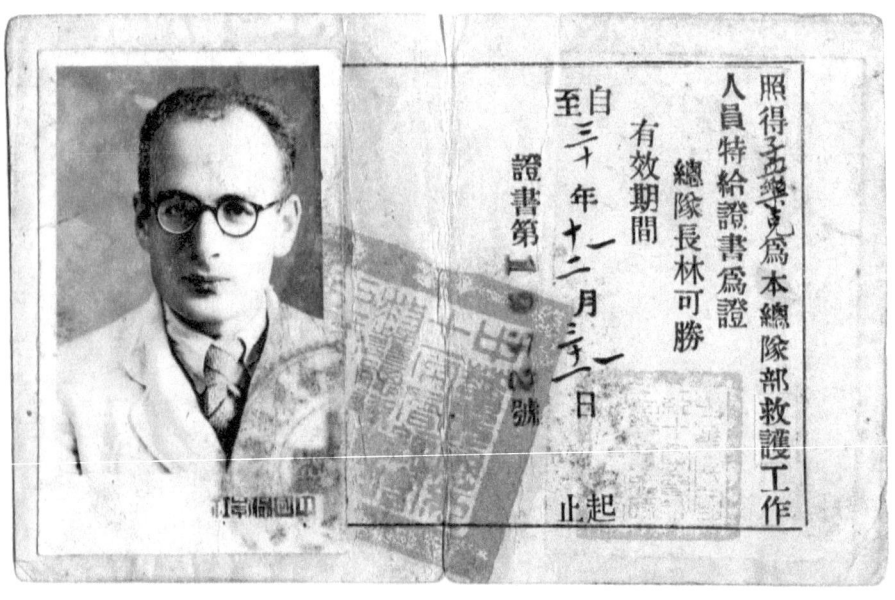

Dr. Erich Mamlok's Chinese Red Cross Medical Relief Corps identity card from 1941 (courtesy Robert Mamlok).

In March 1942, when the Japanese besieged Rangoon, General Chiang Kai-shek sent a Chinese Expeditionary Force to Burma along with a Chinese Red Cross/Medical Relief Corps unit led by Dr. Lin to defend Mandalay and northern Burma. However, despite this and other allied efforts, the Japanese succeeded in cutting off China's last remaining land route, the Burma Road. The allied forces were badly routed in their first Burma campaign. The American Commanding General, Joe Stilwell, and Dr. Lin heroically led military and medical units respectively from Burma to India, barely escaping capture by Japanese forces, which by summer 1942 controlled much of Southeast Asia.

Back in the Chinese Red Cross/Medical Relief Corps' headquarters in Tuyunguan, things were also not going well for the International Medical Relief Corps in 1942. Dr. Coutelle wrote to his wife, Rosa, (now safely back in England with their son Charles) that the Medical Relief Corps' new leadership continued the International Medical Relief Corps' forced inactivity:

> China's war has now been connected with the world and a common worldwide front against aggression has now been established. Maybe—we all hope so—we will have more to do and will be better employed then [sic] up till now. You see, I am still in Kweiyang [Guiyang] and doing nothing. It is now the sixth month! We are all here: Flato, Kaneti, Taubenfligel, Mamlok, Mania [Kamieniecka] Dr. Courtney (the cousin of Patience [Darton]) and I. Waiting—Waiting.[42]

However, the physicians trapped in Tuyunguan continued to care for their patients and each other as well as they could. During this time, Dr. Kriegel contracted a serious form of amoebic dysentery that Dr. Coutelle confirmed with his microscope.[43] In March 1942, the thirty-one-year-old Dr. Barbara Courtney planned to join a Chinese Red Cross/Medical Relief Corps' unit that was to go to Chekiang [Zhejiang] Province to investigate a reported outbreak of plague. Dr. Courtney finally received permission to serve in the field. Each medical staff member assigned to that unit received a vaccination for plague the day before leaving. Despite battling an upper respiratory tract infection, Dr. Courtney received her vaccination, perhaps ill-advisedly, as she did not want to miss the opportunity to join this group.[44] Her friend, Dr. Coutelle, described what ensued:

> The next day she fell ill and died the following night of cerebrospinal meningitis, probably malignant because of coincidence with a plague vaccination. The diagnosis was made early, we had sulphonamide—but all in vain. Courtney came to us from a quite different direction. She was member of the Indian Theosophical Society. In spite of this great difference in outlook she gained quickly our respect and friendship, because she gave us a quiet example of a really simple, modest and absolutely honest life. She showed without words, that her ideal of "universal brotherhood" was really the guide of her life. She became to us a good friend and was liked by every one of us.... We now know that [Mrs. Hilda] Selwyn-Clark tried to discourage her from joining the Chinese Red Cross because of the hard conditions she would find. She also offered instead a place in the Mission Hospital of the International Red Cross. Courtney declined and came over on her own responsibility.... We buried her on a fine hillside opposite the fine mountain range she liked so much.... Her example will be unforgotten and we will continue to work ... and the pain must be transformed in active energy—only in this way we can really honour her memory.[45]

A Chinese physician with the Chinese Red Cross/Medical Relief Corps also shared memories about the life and death of Dr. Courtney:

> She became very friendly with a young Jewish doctor, but she did not allow their friendship to interfere with her work. And one day the Surgeon-General ordered us to prepare a group of doctors to go to the front, and she was among those who were chosen. I have never known a girl so delighted. If the height of her ambition was to work in China, a still higher ambition was to work at the front and tend the wounded. She was radiant with happiness. She was like a flame, absorbing the atmosphere around her, dancing with life and vitality. And then she was struck down with meningitis. It can be a very painful death, and her death was very painful, for at first we could not recognize that it was meningitis—it was unthinkable that she could have the disease. And so in a few days she died.
>
> We buried her high up on the mountains. We carried the heavy wooden coffin up the rocks, stumbling a little because it was a windy day, and there was rain in the air, and we wanted to get the ceremony over quickly; it was too painful, you understand. The coffin was lowered into a shallow grave, we read some prayers and suddenly the young Jewish officer ran forward a little, crying as though he thought he could summon her back from the grave...[46]

Dr. Courtney's tomb in Tuyunguan bears her legacy:

> This memorial is in memory of Dr. Guy Courtney, a British woman doctor who came in support of the Chinese war of resistance against Japan in 1941. Courtney died at her post in 1942 while working to prevent and cure the diseases caused by the germ warfare waged by the Japanese.

With the loss of Dr. Courtney and the continued absence of Dr. Lin, who was still serving with the Chinese Expeditionary Force in Burma, the International Medical Relief Corps' doctors in Tuyunguan were growing increasingly frustrated amidst forced idleness and potential danger. On June 10, 1942, Dr. Coutelle shared the state of the doctors' frustration with his wife Rosa:

> I for myself have nothing agreeable to write. The situation here has become quite tense. I have nothing to do.... At the same time, the propaganda starts against us. We are "lazy Jews," who do not want to work. At the beginning of this year Mania [Kamieniecka] had been complimented out of the lab. In the same way now rumors are spread that she went away by herself, because she is not interested in doing anything ...
>
> Dr. Pan Shi, [Pan Ji] one of the leading man of the Chinese Red Cross (Lin is the head of the Medical Relief Corps of the Chinese Red Cross) frankly told Kaneti: "Oh yes, of course he can sign the petition for passports for us, but he will not do it as he hopes that this will be the end of our work with the Medical Relief Corps." ... [Lin's] absence is being used now to attack us. How far Lin, whose position has considerably weakened in the last year, is able and even willing to support us, is uncertain. It is always going like that; the moment that difficulties or setbacks arise for China, then the defeatists and reactionaries try to attack. And this holds true too for the Chinese Red Cross.
>
> Lin's most bitter enemies are the former Hong Kong directors of the Chinese Red

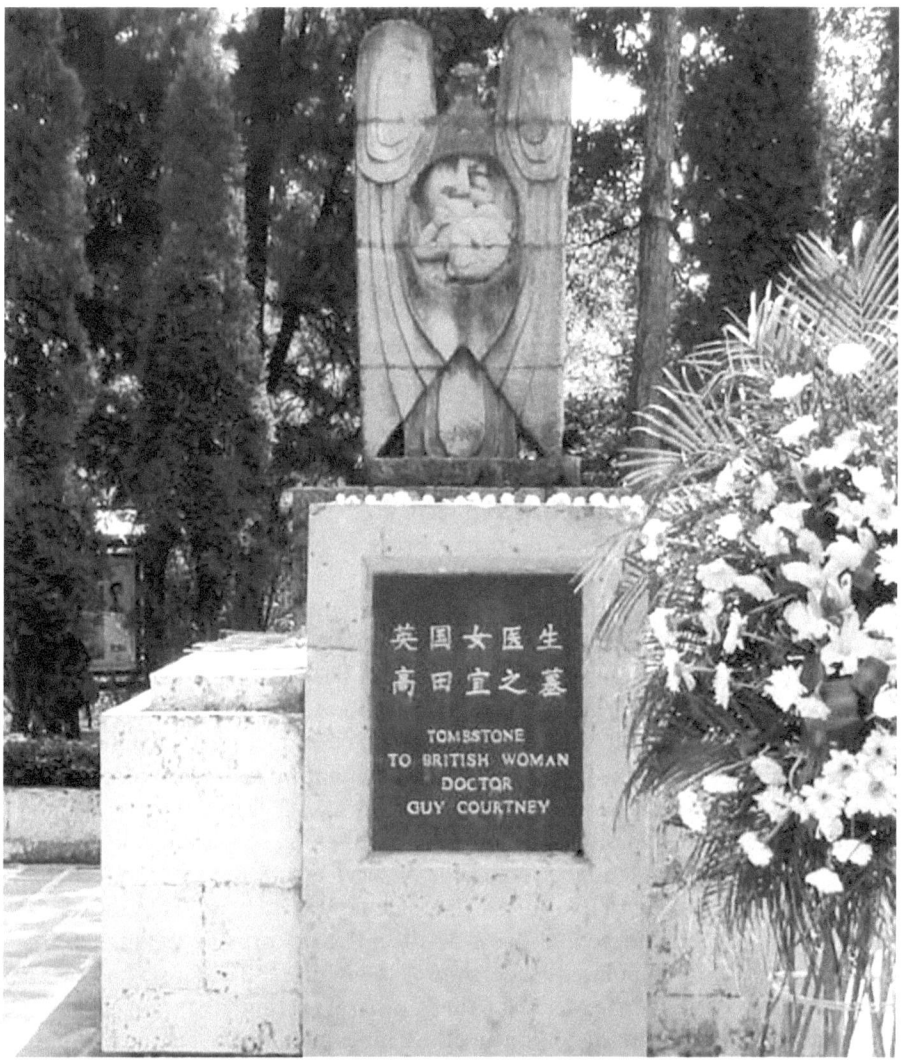

Dr. Barbara Guy Courtney's tombstone at the Tuyunguan Park Memorial to the Chinese Red Cross Medical Relief Corps (near Guiyang, China) (courtesy Robert Mamlok).

Cross [Drs. Wang and Pan Ji] who are now in Chungking [Chongqing]. These are the same men who once sent a letter to the different armies where Chinese Red Cross units were working, stating that the Chinese Red Cross organization was infected with reds and that they should be on guard.[47]

Journalist Israel Epstein (伊斯雷尔·爱泼斯坦, Yisilei'er Aipositan) wrote similarly about the Spanish doctors' inactivity in 1942:

A year previously, one of the proudest possessions of the [Medical] Relief Corps had been a team of foreign doctors who had served in the International Brigade in Spain and had come to China as volunteers after the fall of Madrid. Now they were being removed from front-line jobs and concentrated as virtual prisoners at headquarters. China needed every medical man she could lay hold of but she could not use these "premature antifascists." Their request to be sent to the front behind the enemy lines if the Kuomintang did not want them to work in its own areas was flatly refused.[48]

A few International Medical Relief Corps' physicians who were still able to continue to practice medicine on the front, such as Drs. Leo Kamieniecki and George Schön, attributed their good fortune to the patronage of the more progressive divisional commanders. For example, Dr. Schön, attached to the 18th Division, east of the I'Chang front, continued to speak about the exemplary command of General Lo (羅卓英 Luo Zhuoying). Specifically, he cited General Lo's support for the creation of public health measures for the prevention of the spread of infectious illnesses among his troops.[49] The excellence of General Lo's command was well recognized. He became Commander in Chief of the 1st Route Expeditionary Forces, in Burma, and in 1942 became Chief of Staff to General Joseph Stilwell.

Dr. Schön also lamented the forced inactivity of ten of his fellow International Medical Relief Corps' colleagues in Tuyunguan. He added that Dr. Pan Ji was very hostile to these doctors and tried to intern some of them, especially those of German nationality.[50] Dr. Kent, who also remained on the front, reported back to the Chinese Red Cross' headquarters in August 1942 from the 2nd Group in Taoynan: "There is no fighting but much troop movement. Our unit is frozen in preventative work.... I visited the 67th Army, which was very glad to receive our unit, but then had to move."[51]

In August 1942, after five months of service with the Chinese Expeditionary Force's failed First Burma Campaign, Dr. Lin returned to the headquarters of the Chinese Red Cross/Medical Relief Corps in Tuyunguan. By then, the newly appointed leadership of the Chinese Red Cross had taken complete control of the Medical Relief Corps. With limited patronage in the National Health Administration and the Chinese Red Cross, Dr. Lin had little recourse but to again resign as director of the Chinese Red Cross/Medical Relief Corps. He continued to head the Emergency Medical Service Training School but would resign within a year from that role too. Dr. McClure wrote to a Friends Ambulance Unit in Yunnan about how much worse the Chinese Red Cross became without Dr. Lin:

> For some time there were signs of serious political interference with the work of the Chinese Red Cross and this culminated in Dr. Lin the heart and soul of the medical work, resigning his post as commander of the Medical Relief Corps.... The politicians have been entirely unable to steer the ship and it has been floundering around ever since with Chinese Red Cross units withdrawn from some fronts and deprived of needed

supplies on all fronts and wholesale resignations while all work has been brought to a standstill.[52]

The International Medical Relief Corps' members had witnessed the rise and fall of the Chinese Red Cross/Medical Relief Corps. Like most of their biomedical Medical Relief Corps' colleagues, they initially praised Dr. Lin's leadership and success. When Dr. Lin resigned, the loss of his charismatic and patriotic leadership resulted in the resignation of many of the Chinese Red Cross/Medical Relief Corps' personnel. The Chinese Red Cross/Medical Relief Corps continued to shrivel as funding stagnated, morale plummeted, and inflation climbed.

The factors contributing to Dr. Lin's downfall included administrative jealousy of his success and deep-rooted political distrust of his egalitarian motives. In effect, the Guomindang Nationalist Party's intolerance of medical support for the Chinese Communist Party Armies trumped Dr. Lin's and the Chinese Red Cross/Medical Relief Corps' vision of medical care for all of China.[53] Thus, the International Medical Relief Corps' physicians were again in the all too familiar role of involuntary retention as they hoped for an outlet from their latest political predicament.

III. THE INTERNATIONAL MEDICAL RELIEF CORPS AND THE CHINESE EXPEDITIONARY FORCES: 1943–1945

9. The International Medical Relief Corps and the Chinese Expeditionary Force in Burma and India

In fall of 1942, the International Medical Relief Corps' members' gloomy and uncertain future took an abrupt turn for the better as most departed Tuyunguan and joined the Chinese Expeditionary Force-X in India and Burma. The reasons for this sudden departure are as complicated as the volunteers' arrival. General Joe Stilwell had befriended Dr. Lin during their prewar period in China, and they had met again during the disastrous first Burma campaign. They shared a common vision to allocate medical resources as well as possible and to defeat Japan in the second Burma campaign.

The Allied command was clearly aware of the potential liaison value of the now bilingual, battle-hardened, and endangered International Medical Relief Corps' physicians. After all, their arrival in China had been on the front page of the *New York Times,* and Agnes Smedley had publicized their activity in her widely read book, *The Battle Hymn of China.* In addition, the International Medical Relief Corps' physicians had shared the frustrations of their forced inactivity with the United States and British relief organizations and militaries.

In many ways, the volunteers' departure was a match made in heaven. The Chinese Red Cross, the International Medical Relief Corps, and the U.S. military command were all pleased by the opportunity to place the International Medical Relief Corps' physicians under United States' rather than Chinese command. Furthermore, such new alignment reduced the Chinese Red Cross/Medical Relief Corps' fears that the Spanish doctors would try to join the Chinese Communist Party's army medical services and that negative publicity from the International Medical Relief Corps' physicians' forced inactivity might jeopardize the Chinese Red Cross' future accrual of foreign medical aid. This latter fear was well founded. Due to the persistent diligence and advocacy of Drs. Mary Gilchrist and Rosa Coutelle in Great Britain, the China Medical Aid Committee in London had already sent a representative of the International Red Cross to inspect the plight of the Spanish doctors in Tuyunguan.[1] Dr. Mary Gilchrist, secretary of the China Medical Aid Committee of London, continued her close communication with the Spanish doctors throughout the war, even when it meant typing letters under her desk during the bombing of London.

On November 20, 1942, General Stilwell asked the Chinese military to send eight-to-ten foreign doctors to help the Chinese Army in India (*Chih hui pu*), which was being trained by the United States Army forces in Ramgarh, India.[2] They agreed that the Chinese Red Cross/Medical Relief Corps would send ten doctors to Kunming, in Yunnan province, and that the U.S. military would then fly them to India.[3] On December 8, 1942, basic transfer

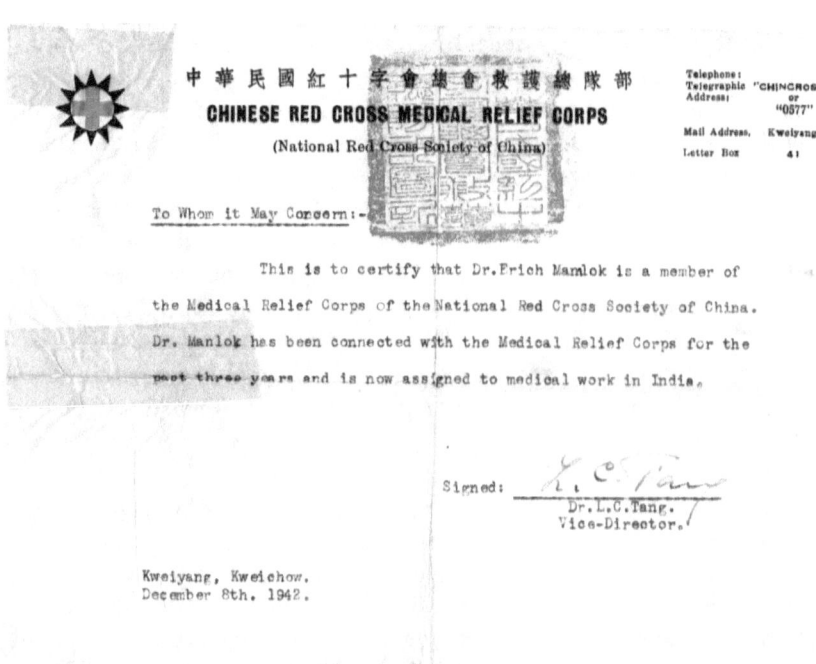

Certificate from the Chinese Red Cross Medical Relief Corps authorizing travel to India to provide medical services to the Chinese Expeditionary Force. Guiyang, China, December 8, 1942 (courtesy Robert Mamlok).

papers were finalized and these International Medical Relief Corps' physicians soon soared south over the Himalaya Mountains.[4]

The departure of most of the International Medical Relief Corps' physicians from China was one of the few events in 1942 that had the approval of both the Generalissimo's Guomindang Nationalist Party and Chairman Mao Zedong and Zhou Enlai's Chinese Communist Party. At this stage of the ongoing anti–Japanese war and looming Chinese civil war, the International Medical Relief Corps' physicians' departure from Tuyunguan became an urgent matter of personal safety. The Spanish doctors again first sought the advice of Zhou Enlai, who convinced them to accept the Americans' proposal. Ominously, Zhou Enlai told these physicians that they "should work against Japan, for many Chinese soldiers, and [they] would also be more secure as [they] were not at the time."[5] Dr. David Iancu described Zhou Enlai's advice:

> I received news from the Chinese Red Cross program, that a group of our doctors are to be sent to military units that were to be trained and armed by Americans to fight the Japanese that invaded Burma and India. At the request of the Red Cross some of our group is to go with these units. We again approached the leadership of the Chinese communist party. With the approval of Zhou En-lai, some doctors, including myself, will go to India, and from there, the newly formed unit, will go to Burma.... We were told that we could go to work with the Chinese units, as before then, possibly to make contact with the communists in those places where we work, but to leave all our party documents in China.[6]

This news of the impending departure traveled slowly to the members of the International Medical Relief Corps still in the field. Dr. Rolf and Joan (Staniforth) Becker wrote that they, too, had received a telegram to go back to Guiyang in December 1942 with a planned departure to India: "It took us over a month traveling over the mountains and down the Yangtze to get back to Chungking [Chongqing], as Rolf was recalled for assignment in Burma. We were disgusted to find out that we arrived just too late. Eight of the foreign doctors had just left.... Rolf will probably now go to the Yunnan front."[7]

Further to the south of Guiyang, in Yunnan Province, Dr. Walter Freudmann recalled the episode that was unfolding:

> The time had come when the doctors who were being kept idle in Guiyang would find employment again. Guiyang was glad to get the European doctors out of China. Our unit in Yunnan was told to go directly to Kunming where we would meet our other colleagues from Guiyang and leave for India by air.... The only document the American command gave us, ignoring all formalities, was a written order for eight doctors of the Chinese Red Cross to go by air to India to the training camp.[8]

Dr. Coutelle described the departure to his wife in a letter on November 11, 1942:

> Nine of us (Taubenfligel, Mamlock, Kriegel, Kisch, Baer, Freudmann, Yancu, Volochin and I and probably Flato too) will go to Kunming and from there by plane to India. We

will work under Allied command among Chinese troops stationed there. Lin sends us there. The whole development came in a real hurry.... How exactly our status will be is not yet clear, but it seems quite certain, that we will have the possibility to work. Lin must be quite happy to get us out of his way.[9]

Dr. Coutelle probably did not know that Dr. Lin, now demoted to the role of a general advisor with the Chinese Red Cross, was probably not responsible for actuating the transfer orders. The transfer orders were signed by Dr. L.C. Tang.

Dr. Iancu similarly recalled that he left Kunming in December 1942 with Drs. Baer, Freudmann, Coutelle, Kriegel, Flato, Taubenfligel, and Volokhine and reached Calcutta on December 31, 1942. Drs. Kisch and Mamlok were the other two International Medical Relief Corps' members who flew with this group to Calcutta. The married couples, the Beckers, Kranzdorfs, Kamienieckis, and Kanetis, remained in China.[10] Drs. Jensen, Kent, Mann, Schön, Jungermann, Marens and Cohn also remained in China at that time. It seems probable that the U.S. command did not wish to employ any of the married couples as Dr. Kisch was the only married physician who could go to India while his wife Edith (Marens), stayed in Tuyunguan.

Frigid temperatures and limited oxygen made these high-altitude flights memorable. In addition to the urgently needed relief physicians, the plane carried a cargo of titanium bars, which served for the physicians' seating. As their plane landed in India, an American psychologist greeted them, and Dr. Coutelle noticed him talking to the pilots. The presence of mental health support was well needed, Dr. Coutelle added, as many of the U.S. pilots would perish during such harrowing transport missions "over the hump" during World War II.[11]

As they left the forced inactivity of Tuyunguan behind, life appeared to be looking up for this group of International Medical Relief Corps' physicians. Dr. Iancu wrote that they merrily celebrated their arrival in Calcutta on New Year's Eve 1942:

> We procured some food and drink and we spent the evening singing our revolutionary songs, as we were doing in China. At midnight, our party was interrupted by some English policemen. They interrogated us, in order to learn who we were, what we were doing on Indian soil, and how we had reached Calcutta. We gave them the requested explanations but they asked for supporting documents. As none of us had identity cards or documents proving our mission, they asked us not to leave the hotel until the next day when we were to clarify all issues. Of course, we didn't want to leave the hotel but this encounter spoiled our party mood so we stopped the party and went to bed. The policemen returned the next day, put us all in a police van and took us to the Calcutta Police headquarters where we underwent separate interrogations. We had nothing to hide and each of us declared who he was and what the purpose was of our arrival in India. Each of us also filled in a statement form that included our citizenship. During the interrogations, an American officer showed up and he gave all the needed clarifi-

cations. The investigating officers showed their indignation to the fact that the Americans had brought foreigners on a territory that didn't belong to them. The English considered themselves full masters of India. We left the Englishman and the American to quarrel about the rights they were contesting.[12]

The British forces in colonial India and the American military command in Burma continued to argue about what to do with the anomaly of Chinese-speaking, enemy alien Europeans who had appeared without official British notice in India. To their credit, the International Medical Relief Corps' physicians looked like a respectable and nonthreatening group and General Stilwell and the American and Chinese forces in Burma desperately needed them. General H.L. Boatner the Chief of Staff of the China-Burma-India forces, reported their dilemma to the commanding general of the Chinese Army and the Chinese Red Cross:

> 10 doctors ordered by the headquarters of the Medical Relief Corps to join the Chinese Army in Ramgarh left China [Kunming] on December 26, 1942, and arrived in Calcutta on December 30, 1942. At Calcutta, five of our doctors, namely Baer, Iancu, Freudmann, Mamlok and Coutelle, were detained by the British authorities for some investigations. The other five, namely Taubenfligel, Kisch, Volokine, Kriegel and Flato, arrived in Ramgarh on January 7, 1943.[13]

This must have seemed like an eternity to Dr. Freudmann, who was to write in his memoirs that "[w]e had to wait in Calcutta for an entire month under the close surveillance of British detectives until an American military officer finally escorted us to Ramgarh by car."[14]

The political furor caused by the International Medical Relief Corps' physicians' transfer to India dragged on for several months. First, the government of India communicated with the British embassy in Chongqing:

> They [the government of India] are considering protest to the Americans against the importation of "enemy aliens" without their prior consent but before doing so would like to know if the British embassy in Chungking or consul general in Kunming were in any way consulted?[15]

Officials in the British embassy replied that the Chinese and the Americans should have arranged things first with the government of India, and hoped that things would straighten out. They noted that the China Medical Aid Committee of London was very interested in the welfare of these doctors and would like to do what they could for them.[16] The British embassy in Chongqing acknowledged that neither the embassy nor the consulate had been informed of the dispatch of the doctors to India, which seemed to have been arranged by U.S. Army authorities in China.[17] On April 13, 1943, the government of India detailed their assessment of the enemy alien International Medical Relief Corps' physicians:

Our reaction was that from a security point of view, the less foreigners we had in India the better.... They arrived in Calcutta with no visas for India but with a letter from Headquarters of the United States' Kunming command, to the effect that they were brought to India at General Stilwell's request. Intelligence reports are to the effect that Coutelle can be said to be positively harmless, that Mamlock is to some extent suspicious and that the other eight are at best not definitely suspect. Nevertheless, all 10 were allowed to go to Ramgarh where they have been absorbed in the Chinese Red Cross.... Meanwhile we would ask that the remaining foreign doctors be not sent to India.[18]

While British, Indian, and American allies negotiated the nebulous fate of the International Medical Relief Corps' five enemy aliens, Dr. Iancu wrote that they could not move within the territory of India unless accompanied by one of the American officers. These five International Medical Relief Corps' members now had time to reflect on their unusual fate. As enemy aliens, they were now living somewhere between their third (Dr. Mamlok) and seventh (Dr. Coutelle) land of exile. Drs. Baer, Coutelle, Freudmann, Flato, and Iancu had already been interned after the Spanish Civil War. Dr. Mamlok, the youngest member of the group, had the dubious honor of being the first International Medical Relief Corps' member interned by the British allies for a second time. He assured his soon-to-be-British-interned companion physicians that his first internment with the British in Hong Kong was not as bad as the French internment camps about which his colleagues shared stories.

In the meantime, the Chinese Consulate General in Calcutta was imploring the Chinese Red Cross/Medical Relief Corps to send a telegram as soon as possible to vouch for the background of the five enemy alien doctors.[19] While these International Medical Relief Corps' physicians languished in India, they wrote to their friends and families, now strewn across four continents. The irony of having again left a country with anti–Fascist unity only to arrive to unanticipated political discord was too apparent. However, the group remained equally and temporarily divided by their national origin. Five were viewed by the British as enemy aliens and five were viewed as physician allies hoping to provide much needed medical service.

Within two weeks, President Franklin Delano Roosevelt and Winston Churchill met in Casablanca to plan the invasion of Europe. Although the war against Japan would drag on for another thirty-one months, the International Medical Relief Corps' members now knew that they were winning in the war against fascism. In addition, the U.S. Military Command and their British Allies worked together to release the enemy alien International Medical Relief Corps' physicians in Calcutta. Despite their internment, the International Medical Relief Corps' New Year was getting off to a good start.

Under the watchful eyes of the British, the group soon traveled 280 miles northwest by train from Calcutta to the small village of Ramgarh in the province of Bihar, India. Camp Ramgarh became the main staging ground for the training and care of the Chinese Expeditionary Force-X. The British originally had established Ramgarh as an Italian prisoner-of-war camp before its use by General Stilwell and the United States Army command. The British housed, fed, and paid the troops in a reverse Lend-Lease[20] agreement while the Americans equipped and trained them.[21] The irony of volunteering to serve in an old internment camp likely gave the much-interned International Medical Relief Corps' physicians a sense of *déjà vu*. However, the facilities were much nicer than what they had endured. The hospital at Ramgarh consisted of twenty-two wards, each in a separate brick building with a tiled roof and cement floor. A central roadway divided the camp in half and double barbed-wire barricades secured its perimeter.[22]

The military objectives were, by all accounts, no small undertaking. In January 1943, General Stilwell assured Chinese General Ho Ying-ch'in (何应钦 Hé Yìngqīn) that he had requested from Washington "procurement of 200,000 rifles, 10,000 2.5 ton trucks, 2,500 weapons carriers and 10,000 jeeps with six months of maintenance equipment."[23] By March 1943, Chiang and Stilwell agreed to train thirty divisions of Chinese troops. More than 100,000 Nationalist army soldiers were to be trained in Ramgarh (the X force) and the rest were to be trained in Kunming (the Y force) and Guilin (the Z force) China.

However, the Chinese military were not initially able to meet these manpower projections. In part, Chiang Kai-shek felt conflicted between the need to appease his new allies by participating in the Northern Burma campaign and wishing to maintain his armies for any future conflict with the Chinese Communist Party. He would prefer to rely on U.S. airpower rather than large-scale ground operations that could significantly diminish his military forces.[24] Correspondence between General George Marshall and China's Finance Minister, Song Ziwen (宋子文 T.V. Soong) in August 1943, confirmed General Stilwell's need to have twenty-three thousand additional Chinese soldiers fill the vacancies in the newly refurbished 22nd and 38th divisions.

However, the Chinese military were also not prepared to meet what the Americans viewed as a minimal standard of health for the Chinese troops. Song Ziwen's representatives wrote that, "the standard of physical requirements of the American authorities is high, only 20–30 percent of recruits available were picked. Therefore, the government must select from 100,000 men to find 30,000 recruits."[25] Despite the Chinese Red Cross/Medical Relief Corps and others' efforts, most Chinese troops continued to suffer from malnutrition and could not meet the Allies' minimum standard of health.

The Allied command tried to initially enlist the International Medical Relief Corps' physicians in Burma as contract surgeons with the U.S. Armed Forces. However, these doctors preferred to retain their civilian status as they again served with the Chinese troops. Dr. Coutelle explained:

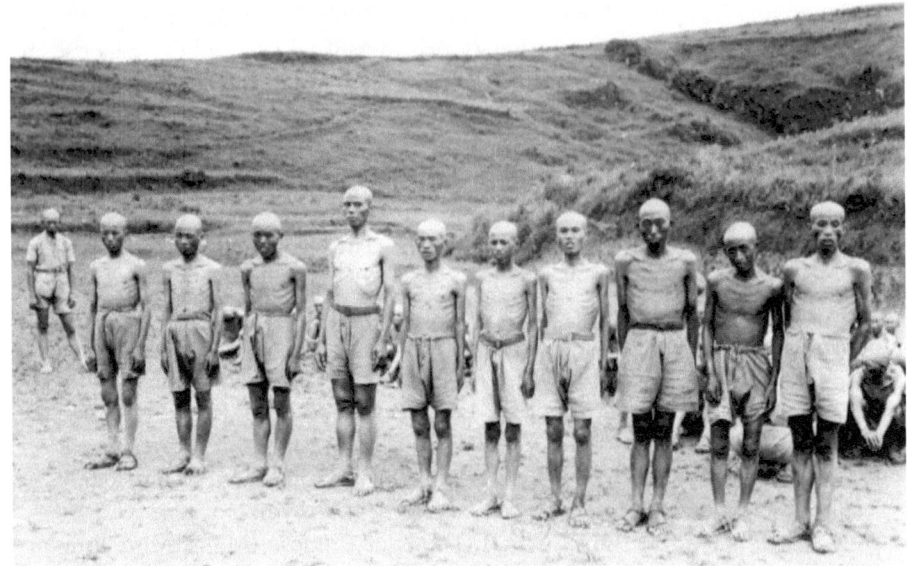

Group of malnourished recruits of the 13th Army Chinese Headquarters rejected for active duty with the Allied command, June 9, 1945 (National Archives: 111-SC-246170).

> Originally, we were to be hired as contract surgeons. That would have given us a much better pay and health insurance against war-related injury. But for this contract we had to agree to stay with the army for as long as was considered necessary. However, since we all wanted to return to our countries immediately at the end of the war in Europe, we refused the contract. Therefore, Stilwell—totally non-bureaucratic—appointed us to "Liaison doctors" (a unique status) with a 14-day notice period on both sides and a salary of $100 [from April 1944—February 1945], later $200.[26]

A grateful General Stilwell continued to do all he could to support the International Medical Relief Corps' physicians' service to the Chinese in their new role as liaison physicians with the U.S. Army. For example, he ordered that "[if the liaison physicians were] captured by the enemy, they should be granted the equivalent status of first lieutenants in the U.S. Army Medical Corps."[27]

In addition, the International Medical Relief Corps' physicians in Burma would receive the U.S. military rations of food, clothing allowances, and medical care that were considerably better than what they received with the Chinese Red Cross in Guiyang. Nevertheless, General Boatner wrote appreciatively to Dr. Kisch: "Such service as you [the medical liaison officers] have performed in the past is not truly measured in monetary values alone, but rather in the true spirit of appreciation shown by all members of the allied service for a job well done."[28]

1 MARCH 1944

CERTIFICATE

This is to certify that DR. ERICH MAMLOK is a
Medical Liaison Officer detailed by Lieutenant General Joseph W. Stilwell
Theater Commander for service with the Chinese Army in India and is under
United States Army military jurisdiction for administration, discipline,
criminal jurisdiction and trial. Reference U.S. Article of War 2(d) and
paragraph 3 Ordinance IVI of 1942 Legislative Department Government of
India. If captured by the enemy he should be granted the equivalent status
of First Lieutenant in the United States Army Medical Corps. Reference
Par 76 Geneva Convention of July 27, 1929 relative to treatment of
Prisoners of War.

For Lieutenant General JOSEPH W. STILWELL:

Wm. E. BERGIN
Brigadier General U S A
Chief of Staff

OFFICIAL:

M. R. Murphy
M. R. MURPHY
Major, F. A.
Adjutant

General Joseph Stillwell notes that if the Medical Liaison physicians serving the Chinese Army in India are captured by the enemy they should be granted the equivalent status of First Lieutenant in the United States Army Medical Corps. March 1, 1944 (courtesy Robert Mamlok).

General Boatner was not the only one who believed the job was well done. Dr. Coutelle reported that the high morale, good organization, and cooperation between the Chinese and American units was impressive. On the other hand, he found the active involvement in jungle combat very hard and exhausting and the fight "to the last man" on the Japanese side very bloody. It is estimated that some eighty thousand Japanese died during the recapture of Burma and that four out of every five of the troops that had started out with General Stilwell during the three-month siege of Myitkyina had been either wounded or killed. Dr. Coutelle also noted that most American soldiers had no political motivation to fight in this war: "It was a job, imposed on them by the Japanese; to be done as well and quickly as possible and to make the best for one's self out of it."[29]

With new contracts and politics aside, the International Medical Relief Corps' physicians began their medical liaison role between the American and Chinese allies. The new allies viewed the standards of nutrition and support for this multinational fighting force quite differently. John Sweeney, a U.S. Army instructor at Ramgarh, summarized the troops' consensus of the living standards in Ramgarh: "For the Americans it was hell and for the Chinese it was heaven."[30]

Among the difficulties for the Americans was an inability of the China-Burma-India command to supply an appreciable diversity of acceptable food to sustain the army. The choice of rations was relatively limited, as this was now the longest military supply line in the world. However, the American soldiers' complaint that the caloric value of the Expeditionary Force Menu "No. 1" ration was inadequate must have amused the International Medical Relief Corps' physicians, for the protein rich 3,945 calories per day were far beyond what the Chinese soldiers and International Medical Relief Corps' physicians were used to.

The shortage of American physicians serving the Allied command in the China-Burma-India region had, in part, a nutritional basis. However, obesity rather than malnutrition excluded the enlistment of many otherwise well-qualified American medical candidates. The scarcity of medical manpower in the China-Burma-India theater became so severe that the American military subsequently waived the exclusion of obese physician recruits. A Ramgarh limerick celebrated this U.S. Army policy change:

> Hi diddle, diddle,
> A corpulent middle,
> And other defects may be waived.
> It means more physicians,
> Can now get commissions,
> The Medical Corps has been saved![31]

The American military's concerns about the recruitment of obese American physicians contrasted strikingly with the nutritional deficiencies of the incoming Chinese troops. For example, an outbreak of beriberi among the Chinese troops at Ramgarh raised considerable alarm.[32] Beriberi's presenting signs of night blindness, glossitis, and osteomalacia had certainly been sightings that were more common for the International Medical Relief Corps' physicians than the corpulent middles of some of their new allies.

Some International Medical Relief Corps' physicians wrote about more than nutritional differences among their new allies. Although some International Medical Relief Corps' physicians had contact with American volunteers during the Spanish Civil War, others were forming their initial impressions of the politically heterogeneous American allies. Dr. Iancu had served with Dr. Barsky's American surgical team in the International Brigades.[33] He wrote that some American soldiers had very reactionary ideas and regarded the Chinese and blacks as inferior races. He recognized that racism was deeply rooted in America in the 1940s but acknowledged that other American soldiers were more progressive and shared his egalitarian views.[34]

Dr. Freudmann wrote more harshly about the limited intellect and racism that he saw: "In a moral sense, the Americans led a rather shallow life, talking mostly about home, the family, movies and love, about girls and erotic conquests and most of all about food. For the 'inferior' Chinese race they had nothing but disdain."[35] Concerns of racism in the U.S. Army forces in the China-Burma-India theater in 1944 were well placed. For example, the commanding officer in the 518th Regiment was seeking a court martial of four men at that time. He wrote that they "constitute an undesirable and dangerous nucleus for the furtherance of racial propaganda and unrest and are impairing the efficiency of the unit ... information obtained within the company indicates that the life of at least one of the officers of this unit is in jeopardy."[36] Others, however, spoke more compassionately about the American allies: "The Americans were under order not to interfere with Chinese discipline. They were often sickened or enraged to see a Chinese soldier casually shot for using a hand grenade to catch fish."[37]

The Northern Burma Offensive

The Northern Burma campaigns started after the monsoons in November 1943. The American, British, and Chinese allies looked forward to ousting the Imperial Japanese Army that had succeeded in closing the Burma Road to China. The mountainous tropical jungles of northern Burma added a memorable and soggy chapter to the saga of these International Medical Relief Corps' physicians: "From March through October 1943, 175 inches of rain fell in the mountains and 100 inches in the valley."[38] Wang Ruifu, an interpreter with the 50th Division of the Chinese Army in India, described the battle terrain:

> We spent most of our time fighting in impenetrable jungles full of wild towering trees with leaves as big as washbasins, and vines and bushes so numerous that they covered the sky. Hot and humid air blew north off the Indian Ocean, which, being trapped by high mountains, turned into torrential rain, making it the wettest area on earth. We

could not build barracks and there was no shelter. We carried a machete to break brambles and thorns when we marched, to cut trees to make temporary shelter and to cut firewood.... The damp atmosphere led to a plethora of insects, mosquitoes and moths flying into your face. Guards needed to wear a mosquito net. We all used insect repellant on the exposed parts of our body and took a yellow pill, Atabrine, to prevent malaria. Our worst natural problem was the leeches.[39]

Dr. Gordon Seagrave popularized the American view of the medical aspects of the northern Burma campaigns in his popular book: *Burma Surgeon*.[40] He also spoke of northern Burma as the ancestral home of the leech:

They were so close together that your eyes had to be focused on the ground to find a place to step without landing on several of them. They seemed to direct themselves by a sense of smell. They would wave their big suckers in the air directly towards you. If you would suddenly move, the leech would immediately sway like a compass needle to be pointed directly at you.[41]

Despite the hardships of a very hostile terrain and the difficulties of molding dissimilar allies into a well-cared-for fighting force, the second Burma campaign was a success. The campaign in Northern Burma was one of the first in which the Chinese forces took the offensive and won a decisive victory.[42] The medical campaign enjoyed a similar success. Colonel Haueh Ying Kwei, a surgeon attached to the 38th Division of the Chinese Army in India in northern Burma, shared his appreciation of the joint medical efforts:

Our national army formed the main forces that launched and sustained the attack. The first engagements occurred in the Hukwang and the Mogaung valleys.[43] ... Throughout this campaign, it was found that the ratio of wounded to killed was roughly two to one. A total of some 13,000 casualties were treated by the joint efforts of Chinese and American medical units. Of these, 60–70 percent have been returned fit to units; about 5 percent are permanently disabled. Evacuation of the wounded and the sick from the division to the rear was the responsibility of the U.S. Army units.... The medical care given on the battlefields and hospitals was excellent.[44]

A *New York Times* correspondent summarized this arrangement as the best medical care that the Chinese military had ever received.[45]

Drs. Bedřich Kisch and Wiktor Taubenfligel joined Drs. Kwei and Seagrave in the Chinese 38th division.[46] Dr. Seagrave shared his admiration for Dr. Taubenfligel during the Hukawung offensive:

Opposite, top: A sentry guides walking Chinese wounded to the Seagrave Clinic (National Archives: 208-FO-OWI-3792). *Bottom:* Much of the improvement in medical care dealt with rapid transport of wounded soldiers. For example, U.S. Army nurse Jeanette C. Gleason treated wounded Chinese soldiers on an evacuation plane on its way back to India in November 1944. This was not without risk. Lieutenant Gleason was once forced to parachute from a damaged plane over the Himalaya Mountains and walked for four days before reaching friendly territory in China (National Archives: 208-FO-OWI-195196).

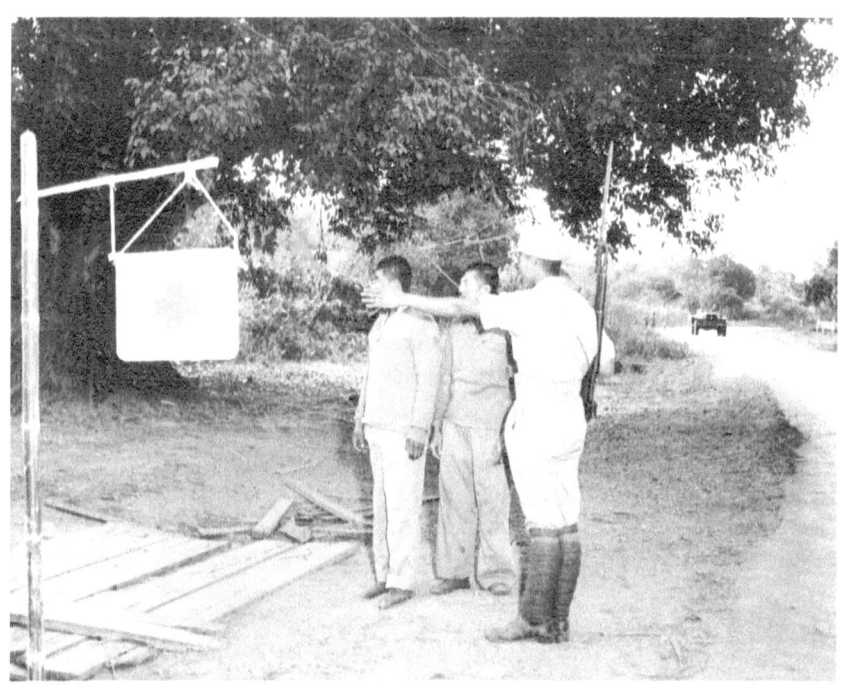

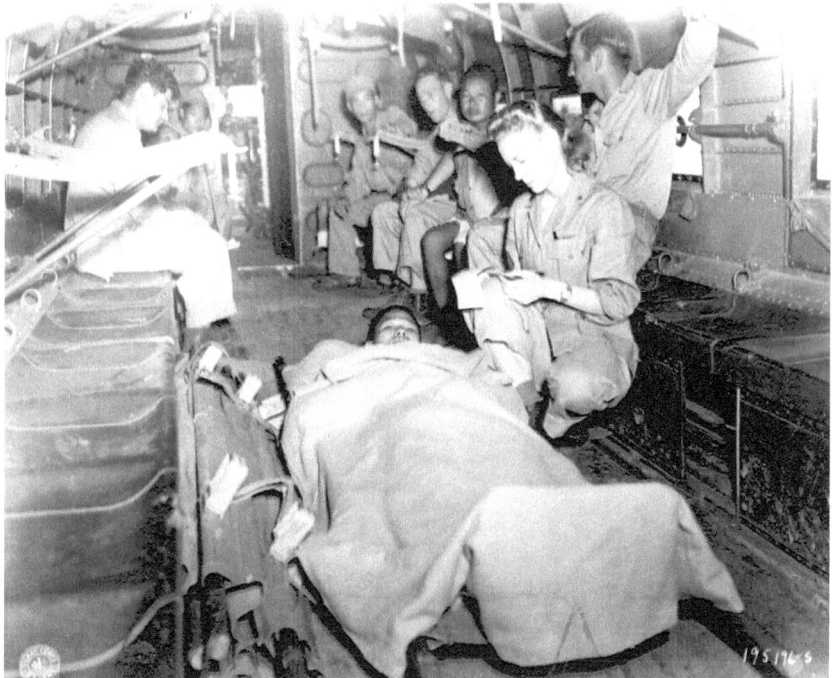

A detachment of our unit was ordered to accompany these troops. Dr. Taubenfligel was a Polish contract surgeon. At the beginning of the war in Spain, he joined a medical unit with the Republican Army and served till the end of the war, after which, with other foreign doctors, German, Czechoslovakian, and Polish, he was evacuated to China. There the group spent troublous years serving the Chinese armies, with little or nothing in the way of equipment and medical supplies. All spoke Chinese well and had learned how to live with the Chinese and like it. Under Stilwell they had been transferred to Ramgarh to work with Major Sigafoos as liaison officers with the Chinese regiments ... Taubenfligel was a grand person to have around. Although he had taken punishment the like of which few American officers have ever experienced, he was never known to complain and had a sense of humor that was heaven to the whole group. At Myitkyina when Colonel Petersen offered me my choice of any liaison medical officer as a permanent addition to our unit, I chose Taubenfligel.[47]

Much as in China, the International Medical Relief Corps' liaison doctors in Burma, such as Dr. Taubenfligel, were attached to different Chinese Army in India divisions throughout the front rather than kept as a single corps. Each division of the Chinese Army in India consisted of three medical corps officers and two liaison doctors.[48] In the spring of 1944, Dr. Walter Freudmann

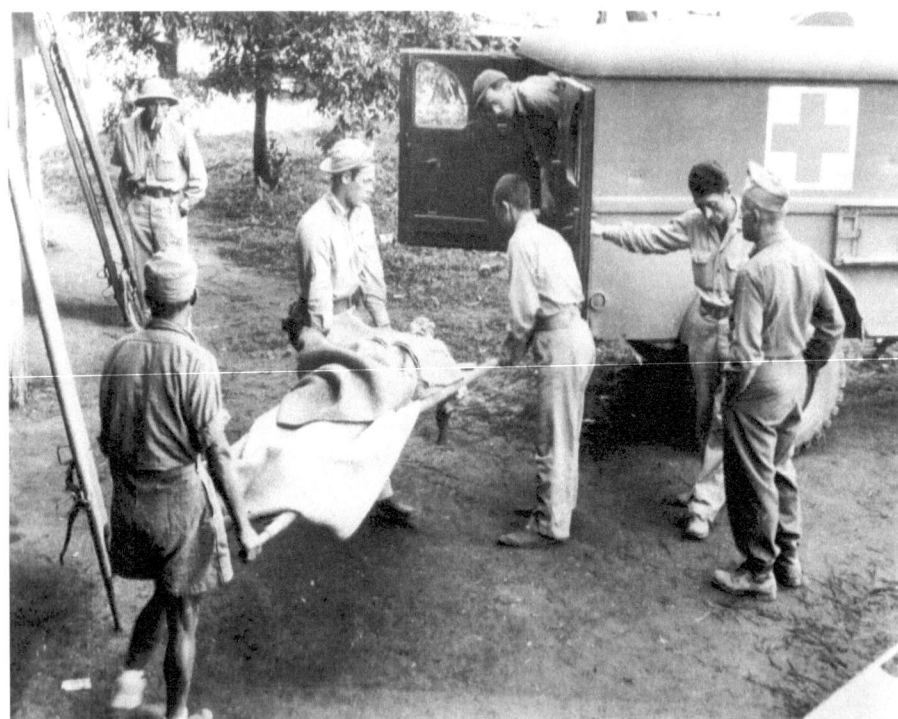

Drs. Seagrave (far right) and Taubenfligel (second from right) evacuating a wounded Chinese soldier in Burma, circa 1943–1944 (National Archives: 208-FO-OWI-3785).

was attached to a battalion in the jungle, and later to the 5th Artillery Regiment. From May 1944 to January 1945, Dr. Franta Kriegel accompanied a motorized unit. Dr. Carl Coutelle served in the 112th Regiment, also from May 1944 to January 1945; and from July 1945 until the end of the war, he served with the hospital services of the 50th Division. Although hospitals officially had Chinese doctors as directors, Dr. Volokhine served as medical director of the Chinese Convalescent Hospital.[49]

In Burma, the International Medical Relief Corps' physicians again endured some of the forced inactivity that they encountered in Tuyunguan. Perhaps this was due to the diplomatic furor created by the transfer of the enemy aliens from China to India without the knowledge of the Indian government. Thus, the movement of the International Medical Relief Corps' physicians in Burma was restricted. Dr. Mary Gilchrist of the China Medical Aid Committee in London shared this concern with the British Foreign Office secretary, A.L. Scott, on April 10, 1943:

> Although they are working with the Chinese Red Cross with the Chinese troops under U.S. command, those [International Medical Relief Corps' members] that are "enemy aliens" are not all wed to move about with their units and their work is greatly hampered in consequence. The American commanders say it is by the order of India. Dr. Iancu, a Romanian, had to be replaced by a Pole, Dr. Taubenfligel, when his unit moved camp. Could the government of India be asked to give our men some form of certificate of status or registration so that they could move with troops with whom they are working as medical officers? ... It is all very disheartening this constant interruption of work of medical men, who are keen to help, and of whose skill there is now such a shortage.[50]

Most of the enemy-alien-liaison physicians managed to remain on the battlefront. Dr. Erich Mamlok served under General Liao Yao-hsiang [廖耀湘 Yao Shiang] in the 65th regiment of the Chinese 22nd Division from December 1943 through May 1944. He joined the 65th Regiment in the Hukawung Valley and accompanied them to Warazup in the Mogaung (Möngkawng) Valley. The Chinese 22nd Division's task was to sweep south through the "inconceivably thick and trackless Taro Plain." By February 1944, through heavy fighting, the Taro Plain was freed of Japanese forces.[51]

Dr. Mamlok's years of marching through China with his *pugai* and cloth slippers had not prepared him well for the treacherous jungle warfare of Burma. During a bloody campaign in the Mogaung Valley, he broke his entrapped ankle under a tree root and needed an emergency air evacuation to a base hospital in India. Compared to the International Medical Relief Corps' days on the Changsha and Hengyang fronts, transportation was much improved. Dr. Mamlok was flown to India in a Douglas C-47 Skytrain: "Only the pilots were given oxygen and when I regained consciousness, it was an amazing contrast from the thick green vegetation of the jungle to the dusty plains."[52] He was able to return to combat in northern Burma in 1944.

By late January 1945, the X and Y forces linked up, reopened the Burma Road in February, and reached Lashio in mid–March thus ending the five-year long Japanese blockade of the Burma Road.[53] The following month, Drs. Mamlok and Freudmann were reunited and shipped out together to the 1st Chinese Convalescent Hospital (Sheng), near the Chinese border, by order of Colonel Waldemar F. Breidster.[54]

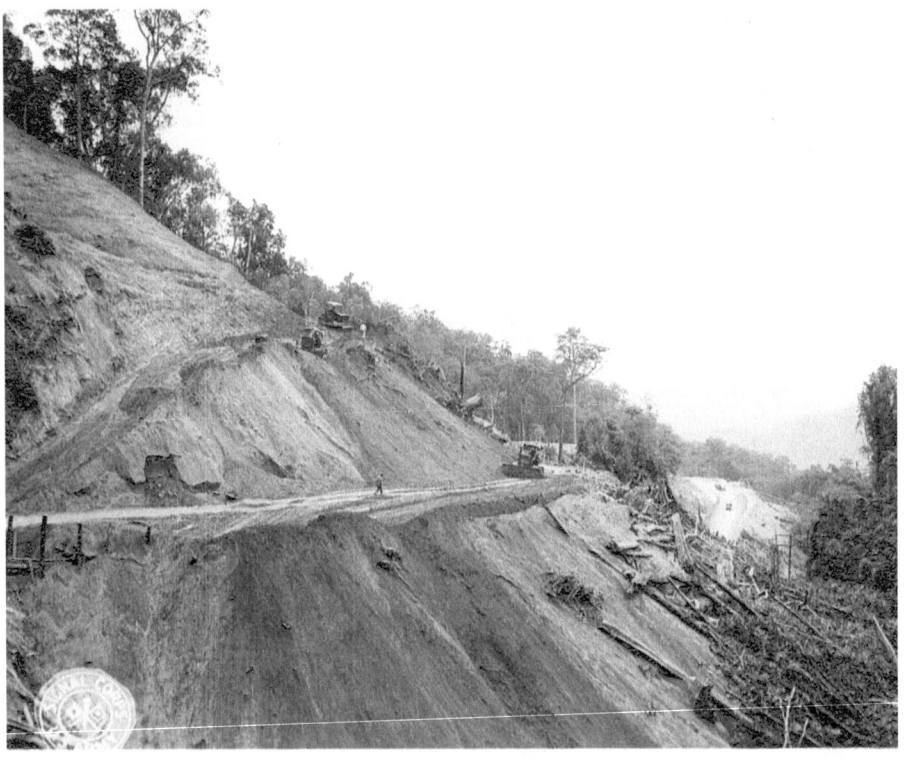

Along the Ledo Road, April 28, 1945. Bulldozers are shown making a new cut at the 96-mile mark on the Stilwell Road in Burma (National Archives: 111- SC-273003).

General George Marshall described the intense battles of the northern Burma offensive as the most difficult campaign of World War II.[55] Under these grueling circumstances, the American military command repeatedly recognized the International Medical Relief Corps' physicians for their heroic efforts. Colonel Harry Bullis of the Northern Combat Area Command wrote, for example, that:

> Mamlok performed his duties at a variety of assignments, including combat in a highly commendable manner. He has demonstrated diligence and ability in his work and is highly regarded by his associates for his professional knowledge. His character is excel-

lent and he is a thoroughly reliable and loyal individual. His entire service has been completely honorable.[56]

In awarding Dr. Mamlok the Emblem of Meritorious Civilian Service, General Stilwell thanked him for "helping to establish a high respect for the United States Medical Department among the Chinese units with which he served."[57]

General Stilwell's award of the Emblem of Meritorious Civilian Service to Dr. Erich Mamlok, October 25, 1944. United States Army Headquarters (CBI) (courtesy Robert Mamlok).

Colonel Bullis offered similar praise about Dr. Bedřich Kisch's diligence under combat and expressed high regard for "his professional knowledge, reliability and loyalty."[58] Colonel Rothwell Brown, commander of the Chinese Tank Unit, praised Dr. Franta Kriegel:

> We are fortunate to have Doc Kriegel. He doesn't know the meaning of fear. In the middle of the Walawbum fighting, he patched up 40 or 50 wounded … he speaks 8 languages, but not Chinese despite the fact the Chinese say he speaks Mandarin beautifully. Stockily built and barrel chested, Kriegel is heavily browned from extensive outdoor living. He does not mind the jungle hardships and his favorite topic of conversation is the courage of the Chinese soldiers. Chinese soldiers are grand and brave. They are patient and appreciative and when they come in wounded, they behave like men even though most of them are boys.[59]

Chinese Army in India Surgeon General Dr. Ping H. Siao asked Dr. Kriegel to help train the Chinese physicians in American hospitals, noting that "[s]uch training is of great importance as the Chinese medical officers

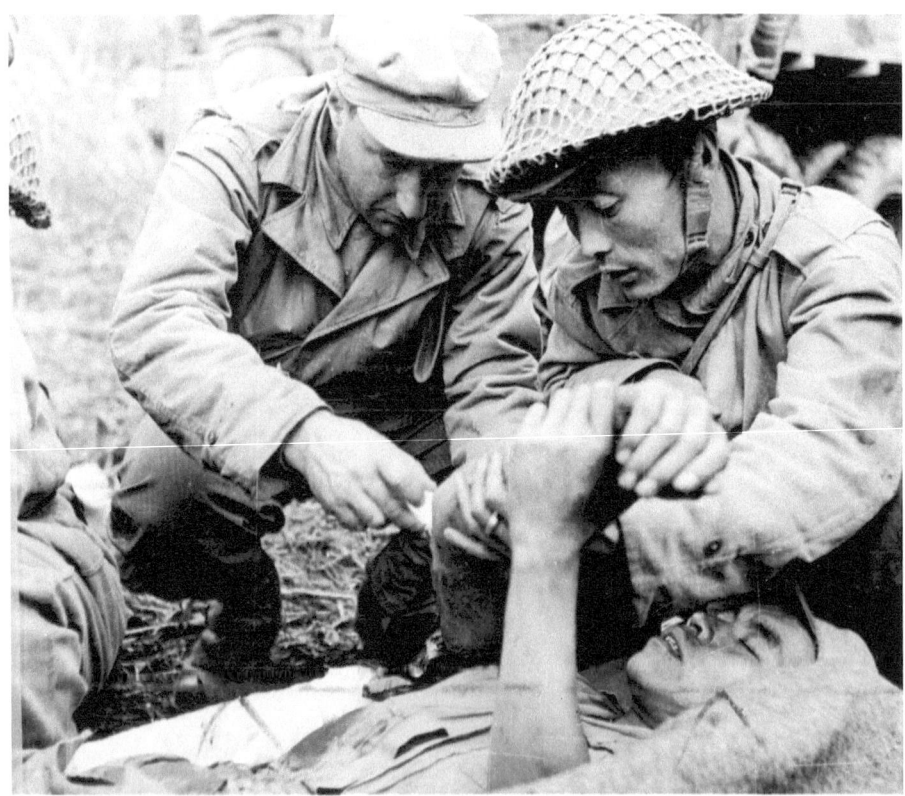

Wounded Chinese infantryman being treated by the Polish Chinese Contract Surgeon (Dr. Frantisek Kriegel), March 4, 1944 (National Archives: 208-FA-24347).

```
                    HEADQUARTERS                    WFB/wam
                CHINESE ARMY IN INDIA
                    A. P. O. 689


200.6 (6 Oct 45)                             6 October 1945.


SUBJECT:   Recommendation for Award of the Asiatic-Pacific
           Theater Ribbon.

TO     :   Commanding General
           United States Forces
           India-Burma Theater
           A.P.O. 885
```

    1. It is recommended that Dr. Erich R. Mamlok, a Contract Surgeon, be awarded the Asiatic-Pacific Theater Ribbon.

    2. Dr. Mamlok served with the 65th Regt., 22 Div., (Chinese) during the period December 1943 through May 44, joining them at Taro in the Hugong Valley and accompaning the organization to Warazup in the Mogaung Valley. After sharing the hardships and also the dangers involved by combat duty, he was evacuated because of a broken leg.

    3. Prior to issue of Circular 113, your headquarters, dated 9 Sep 44, this ribbon was authorized to Dr. Franz Kriegel and Dr. Victor Taubenfligel, and in view of this fact it appears only just that a similar award be made to Dr. Mamlok.

    4. In view of the imminent deactivation of this headquarters, it is requested that a reply covering your decision be sent by radio.

        FOR THE COMMANDING GENERAL:

                              W. F. BREIDSTER
                              Colonel, G.S.C.,
                              Chief of Staff.

Award of the Asiatic-Pacific theater ribbon to Drs. Wiktor Taubenfligel, Frantisek Kriegel, and Erich Mamlok, Chinese Army in India Headquarters, October 6, 1945 (courtesy Robert Mamlok).

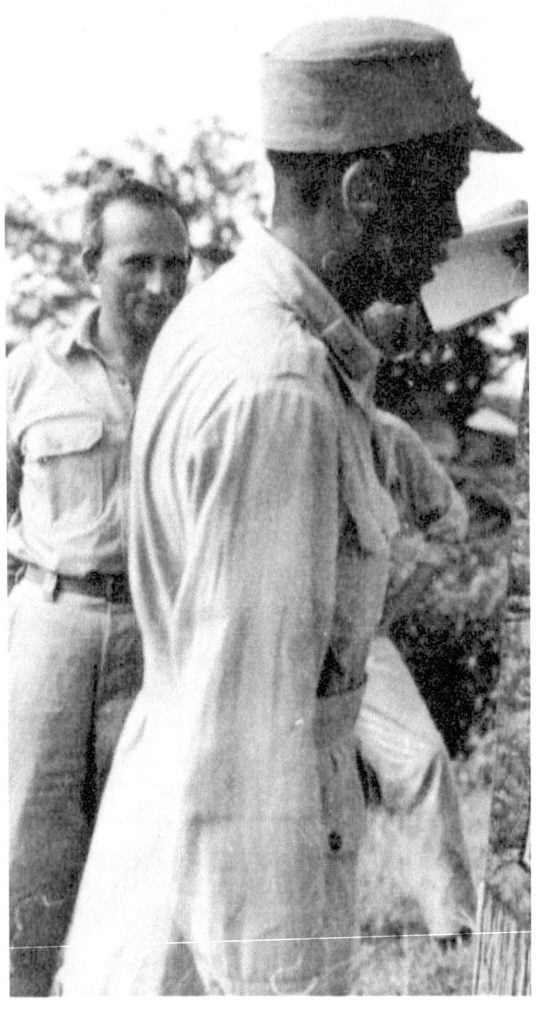

Dr. Stanislaw Flato at an award ceremony of the 65th and 40th portable surgical hospitals of the Chinese Expeditionary Force's 22nd division, August 13, 1944 (National Archives: 111-SC-262576).

are not at present able to main high standards of medical service."[60] It is not surprising that Dr. Kriegel also received "the Emblem of Meritorious Civilian Service of the United States of America for outstanding service during the period August 8, 1943–June 1, 1944."[61] In addition, the U.S. Forces awarded the Asiatic-Pacific theater ribbon to Drs. Taubenfligel, Mamlok, and Kriegel.[62] By the end of the war, almost all of the contract surgeons received letters of congratulations and awards for their work with the U.S. Army.[63]

10. The International Medical Relief Corps and the Chinese Expeditionary Force in China

Similar conjoint efforts among the Americans, British, and Chinese were to play out in the southern Chinese province of Yunnan. Most of the remaining International Medical Relief Corps' members in China now served there together with the Chinese Expeditionary Force-Y. In October 1943, a major assault to reopen the Burma Road[1] began in concert with the Chinese Expeditionary Force-Y (from the east), the Chinese Expeditionary Force-X (from the south), and the British XIV Army (from the west). The Chinese Expeditionary Force-Y maintained their headquarters in Kunming in Yunnan Province, at the Chinese terminus of the Burma Road. There, as in Camp Ramgarh, Chinese troops were trained and treated by the Allied command.[2]

In 1943, the Chinese Red Cross staffed twenty-four surgical teams with the Chinese Army in Yunnan Province. Three of these teams were foreign and staffed by Friends Ambulance Units and British Red Cross personnel. When Drs. Lin and General Loo Chih-teh (卢致德 Lu Zhide or C.T. Loo), the Surgeon General of China, asked the Friends Ambulance Units to equip these three mobile surgical teams, John Rich, the American Friends Service Committee representative, expressed his continuing concerns:

> This means much closer affiliation with the Chinese Red Cross. At this stage of the negotiation, the Friends of the Ambulance Units feels that it has no choice but to go into the scheme. Lin is now an advisor to the Chinese Red Cross and in a strong position. Unfortunately, he and McClure are old opponents, which may cause problems. Also, where are the doctors for the task? The present medical staff is barely sufficient and will have to be augmented by British Red Cross personnel.[3]

In addition, a wary Dr. McClure wrote in March 1943:

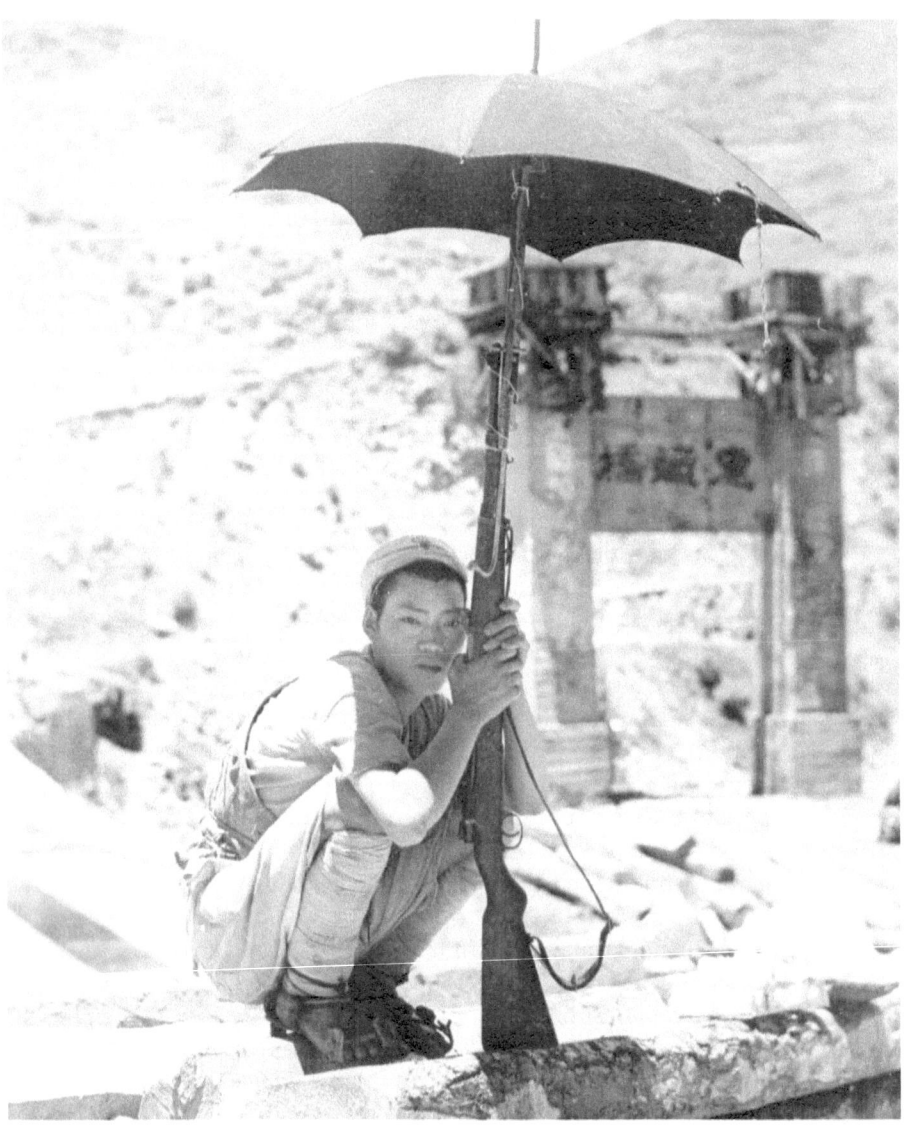

A Chinese Expeditionary Force soldier shading himself from the hot sun with an umbrella tied to his rifle near the Hwitung Bridge over the Salween River, September 16, 1944 (National Archives: 111-SC-193765).

The Chinese Red Cross has never made much of a job of working with foreigners within their organization. They have had 19 doctors from the Spanish war that have never averaged more than 6 months' work each year and often have been one year cooling their heels. We were not keen under these circumstances and knowing their record to put ourselves in the same position.[4]

Despite the Friends Ambulance Units' reservations, U.S. military, the International Relief Committee, the Chinese Red Cross, and the International Medical Relief Corps' physicians succeeded in becoming interdependent and linked together under the Allied command.[5] Dr. McClure noted that, in the Salween gorge near Paoshan, Yunnan, Friends Ambulance Units and the International Medical Relief Corps' physicians found a similar set of challenges: "malaria, typhus, scabies, beriberi, dysentery, trachoma and a woeful absence of any medical knowledge among the corpsmen."[6]

As the Allied command's presence grew in subtropical southern China, the International Medical Relief Corps' physicians became an important source of medical advice. After all, they were among the very few Western physicians who had several years of experience mastering the limited and complicated medical structure and politics of the Army Medical Corps and Chinese Red Cross. Dr. McClure wrote from Mengtze (Mengze) in southern Yunnan Province about his visit to Dr. Kranzdorf's Chinese Red Cross Unit:

> He is a Romanian and is married to a Romanian wife who is in the Chinese Red Cross too. He knows his skin work and has given us some interesting notes on methods that

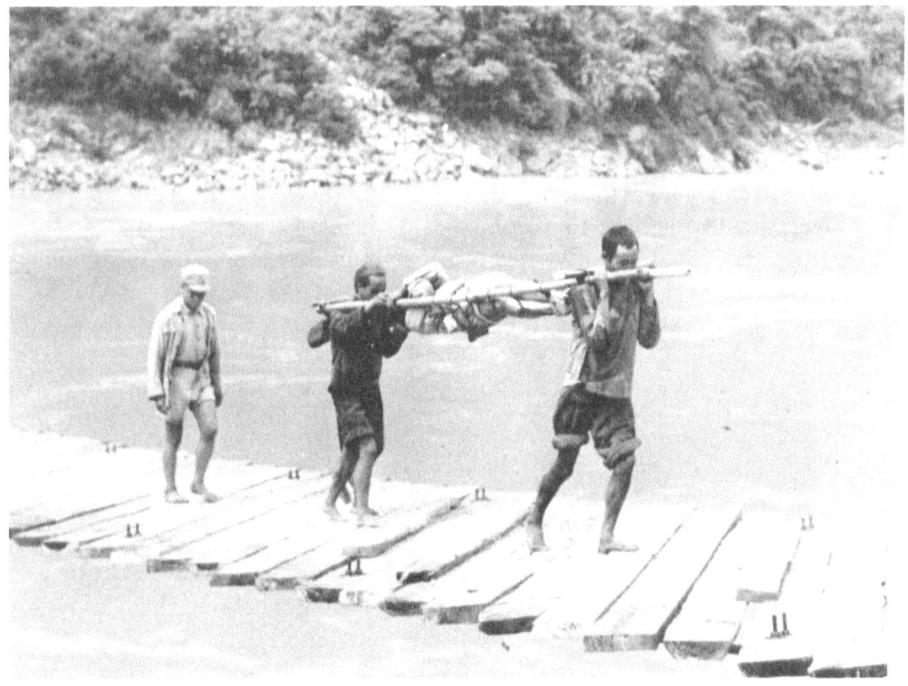

Transporting a wounded Chinese soldier over the Salween Gorge for treatment by the Chinese Expeditionary Y Force medical staff, September 8, 1944 (National Archives: 111-SC-193370).

he uses. I asked him a lot of questions on how he gets things worked and he certainly has more luck with local officials than any I have. When we know what local officials do for the others, it allows us to speak with authority when we ask for things for our teams.... Kransdorf being a skin and v.d. [venereal disease] specialist has wide experience in some of these things and has worked out methods that are very applicable for China. He has not 914 to treat syphilis, so he has worked out the following method with Mercury bichloride.[7] I think these things could be easily made up in the field and should be kept around to all of our teams as successful alternatives to 914 in syphilis. Given that there is almost no limit to the anti-syphilis work that our teams could take on.[8]

In June 1943, Dr. McClure again sought out the council of the International Medical Relief Corps' units attached to the Chinese Expeditionary Force-Y command in Yunnan Province: "We met Dr. Becker in Tsuyung [an airfield near Chuxiong City] and he gave us a lot of information on how to go about becoming settled into Chinese Army Hospitals. He was, on the whole, very encouraging.... At MiTu in Yunnan, we met Dr. Kent who was most cordial."[9]

Much as with the International Medical Relief Corps' physicians attached to the Chinese Expeditionary Force-X in Burma, the International Medical Relief Corps' members in Yunnan Province, such as Dr. Becker, welcomed the alliance of American, British, and Chinese forces. Dr. Becker referred to this time as the most prolific and medically satisfactory period of his activities in China. He described the Chinese division doctor as being grateful for his help and added that he supported him in every way and does not begrudge the fact that he himself is not medically trained.[10]

During 1943–45, the International Medical Relief Corps' members were spread out throughout the China-Burma-India theater. Dr. Fritz Jensen returned to Chongqing after spending two months in the southern Yunnan and Guangxi Provinces.[11] Mrs. Joan (Staniforth) Becker, who had previously worked in Tuyunguan as an administrative assistant to Dr. Lin, also moved to Chongqing:

> I took a job with the Press Attaché office of the British Embassy in Chungking [Chongqing]. As my little contribution to China, I am going to be helping Madame Sun Yat-sen with the Chinese Defence League.... I do not like living in Chungking [Chongqing] though as it is painfully evident that everything China gets from abroad is dissipated here in Chungking [Chongqing] while the rest of China suffers.[12]

Dr. Adele Cohn was in Tuyunguan complaining about the brutal Chinese winters and her increasingly untenable professional situation, while Dr. Wilhelm Mann spoke of the loneliness that resulted from the sudden departure in late 1942 of the ten International Medical Relief Corps' members to Ramgarh.[13] By April 1943, only a few of the International Medical Relief Corps' members were left in Tuyunguan. Dr. Schön was now representing the group.[14] When John Rich visited Tuyunguan in June 1943, he described his encounter with the International Medical Relief Corps' members who remained there:

> Dr. [Edith (Marens)] Kisch was a vivacious Jewish-German refugee, wife of one of the "Spanish doctors" [Dr. Bedřich Kisch] now in India ... [I also met] Dr. Kaneti, a young Bulgarian Jew trained in Sofia. He is an attractive man, uncomplaining and confident. His attractive little Chinese wife was also present. Later in the day, I was to meet three more of these men who served as doctors in the International Brigade in Spain.... They have had a long uphill fight to find a place. Now they seem to be better accepted.... We strolled to Lin's quarters and were joined by Lin's secretary, Mrs. [Joan Staniforth] Becker, an English girl married to one of the "Spanish doctors." Lin was hospitable and frank in his conversation. We chatted about the use of extra Friends of the Ambulance Units' men ... and they confirmed our agreement to send doctors and vocational training experts.... I then adjourned to the home of Dr. Cohn, an American woman doctor sent out by the American Bureau for Medical Aid to China to specialize in tuberculosis. She is a "shock-headed" person with a deep concern to help the soldiers and a fine scorn for the inadequate and inefficient attention given them. After two years, she is disillusioned and critical.[15]

Dr. Cohn described her sense of isolation, political turmoil, and homesickness from Tuyunguan in 1943:

> Dr. Lin left to Chungking [Chongqing] a few days ago to face another tribunal and we are hoping the business will be completed quickly. It seems that he has to waste so much perfectly good time clearing himself. I am truly sick of the whole business of politics and petty jealousy and I still feel that Lin is honest.... I want to come home as I do not have enough to do here.[16]

Dr. Cohn's conviction in speaking out against the corruption, inequality, and underutilization of the foreign physicians would come under increased scrutiny. The president of the American Bureau for Medical Aid to China, Helen Stevens, summarized Rich's subsequent recommendations to the American Bureau for Medical Aid to China's Board of Directors:

> If she [Dr. Cohn] comes back to this country [America] we will have "our hands full" ... she is extremely outspoken and has nothing but criticism of China ... she is a frustrated woman and ... it is going to be extremely difficult to keep her from talking in an unfortunate way when she comes back to this country ... in some ways it is important for Dr. Cohn to get out of China now but ... it would be equally unfortunate for her to come back to this country "bursting to talk." ... He suggested that American Bureau for Medical Aid to China see whether she could be sent to India.[17]

As the American Bureau for Medical Aid to China debated the affect that Dr. Cohn's criticism could have on their fundraising, she continued her work with the Chinese Red Cross/Medical Relief Corps in Tuyunguan and subsequently with the Chinese Red Cross in Chongqing. Dr. Lin, still a general advisor with the Chinese Red Cross, left Tuyunguan in April 1943, to serve with the Chinese Expeditionary Force-Y in Yunnan Province in south

China. Much as the American Bureau for Medical Aid to China had shared their concerns about Dr. Cohn, Dr. McClure of the Friends Ambulance Units continued to share his concerns about Dr. Lin with Dr. Van Slyke of the American Bureau for Medical Aid to China:

> My opinion has changed. He was a long time in getting back from India. When he returned, political opposition to him had grown so he felt he had to resign. Although this looks like a dirty trick of stabbing a man in the back while he was gone, there is more to the story.... His strengths are his courage, energy and technical medical knowledge. He lacks organization ability, in that he is number one and when he is away, nothing happens. He is subject to fixed ideas that he will not let go. At this time, he is more interested in running a medical college than relief work on the front. He is ruthless in getting funds earmarked for his goals.... Hence Lin's new position dealing with field work and having nothing to do with administration and money appears well chosen. We hope to be coming under his direction for this. But it would sabotage plans if Lin were to get hands on money directly.[18]

Around the same time (March 1943), the American Friends Service Committee leadership expressed a strikingly similar ambivalence toward Dr. McClure's leadership:

> McClure does not measure up as a Commandant but they [the Friends Ambulance Units men] admire his great qualities of enthusiasm and drive and abilities as a surgeon. They admit that they could have never started without him. Now he is a problem. He inclines to make commitments without clear-cut terms and tends to overstate the situation and the capacity of the Unit to fulfill agreements. His recklessness partly explains the checks set in by the Executive committee. Perhaps the time has come for him to assume charge of the medical program and surrender the title of Commandant. It is not a simple decision; he has wide connections in China and there is no assurance he would stick to the medical end of the work.... The idea is growing that Bob [McClure] should remain with the unit as a technical consultant. He serves an exceedingly valuable purpose in sparking the group into new lines of thought and his knowledge of China is profound although his judgment is too sanguine and he is often too willing to act on superficial knowledge of working relationships.[19]

Almost everyone admired the goals of humanitarian medical aid that passionate and strong-willed physicians like Drs. Lin, McClure, and Cohn had strived for in the past several years. However, their supporting organizations remained very worried that these doctors' independent and often outspoken character would hamper their fundraising, administrative chain of command, and political agenda. For better or worse, the International Medical Relief Corps' physicians and friends had the confidence to place their personal vision ahead of the vision of the institutes that they served. In retrospect, their vision was usually right.

In summer 1943, combat continued in Burma and on the south China border. Most International Medical Relief Corps' physicians who remained in China continued to serve on the southern front in Yunnan Province with

Dr. Lin and the Chinese Expeditionary Force-Y. Dr. Jungermann (41st Unit leader), Dr. Becker (21st Unit leader), and Dr. Kent (22nd Unit leader) were stationed in Sinagyun with the Chinese 2nd Army. Dr. Kamieniecki (51st Unit leader) was stationed in Baoshan with the 71st Arm. Dr. Kaneti (12th Unit leader) was in Venshan with the 5th Army, and Dr. Kranzdorf (31st Unit leader) was in Mungtzu with the 1st Army Group.[20] Dr. Becker noted that the "team is reinforced by a Polish nurse [Mania Kamieniecka], the wife of a doctor, who took over the modest laboratory and an Austrian medical student [Edith (Marens) Kisch], both former members of the medical corps of the International Brigades."[21]

Gisela Kranzdorf was probably also assigned to help her husband in Unit 31 in Mungtzu in Yunnan province in 1943. She would die there at the age of thirty-nine years of typhoid fever during an outbreak in 1944.[22] Gisela Kranzdorf was buried on March 13, 1944, in the cemetery of Jianshui, Yunnan Province.[23] Her broken-hearted husband, Iacob, survived his bout of typhoid fever and continued to work with the Chinese Red Cross in Yunnan under difficult emotional and material conditions. Dr. McClure visited the widowed Dr. Kranzdorf four months later:

> Dr. Kranzdorf's Chinese Red Cross station was in an old delousing station. The team lives with pigs in their building and lives very much like the pigs. They claim that they are not getting pay nor enough supplies. Kranzdorf is doing more and more on less and less. He sees more than 100 cases per day in the sloppiest of styles. He gives out lots of malaria drugs and never uses the microscope. He says he has no time and I think he is right.... Both he and Becker dress all surgical cases with reclaimed dressings for the U.S. hospital uses its dressings only once.[24]

The medical facilities had also not improved very much back at the Chinese Red Cross' headquarters. In November 1943, Dr. Cohn wrote to Helen Stevens at the American Bureau for Medical Aid to China that she would be going to Chongqing to take over the job of the tuberculosis sanatorium in Koloshan, run by the Methodist Union Mission. She noted that Arthur Kohlberg had written that this would end her American Bureau for Medical Aid to China mission. In severing her ties with the American Bureau for Medical Aid to China, Dr. Cohn wrote that "I do not feel that American Bureau for Medical Aid to China's investments have given adequate returns." Her assessment of the direction of the Chinese Red Cross and the Emergency Medical Service Training School without Dr. Lin's leadership were similarly unflattering:

> It is a pity that Lin has been marginalized.... Despite his grandiose, always expensive ideas, he has accomplished much and I believe he can do more for China than any other man. But the foreign press and American Bureau for Medical Aid to China in particular have spoiled Lin and he is a bit of a megalomaniac. I believe ... the only real effort being made at the Emergency Medical Service Training School is gardening, at

least three department heads putting more thought and energy into what vegetables they should plant than in their wards or departments.[25]

Dr. Cohn was not the only one who had a negative impression of the Emergency Medical Service Training School. Dr. Walter Lurje, a less well-known German born head of the Chinese Red Cross/Medical Relief Corps' 73rd unit shared Dr. Cohn's views. He wrote a scathing report to Dr. Jung (荣独山 Rong Dushan) about the Emergency Medical Service Training School graduates that he encountered:

> For your fine boys, this food is not good enough ... and now they demand to have a servant! To be lazy, impertinent and conceited, that is all they learn in Kweiyang [Guiyang]. Really, if the Generalissimo would give a prize for the best irrational work in whole China—you would merit it for your fine training school.[26]

With a diminished role for the Chinese Red Cross/Medical Relief Corps in southwest China in the spring of 1944, several International Medical Relief Corps' members sought alternate paths to serve the Chinese population. Dr. Cohn wrote in her diary that Dr. Schön also worked two days a week at the Guiyang Prison. Dr. Bob McClure described his visit to Schön's prison infirmary in his correspondence from March 28, 1944:

> I was invited by Dr. Schoen [Somogyi] one morning to join his rounds. The conditions vary considerably based on the individual patient. There is a tremendous contrast between the small hovels about the size of a Kutsing hostel bedroom housing 12–13 men with no furniture and the clean whitewashed well furnished rooms of the wealthy merchants and high ranking army officers.... The conditions of the ordinary soldier prisoners were terrible as they have no local friends to take any interest in them. Should any of their scanty clothing get worn out or lost, they just have to stay in bed in the cold weather; a number had no shirts and others no trousers. When they work outside the prisons, they have iron bands tied around their necks and two or three prisoners are connected by light chains. At the moment, there are 700 prisoners, including 100 women and some of them have their children with them. The chief diseases are malaria, relapsing fever, dysentery, and typhus. The death rate is one to two a day. It is no use continuing on the description of these prison conditions for Dickens did it most effectively long ago.[27]

When Michael Harris of the Friends Ambulance Units met with Dr. Mann at the Chemical Laboratory of the Emergency Medical Service Training School in Tuyunguan, Dr. Mann was also looking for other professional opportunities:

> Herr Mann is extremely keen to help us and gave me useful data on how to obtain absolute alcohol from commercial alcohol etc. ... He is now experimenting and working out some interesting data on a sample of lubricating oil from Friends of the Ambulance Units' stocks. When training in Germany, Herr Mann worked for some time in the labs of a large oil firm, and so is familiar with the properties of lubricating oils.[28]

The International Medical Relief Corps' physicians were now entering their sixth year in China. They longed to learn of the fate of their war-torn homelands and families that most had heard little, or more ominously, nothing from since they had left for China. They fought the feelings of homesickness, loneliness, and isolation with their efforts to remain engaged with their medical mission. At the same time, they all hoped for a quick conclusion to the war in Asia.

However, the end of the war was not in sight. On April 17, 1944, the Japanese began Operation Ichigo, their largest and last major offensive in China. Japan launched this desperate military campaign, with more than half a million men, because of its dwindling supply of raw materials brought on by the progressive destruction of the Japanese merchant fleet. Japan hoped it could link troops and supplies from China and Southeast Asia to Korea and Japan and remove the threat of allied airbases in China.

As the Imperial Japanese Army pushed rapidly into central China, the Generalissimo and General Stilwell continued to debate the wisdom of trying to remove the Japanese from Burma rather than maintaining resistance against a Japanese advance that was now threatening Guiyang and even the wartime capital of Chongqing. As the Chinese armies in central China were routed, Generalissimo Chiang Kai-shek's worries were mounting: "He did not know from whom next to expect bad news—his American allies, his Japanese enemies, his temporary warlord allies, his adversaries in the Guomindang Nationalist Party, the Chinese communists or the Soviets."[29]

Meanwhile, by the summer of 1944, things were going better for the Allies in Europe and for Dr. Cohn in Guiyang. On June 6, the Allies landed on the beaches of Normandy, and Dr. Cohn landed a new medical assignment. She had initially, and dejectedly, booked passage for a return to America, but then she had a remarkable turn of fortune. A Chinese physician inquired about some medical books she had put up for sale. He was most sympathetic to her plight and thought that, before she left China for good, she might wish to talk to Dr. H.H. Kung (孔祥熙 Kung Hsiang-hsi or Kong Xiangxi), the man for whom he served as personal physician.

Dr. Kung was, after all, the Minister of Finance and Governor of the Central Bank of China at that time, in addition to being a seventy-fifth-generation descendant of Confucius and married to Soong Ai-ling, the eldest of the three Soong sisters. He convinced Dr. Cohn to stay in Chongqing and financed a Chinese Red Cross-affiliated outpatient tuberculosis clinic that she directed. Bolstered by the close emotional support of her British companion, Philip Wright, whom she had married on May 30, and by Kung's financial support, Dr. (Cohn) Wright entered the medically most productive phase of her stay in China.[30]

In May 1944, Dr. Lin's role also improved as he took a position with the

American Bureau for Medical Aid to China while he worked in an advisory role with the Chinese Red Cross. He continued to tell the American Bureau for Medical Aid to China that China's greatest medical need was the development of skilled medical personnel, trained in the swiftest time possible. The shortage of physicians remained critical, especially in the Chinese Communist Party-controlled regions. In Yan´an, the 120th Bethune International Peace Hospital of the Eighth Route Army had only nine physicians in September 1944. Five of these had originally come from the Indian Medical Unit in China, which ran their surgical division.[31] The German physician, Dr. Hans Müller, noted that only he and one Japanese doctor had foreign training in a hospital that served the Chinese Communist Party forces:

> Training in the medical school is very elementary as there are practically no qualified teachers. The people who do surgery on the front have learned by long practice and have no theory.... We have no X rays, or microscopes, but much malaria with no quinine.... Morphine is easy to get because the Japanese distribute ampules far and wide among the people to make addicts of them. Sulfa drugs cannot be bought and no drugs reached us from 1939 until the present.[32]

Modern medical manpower was just as scarce in the Chinese Communist Party's New Fourth Army. Its Surgeon General, C.C. Sheng, later estimated that they had fewer than 60 qualified physicians serving more than 90 million people.[33]

In October 1944, the persistent displeasure of the Guomindang Nationalist Party leadership resulted in General Stilwell's recall.[34] Brooks Atkinson, a journalist with the *New York Times*, shared the same concerns of maltreatment and corruption that the International Medical Relief Corps' physicians had voiced for several years.

> China's war against Japan has been handicapped by internal discord between the Chungking [Chongqing] government of Chiang Kai-shek and the so called Chinese communists, and between Chiang Kai-shek and some of his generals, by corruption, in which Chiang has no personal share but which he is unable to prevent; and by Chiang's final refusal to entrust General Stilwell with full command.... The United States lost a battle, and the Chinese may have lost one too when Stilwell was recalled.... Intrigue, ambition, jealousy and dishonesty have been in high places, but the underfed, ill-armed often badly led Chinese soldier has marched suffered and died for his country with a heroism unsurpassed in any nation's history.... No matter what happens, we cannot fail in our friendship for the Chinese people.[35]

Negative portrayals of the conditions in Guomindang Nationalist Party-controlled China and the circumstances surrounding General Stilwell's dismissal were not limited to the *New York Times*. Many other members of the Western press wrote critical appraisals of China that were far removed from the special paternal relationship that Henry Luce and the United China Relief had envisioned.[36] In China, Mme. Sun Yat-sen wrote that "Stilwell has done more to help the Chinese people than any individual I know since the war. You can imagine how depressed I am at his departure."[37]

Stilwell also was remembered as a true friend of the International Medical Relief Corps. Dr. Charles Coutelle recalled that "My father never made a secret of his time with Stilwell of whom he always spoke with high regards. He also regarded this as the most effective time in the Far East."[38] Dr. Mamlok also looked back on his medical service to the Chinese in Burma and India as the most meaningful period of his six years in Asia.[39]

Within weeks of Stilwell's dismissal, a war-weary world continued to face the reality of large-scale Japanese and German counter-offensives in 1944. The final major Japanese offensive in central China, Operation Ichigo, resulted in the capture of Changsha and Guilin as Japanese forces again pushed toward the west. Later that year, in what would turn out to be the final major German offensive, the Battle of the Bulge, would play out in the Ardennes.

General Wedemeyer reported from China that by November 1944, the Japanese had reached to within sixty-five miles of Guiyang.[40] In December, the evacuation of the Chinese Red Cross/Medical Relief Corps from Guiyang was in place, ahead of the anticipated Japanese onslaught. However, as Christmas approached, both the Chinese Red Cross/Medical Relief Corps' evacuation and the Japanese assault bogged down in the coldest weather in seven years of war.[41] Much like the German Operation Barbarossa into the Soviet Union three years earlier, the bitter Chinese winter helped to stop the Japanese advance.[42] An enduring lesson of World War II is that neither the Germans nor the Japanese were ready or able to wage wars of attrition on large, cold landmasses.

While the severe winter helped to stop the Japanese advance in 1944, it had previously made life miserable for Dr. Cohn. "The past few days we have had below zero weather," she wrote.

> I awaken each morning to barn like cold. My washcloth has been frozen solid and even the oil in my lamp has frozen one evening! Thank heaven that I have enough warm clothing and that I am not ashamed that I shed little of my waking clothes when I go to bed; everyone does the same.[43]

Dr. (Cohn) Wright was not the only one affected by the severe cold. Dr. Mann wrote from Tuyunguan that it

> is snowing outside and it is terribly cold in my room. The test tubes contain ice in my lab. I can turn them over and nothing flows. Every morning it takes great effort to lift my blanket and crawl out of my beloved bed. I have some frostbite on my hand for the first time in my life. How I envy your warm large fireplace. I have just a few charcoal pieces under my desk so that my fingers do not become too stiff.[44]

Dr. (Cohn) Wright created a busy, wartime program for TB management by establishing an outpatient ambulatory pneumothorax induction clinic.[45]

She noted that until January 1, 1945, she worked alone in the clinic; then, a fellow International Medical Relief Corps' physician whom she had met in Tuyunguan came to help: "Now that I have Dr. Schon [Schön] to help with pneumothorax induction, I accept more cases than have been started in other places."[46] By April 1945, she noted how increasingly busy she was, but she did not mind being exhausted. With Dr. Wright's support, Dr. Schön's help in the clinic, and the presence of Allied forces in Chongqing, she felt that her efforts at the clinic were going well and proudly noted that the Chinese Red Cross' TB clinic was the only one of its kind in China. Dr. Wright had seen as many cases in Chongqing as in an entire year in Guiyang: 3,100 patients in the first

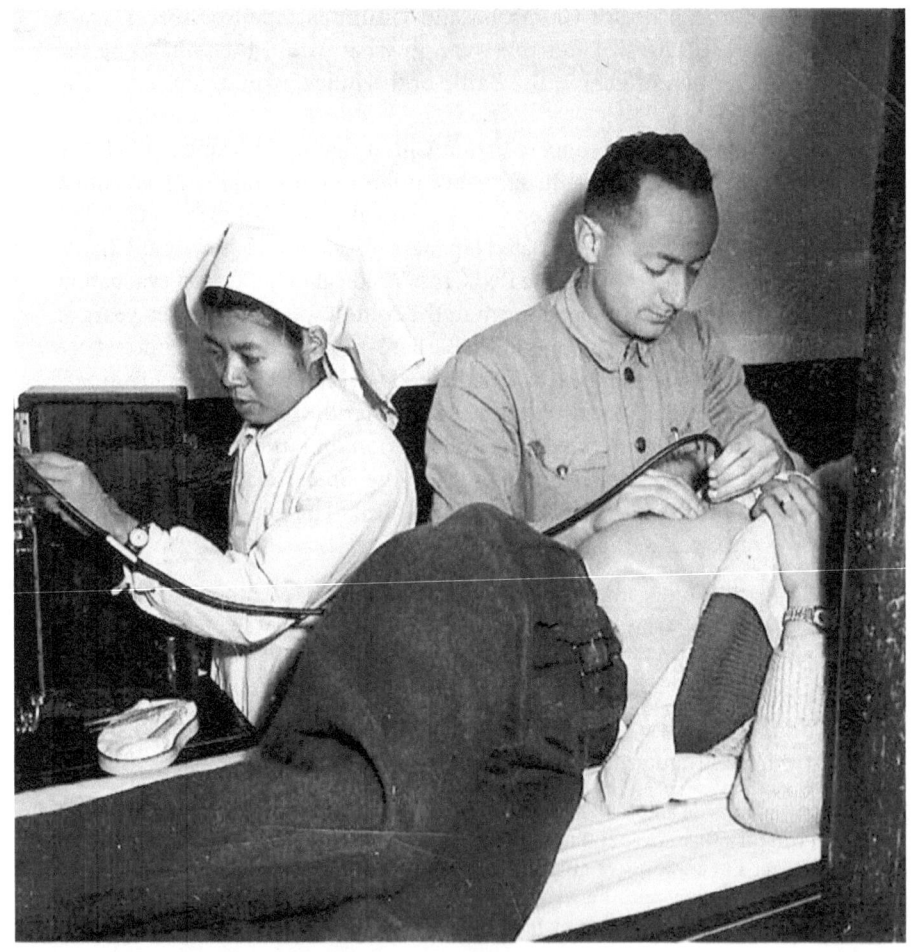

Dr. Georg Schön inducing a pneumothorax in Dr. Adele Cohn's outpatient TB clinic in Chongqing, China, 1945 (courtesy Max Wright).

four and a half months. She achieved her goal of improving tuberculosis management in wartime China.⁴⁷

As spring appeared, the Japanese advance stalled and internationalism moved forward on several fronts. On April 25, 1945, representatives from forty-six nations met in San Francisco to sign the charter of a new organization, the United Nations. That same day, Dr. Fritz Jensen married Wang Wu-An in Zhou Enlai's house. Professor Joseph Needham (李约瑟 Li Yue se), the Director of the Sino-British cooperative in Chongqing, noted in his wedding speech that this meeting of East and West in Chongqing was a good sign for the world.⁴⁸ Another good sign appeared two weeks later. On Friday, May 8, victory in Europe (VE day) was declared. Joan (Staniforth) Becker wrote to her mother:

> You must all be feeling wonderful today—VE day! We are having no celebrations here and most people are not especially moved by it. The Americans out here will not do any real celebrations until the Pacific War is finished and the Chinese are not really very much interested. For us of course it holds out more hope of moving on out of here.⁴⁹

In China, General Wiedemeyer's Alpha Plan continued to revamp the Chinese training and combat-command-supporting services that opposed the Japanese advance in central China. During this reorganization, Dr. Lin became Surgeon General of the Chinese Army Medical Administration and was appointed as the chair of the Commission on Medical Education. In addition, the American Bureau for Medical Aid to China supported him with $100,000 from the National War Fund through the United China Relief.⁵⁰

By June 1945, the Japanese were in general retreat in central China and the end of the Sino-Japanese war was in sight. Some of Dr. Lin's tasks in June 1945 included beginning to bid farewell, from his new office in Chongqing, to some of the International Medical Relief Corps' members. "Dr. Adele Cohn Wright," he wrote to American Bureau for Medical Aid to China, had

> just left China for India en route to England when your letter came. I was therefore not able to contact her about her passage home, or the funds in Hong Kong. She will be going on to the states after a few months in England when you can settle all accounts with her personally.⁵¹

Dr. (Cohn) Wright, the only American physician sent to wartime China by the American Bureau for Medical Aid to China, was on her way home. At the same time, Dr. Lin acknowledged the departure of Joan (Staniforth) Becker from the Chinese Red Cross: "[She] stayed half a month and then joined her husband [Dr. Rolf Becker], who was appointed to the motor school, she herself being given a secretarial post by the U.S. Army in the school."⁵² It would be several years before the couple would return to Europe.

Back in Burma and India, many International Medical Relief Corps' physicians also were starting to think about how they might return to their newly liberated homelands. The China Medical Aid Committee of London began to plan their repatriation. But, it was more than just a matter of shipping them home. Money was needed to fund their return trips. On April 6, 1945, Dr. Mary Gilchrist wrote to the Chinese Embassy:

> The China Medical Aid Committee was responsible for sending out nine doctors to China. In addition 10 doctors were sponsored by the Norwegian committee.[53] The Foreign Auxiliary had saved a portion of their salary each month for their return travel. After 1941 no news was received from the Foreign Auxiliary on the money until 1943. Dr. Lin then asked the British Embassy in Chungking [Chongqing] for help. The British Embassy referred this to the Foreign Office that then asked us to help. The Foreign Office then told us to tell Dr. Lin that he should approach the U.S. authorities for help and try to find Hilda Selwyn Clarke to authorize the money withdrawal.[54]

The British, United States, Chinese, and Indian governments had the complex task of repatriating the International Medical Relief Corps' physicians who were in Burma. On June 8, 1945, the U.S. Foreign Service wrote to the United Kingdom's Foreign Service requesting repatriation of eight of the contract surgeons associated with the China Medical Aid Committee of London: Drs. Kriegel, Taubenfligel, Iancu, Baer, Kisch, Coutelle, Freudmann, and Volokhine.

> The U.S. Consulate is in contact with the French Consulate as Kriegel, Taubenfligel, Baer and Iancu wish to travel there. They [the French] have not replied. Our group believes they should be first returned to the UK, to await transportation to their respective homelands when the opportunity offers.[55]

On July 24, 1945, the Government of India asked the Foreign Office of the United Kingdom if "HM [Her Majesty's] government has any objection to having the International Medical Relief Corps' physicians return to GB?"[56] The United Kingdom's Foreign Office replied, "I don't think that the passport department of the UK will need to come into play. The government of India will issue visas."

On August 8, 1945, the External Affairs Office of the Government of India wrote back to the Foreign Office of the United Kingdom: "They are also in receipt from US request of June 8, 1945, of repatriating these physicians to GB. They are asking GB if they have any objection to granting them a visa."[57] With the continued support of the China Medical Aid Committee of London, these physicians had cleared the visa and immigration hurdles and would soon be on their way.

Repatriation was less certain for Dr. Mamlok, the one International Medical Relief Corps' liaison physician with the Chinese Army in India not originally sent to China by the China Medical Aid Committees. He was assisted separately by the United States and Chinese governments. In June 1945, Dr.

中 華 民 國 紅 十 字 會 總 會 救 護 總 隊 部

CHINESE RED CROSS MEDICAL RELIEF CORPS

(National Red Cross Society of China)

Telephone:
Telegraphic "CHINCROSS"
Address: or
"0577"
Mail Address, Kweiyang
Letter Box 41

Kweiyang, 15, June, 1945.

To whom it may concern:

This is to certify that Dr. Erich Mamlock, a German doctor, join our medical work of the Medical Relief Corps of the Chinese Red Cross from Oct. 1939 to June 1945 and now we approve his return to his native country.

Yours truly

L. C. Tang

Vice Director of M.R.C.

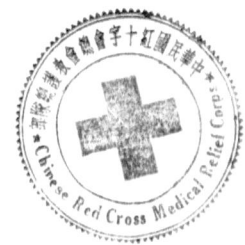

Release of the IMRC physician, Dr. Erich Mamlok from his service to the Chinese Red Cross Medical Relief Corps from October 1939 to June 1945, Guiyang, China, June 15, 1945 (courtesy Robert Mamlok).

L. Tang, the vice president of the Chinese Red Cross/Medical Relief Corps, approved Dr. Mamlok's return to Germany after six years of medical service with the Chinese Red Cross. Later that month, General H.L. Boatner enabled Dr. Mamlok to return home. He wrote:

> Dr. Mamlok is an employee of the U.S. government. He is negotiating with us to discontinue his present employment with us and to return to Germany via India. In view of his outstanding and faithful service to the United States Government, it is requested that all agencies of that government extend to him appropriate facilities and courtesies.[58]

The International Medical Relief Corps' physicians who remained in China dealt with a different set of circumstances. On the one hand, domestic travel for the International Medical Relief Corps' members still left in China became less restrictive and perilous. For example, in July 1945, Dr. Jensen accepted a medical field officer position with United Nations Relief and

Rehabilitation Administration and relocated with his bride of three months to the coastal province of Kiangsu [Jiangsu], north of Shanghai.[59]

On the other hand, the mechanism for repatriation and international travel remained unclear. On August 6, 1945, an American B-29 bomber, the *Enola Gay*, dropped a 9,700-pound bomb nicknamed "Little Boy" on Hiroshima, immediately killing more than 70,000 people. Three days later, a second atomic bomb, "Fat Man," fell on Nagasaki, and resulted in more than 40,000 deaths. As the Pacific war ended, the International Medical Relief Corps' physicians tried, with difficulty, to comprehend what it meant that the atomic age was upon them.

After several years in remote settings, the International Medical Relief Corps' members were far removed from advancements in nuclear physics. Dr. Mamlok asked what "an abomic bomb" was.

With the surrender of Japan on September 2, 1945, some International Medical Relief Corps' members wanted to return to Europe and North America as soon as possible. Others wished to stay in China, and some were conflicted about returning to their homelands. Dr. Mamlok, for example, was still wavering on what to do. He had applied to United Nations Relief and Rehabilitation Administration (which coveted Chinese-speaking Western physicians) for a position as a field medical officer. His application to United Nations Relief and Rehabilitation Administration was returned with the hard-to-answer questions about what he was doing in China and why he had no discernible citizenship in any nation at that time.[60] Dr. (Cohn) Wright also had mixed feelings about her future. "I dread leaving this life which is beautiful and simple (when not overpowering with natural catastrophes)," she wrote, "and I hate to think of leaving all my patients."[61]

The International Medical Relief Corps' physicians who had served with the Chinese Expeditionary Force-X in India and Burma would be the first of the repatriated European doctors. Dr. Coutelle wrote of flying with Drs. Baer, Freudmann, Iancu, Kriegel, Mamlok, and Taubenfligel on a U.S. military transport plane from Calcutta to Frankfurt in October 1945:

> From Calcutta the flight went to Ankara. Then the pilots flew—without restriction by any regulation—to Cairo, made a few turns over the pyramids and the Sphinx, which looked from above, quite different from the usual pictures, like an elongated beast—ready to jump. We flew over the Aegean Sea—an enchanting picture with its many islands—flew around the Acropolis and landed at night in Rome. This night is unforgettable to me. Our Julio [Dr. Wictor Taubenfligel], who had studied here-got us the necessary taxis with U.S. dollars and took us to all the sights—the Coliseum, Roman Forum—they were illuminated by moonlight, giving us a hint of the former grandeur of the city. The next day we landed in Frankfurt—reunion with Germany after 13 years.[62]

The remainder of the contract surgeons slowly made their way back to their native lands. On September 5, 1945, Dr. Kisch was in Trieste after having

VIA AIR MAIL   24 September 1945

Erich Mamlok Esq
CCC, A.P.O. 62F
c/o Post Master
N.Y. City.

Dear Sir:

You are under consideration for the position of Field Medical Officer with the UNRRA China Office.

However, our files are incomplete in that we do not have a personal history statement from you. Therefore, a definite decision cannot be made and we cannot offer you a specific assignment until our records are complete.

Please complete the attached form and mail to this office at the earliest possible moment in order that action may be expedited. In addition to the foregoing, it will be necessary that we have a statement from you stating the reasons as to why you do not have citizenship in any nation. Furthermore, we would like to know the particulars in regard to your being in China and we will need a statement as to whether or not you have received salary payments in foreign exchange.

Your earliest attention to these matters will aid us greatly in making a speedy decision in your case.

                                Yours faithfully,

                                Paul M. Elza
                                Acting Personnel Officer.

Why do you not have citizenship in any nation? UNRRA question to Dr. Erich Mamlok on his job application, September 24, 1945 (courtesy Robert Mamlok).

flown on a U.S. air transport command flight from Calcutta.[63] He received a visa to Great Britain and practiced medicine briefly in England before returning to Prague. In November 1945, Drs. Taubenfligel and Kriegel traveled together by car to Warsaw.[64] Dr. Iancu took a train to Vienna and received permission from Soviet troops to return to Bucharest.[65] He returned home after nine years on the front.

Dr. Arnold Theo "Teddy" Wantoch was not so fortunate. He died on December 12, 1945, in the lung station of the Canadian mission hospital in Chongqing, of pulmonary tuberculosis, at thirty-three years of age.[66] Much like Drs. Bethune, Kotnis, and Courtney, and Gisela Kranzdorf, the poor nutrition, limited medical care, and harsh conditions of wartime China undoubtedly contributed to his demise. A few weeks prior to his death, the British embassy, acting on his behalf, asked the British Foreign Office to request that the United Aid to China relief organization release the £300 that Wantoch had accrued to his brother in London.[67] In November 1946, Wantoch's wife, Susanne, returned by herself to Austria via England on the steamship *Largs Bay*.[68]

Most of the International Medical Relief Corps' members who remained in China with their spouses, including Drs. Becker, Jensen, Jungermann, Kamieniecki, Kent, Kranzdorf, and Schön, joined the United Nations Relief and Rehabilitation Administration and stayed in China until 1947. Although Dr. Rolf and Joan Becker had hoped to travel to England from India in 1945, this was not to be. Dr. Rolf Becker remained in China and described his travels in the Chinese Communist Party-controlled areas immediately after the war:

> The postwar presents us with a new situation. The Japanese have been defeated, but in the country there is uproar, big decisions had to be made. The majority of the Chinese people are convinced that the state that existed under the Kuomintang regime cannot persist. I saw for the first time the big cities of the East, Shanghai and later the old Beijing. Located just outside of Beijing and other major cities, the people are preparing to overthrow the old regime. Senior officers of the National Army assure me that they would not fight in a civil war. The people are hungry. From abroad shipments of food arrived. Our mission is to ensure that at least part of these relief supplies arrived in the liberated areas managed by the communists. In the summer of 1946, it is possible to send a transport ship with food and medical supplies from Shanghai to Chefoo or Jentai, the administrative seat of the liberated territory of Shantung [Shandong] peninsula. I accompanied the ship and stayed on as a medical assistant.[69]

Dr. Kent also served with United Nations Relief and Rehabilitation Administration and traveled from central China to Inner Mongolia [Neimenggu] as a medical field officer and regional medical director. He spoke of his future wife, Edith (Marens) Marcus as the only medical personnel working for the Chinese National Relief and Rehabilitation Agency in 1946.[70]

Dr. Jungermann served as a regional medical officer for United Nations Relief and Rehabilitation Administration in Mukden, Manchuria, and later in January of 1948, resigned from United Nations Relief and Rehabilitation Administration in Shanghai.[71] Drs. Schön, Kamieniecki, and Kranzdorf joined the United Nations Relief and Rehabilitation Administration in Kunming in 1945. Dr. Schön served with United Nations Relief and Rehabilitation Administration in the Catholic Mission in Hunan and later in Tsingtao in Anhwei [Anhui] province until 1947.[72]

Dr. Kamieniecki continued to advocate for better medical care for the much-underserved orphans and refugee centers he served in Hengyang up to 1947.[73] Dr. Mann worked with the Chinese Academy of Sciences and was the last of the International Medical Relief Corps' members to leave China, in 1964. However, the China Medical Aid Committee of London had already concluded its support of the Spanish doctors in March 1946:

> With the end of the war with Japan, the problem of repatriation arose for that was still the moral responsibility of the committee. The visas and passports presented endless obstacles.... Fortunately, seven had been adopted by the American-Chinese Army in Burma, and when hostilities ceased, the Americans shipped them to Europe and they reached their native lands. The committee went on to note that one had found employment for himself and that the other eleven had been enrolled in United Nations Relief and Rehabilitation Administration.[74]

As the International Medical Relief Corps' members' wartime work in the China-Burma-India arena ended, they reflected on the unpredictability of their survival, accomplishments, and future options. In a span of more than six years, much had indeed changed. Many in the International Medical Relief Corps would finally be able to shed their refugee and enemy alien status. Although their homelands lay battered by the fallacy of fascism, the hope of reuniting with friends and family was drawing nearer. Would they be welcomed back as heroes among thousands of raised fists in the fight against fascism?

11. The International Medical Relief Corps' Epilogue: 1945-2012

Many physicians who returned to their native lands would find that the persecution and intolerance that drove them into exile many years earlier remained. For these doctors, their journey had not yet ended, and they would continue their search for a welcome place to live. By the time ten descendant families of the International Medical Relief Corps' physicians gathered in China for a 2015 anniversary, 75 percent no longer resided in the land of their International Medical Relief Corps' ancestor's birth.

Despite the best of intentions, the Polish International Medical Relief Corps members' political, religious, and military background continued to place them at risk in their native land. For example, the rise of anti-Semitism in Poland in 1952 culminated in Dr. Wolf Jungermann's eighteen-month imprisonment in the Warsaw Political Prison Number 1. He was falsely accused of being an enemy of the state and spy. When he was released, he was told it was a misunderstanding and he was given back his old job and $100 in compensation.[1] Dr. Wolf Jungermann's American-born wife, Kendell (Knutson) Jungermann, and their daughters, Karin and Michele, emigrated from Poland to the United States in November 1956. Although Dr. Jungermann had long since given up his past communist ideology, he could not obtain a visa to the United States, and immigrated in 1960 to Israel, where he would work in Haifa as a port health officer.[2] He reunited with his family in Oklahoma in August 1966. Dr. Jungermann, now known as Dr. Jungery, continued to practice medicine in the United States until the age of seventy and died at the age of 80 in Oklahoma City in 1989.[3] His daughter Dr. Michele Jungery became a parasitologist and worked at the Department of Tropical Health, at Harvard School of Public Health. She continued to make significant contributions to our understanding of the scourge of malaria that her father and his colleagues fought against in wartime China.[4]

Vilified unfairly as scoundrels, Drs. Wiktor Taubenfligel and Stanislaw Flato were also imprisoned by the Polish government in the 1950s. After his release, Dr. Taubenfligel worked as a Professor of Surgery in Gdansk, Poland. In 1968, he left Poland through Austria to Canada, along with his son, George. Wiktor's daughter, Ewa, immigrated to Canada two years later. The multilingual Dr. Taubenfligel's earlier medical studies in Italy helped him serve the Italian-Canadian community in Toronto where he continued to practice medicine until the age of eighty.[5]

Dr. Stanislaw Flato served in the Polish Army after his return to Poland but was also arrested in 1952. He was released from prison during the first visit to Poland by Prime Minister Zhou Enlai in 1954. Zhou Enlai asked about the fate of a Polish doctor who provided medical help to his sick wife in Chongqing during the war with Japan. Within twenty-four hours of this conversation, Dr. Flato was released from solitary confinement.[6] He would go on to serve in the Polish diplomatic corps in China until a new wave of anti-Semitism arose following the Six-Day (Arab-Israeli) War of 1967. Dr. Flato died in Berlin in 1971 and is survived by his son, Jurek, and daughter, Krystyna, who subsequently immigrated to Sweden.

The decision to leave or remain in their native land divided the German-born International Medical Relief Corps' members. Dr. Erich Mamlok returned to the American Occupied Zone of Berlin in 1945. His remaining family members in Germany perished in Treblinka, though his parents survived in Uruguay.[7] Dr. Mamlok worked as the chief health officer of the anti-epidemiology unit of the German State Board of Health in Berlin until 1949, when he immigrated to the United States. He believed that the potential for building a better world would be far greater in America than in Germany.[8] Dr. Mamlok considered his period of tuberculosis research in New York as the most meaningful time of his professional life.[9] In 1952, he married a German-Jewish nurse, Helga Rosemarie Mottek, in New York. She spent World War II as a nurse in the Jewish Hospital of Berlin and immigrated to the United States in 1947.[10] Dr. Mamlok died in 1991 and is survived by his son, Dr. Robert Mamlok, and daughter, Susan Fisher, in the United States.

Dr. Erich Mamlok's compatriot, Dr. Walter Lurje, also immigrated to the United States after the war. In 1946, he was still communicating with the journalists Anna [Martens] Wang and Agnes Smedley about conditions in China.[11] In 1952, he resumed his career as a psychiatrist, in Texas at the Rusk Institute.[12]

Dr. Rolf Becker returned to East Germany in May 1948 and initially worked as a district medical officer in Brandenburg/Havel. He later served in a variety of positions, including director of the Ministry of Public Health in Saxony-Anhalt (until September 1952), medical consultant in a mining company and at a rolling-stock manufacturing company, district medical officer in Ribnitz-Damgarten (in 1954), and finally chief medical officer of the Maritime Medical service of the German Democratic Republic (in 1959). Divorced from his wife Joan Staniforth in 1950, he later remarried. He died in December 1999 and is survived by his son, Bernard, his and Joan Staniforth's daughter, Josephine, and his and his second wife, Judith's daughter, Kathrin.[13]

Dr. Carl Coutelle also returned to East Germany, reuniting after seven years of separation, with his wife, Rosa and now six-year-old son, Charles. He initially worked in Berlin for the East German Central Healthcare Administration, which he left in 1949 to train as a pathologist. He became a professor at the Charité Hospital Medical School Berlin in 1959, and chair of the Department of Pathology at the University of Halle in 1963. He died at the age of eighty-five on June 24, 1993, in Berlin.[14] He is survived by his son, Dr. Charles Coutelle, an emeritus professor of gene therapy at the Imperial College of London.

Dr. Wilhelm Mann continued his training and worked as an academic biochemist for many years in Shanghai at the Chinese Academy of Sciences. His work in China ended with the forced closure of all laboratories during the so-called Cultural Revolution. In 1964, he became the last of the International Medical Relief Corps' members to return to their native land. He reunited with his friend from Guiyang, Dr. Carl Coutelle, and then worked as part of the medical faculty of the Humboldt University in Berlin. In 1972, he married Anna Vera Hedwig Hugnin. He died in Berlin on September 23, 2012. At the age of ninety-seven, he was the last surviving member of the International Medical Relief Corps.[15]

In 1945, Dr. Herbert Baer returned to Berlin, Germany, with Drs. Coutelle and Mamlok. Dr. Baer would serve in the former Soviet Occupation Zone with Dr. Coutelle and, later, Dr. Becker. Dr. Baer's immediate family reunions in Germany were not to be. His brother had died in the war, and, of his three sisters, two were killed in Auschwitz in 1943; only one sister survived and fled to Britain.[16] Dr. Baer continued his work in public health for the Central Healthcare Administration (*Zentralverwaltung für Gesundheitswesen*) in the Soviet Occupation Zone of Germany. On August 29, 1946, at the age of forty-eight, he died in a motor vehicle accident. The circumstances surrounding the accident remain unclear.[17] The first rural outpatient clinic of the German Democratic Republic in Golssen was later named after him.[18]

Several other physicians returned to their native countries and spent the rest of their lives striving to improve their war-ravaged lands. This included the Austrian doctors Fritz Jensen, Heinrich Kent, Edith Kent, and Walter Freudmann. Three of the Austrian International Medical Relief Corps' members died of unnatural causes at a relatively young age. Dr. Jensen was murdered. Dr. Kent committed suicide, and the cause of the death of Susanne Wantoch remains unclear.

Dr. Fritz Jensen returned to Vienna in December 1947 but soon stopped practicing medicine, becoming instead a journalist in Asia. He moved back to China in 1953 with his wife, Wang Wu-An, and their adopted son, Mischa. On April 11, 1955, on a flight from Beijing to the Asiatic-African conference in Bandung, Indonesia, his aircraft exploded into the sea near Sarawak, Malaysia.[19] Saboteurs who were trying to assassinate the People's Republic of China's first premier and the Spanish doctors' old friend, Zhou Enlai, mistakenly targeted Dr. Jensen's aircraft.

Dr. Heinrich Kent's friend, Dr. Moses Ausubel, wrote to the Spanish Civil War nurse, Fredericka Martin that, despite his selfless accomplishments, Dr. Kent may have been a troubled man:

> While Dr. Kent was in China, he tried to kill himself with injections of morphine. He was taken to an American military hospital and saved.... The American psychiatrist who cared for him said, "This time we saved him. But he'll try again. Next time he'll succeed." It was eleven years before he tried again and succeeded.[20]

Dr. Kent died in Vienna on December 4, 1961.

Dr. Edith (Marens) Kent completed medical school in Austria, where she remained. After the death of her husband, Heinrich, she tried unsuccessfully to immigrate to the United States to join her sister and son, but was denied entrance due to her Communist Party membership. Dr. Edith (Marens) Kent died in Vienna on December 24, 1981, at the age of seventy-three.[21]

Susanne Wantoch returned to Austria in November 1946, after her husband died in Chongqing, China, in December 1945. In 1957, she traveled to the Austrian Alps, near where she and Teddy Wantoch had wed hastily prior to their travel to China in 1939. When her body was found at the mountain base the following spring, it was unclear if her death was an accident.[22]

Dr. Walter Freudmann returned to Vienna in 1946 and worked as a doctor in Vienna's multicultural 10th district. The Nazis had murdered his parents in 1942, and his brother died as a freedom fighter in Paris in 1943. He married a Roman Catholic, Margaretha (Greta) (last name unknown), and they had one adopted child, Eva.[23] Dr. Freudmann's family wrote that the conflict between the Soviet Union and China disturbed him greatly: "He took the side of the Chinese communists and left the Communist Party of Austria. But till his death, he kept in touch with his comrades-in-arms from Spain and China, wherever they had ended up."[24] Dr. Freudmann died in Vienna in 1993, at the age of eighty-two.

The two Czech physicians, Drs. Bedřich Kisch and Franta Kriegel, also returned to their native land. Dr. Bedřich Kisch, the senior trauma surgeon of the International Medical Relief Corps, returned to Czechoslovakia after a brief stay in the United Kingdom. In the early 1950s, he returned to Asia and provided medical services in Vietnam.[25] He developed contact dermatitis and ceased to practice medicine before he died at the age of seventy-four on September 13, 1968, three weeks after the occupation of Czechoslovakia by Soviet troops.

Dr. Franta Kriegel quickly rose through the ranks of the Czechoslovakian medical system and became the Deputy Minister of Health in 1949. He barely escaped arrest in the early 1950s when he was "rehabilitated." Dr. Kriegel, whose independent thought had already been of concern to the communist party in Spain in 1939, became a Czechoslovakian hero for his resistance to the Warsaw Pact invasion of Czechoslovakia during the Prague spring of 1968. Dr. Kriegel was the only Czech political leader who refused to capitulate to Brezhnev. "Send me to Siberia or shoot me dead," he replied.[26] He survived that confrontation and worked in Cuba on the development of the Cuban healthcare system in the early 1960s. He died, a national hero, on December 3, 1979, at the age of seventy-one.[27]

The two Romanian physicians, Drs. David Iancu and Iacob Kranzdorf, returned to Romania. At the end of the war, Dr. David Iancu became a physician in the Romanian Army. He married nurse Marie Grünberg in 1947. They had three daughters, Tania, Anca-Lia, and Nadia, and one son, Andrei. Tania lives in Bucharest, Romania; Nadia and Andrei immigrated to Canada, and Anca-Lia immigrated to the United States. Dr. Iancu died in 1990, at the age of eighty.

In 1948, Dr. Iacob Kranzdorf (Bucur Clejan) returned to Romania with his Chinese-born wife, Zhao Jingpu (Nelly Clejan), whom he had married in 1946. He worked in the Romanian Health Ministry and died in 1976. His widow returned to Shanghai, China, in 1986 and lived until 2014. Dr. Kranzdorf's relatives emigrated between 1970 and 1986 from Romania to Israel, Canada, and the United States.

The Bulgarian physician, Dr. Ianto Kaneti, repatriated with his Chinese wife, Zhang Sunfen, and their first son, *Baozhong*, to Sofia, Bulgaria. Dr. Kaneti worked as a radiologist, and Zhang Sunfen as a translator at the Chinese Embassy in Sofia. Dr. Kaneti returned to Asia as a military physician, with Ho Chi Minh's Vietminh. The Chinese government has recognized him as a hero of the People's Republic of China. He died in 2004 at age ninety-four and is survived by his two sons, Jose and Viktor, who live in Bulgaria.[28]

Dr. Schön worked with the United Nations Relief and Rehabilitation Administration in China until 1947. In China, he married Delin Zhu (Csu Te Lin Éva) in the German Evangelical Church in Shanghai in 1947.[29] She was the oldest of two brothers and three sisters and worked together with

Dr. Schön at the Chinese Red Cross headquarters.[30] The couple returned to Budapest, Hungary in 1947, where Dr. Schön was known as György Somogyi. He worked in the National Institute of Public Health and later in the National Institute of Rheumatology and Physiotherapy. His wife taught Chinese at the Eotvos Lorand University in Budapest and died of tetanus in 1954. His two sons survive him, Dr. Joseph Somogyi in Berlin, Germany, and Peter Somogyi in Brussels, Belgium.[31] Dr. György Somogyi died in 1977, at the age of sixty-five.

Little is known about the postwar fates of Mania Kamieniecki, Dr. Leon Kamieniecki, and Dr. Alexander Volokhine. The Kamienieckis returned after the war to Lithuania, then part of the USSR. They shared the good news of the birth of their first child with Dr. Rolf Becker in September 1947. Dr. Somogyi visited with Dr. Kamieniecki in Moscow in 1960.[32] Dr. Alexander Volokhine probably returned to the Soviet Union after the war, though his fate also remains unknown to this author.

American doctor Adele (Cohn) Wright's post–China experience took her from England to Jamaica, where she continued her work in tuberculosis. She immigrated with her husband,

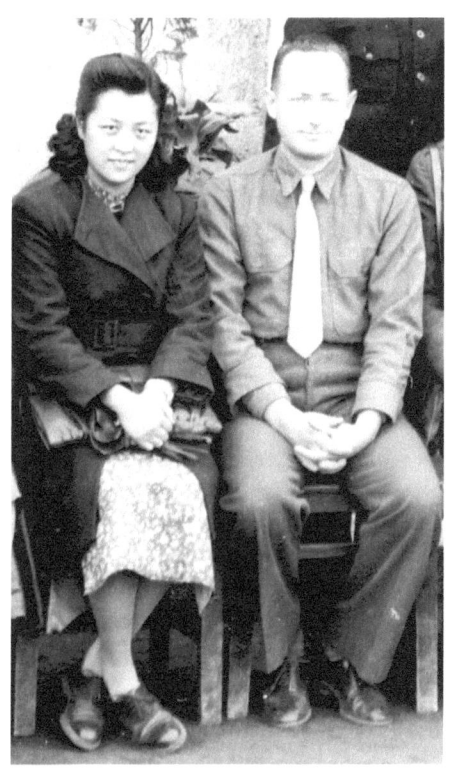

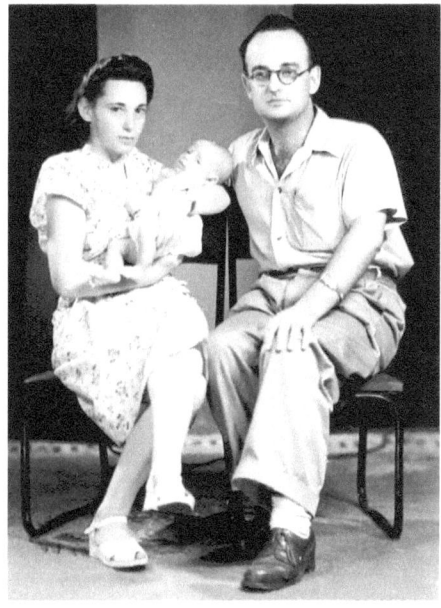

Top: Dr. George Schoen, age 35 and his wife, Delin Zhu (Csu Te Lin Éva), age 27 working with UNRRA in Shanghai in 1947 (courtesy Peter and Joseph Somogyi). *Bottom:* Dr. Leon and Mrs. Miriam Kamieniecki with their newborn child, September 3, 1947 (courtesy Bernard Becker).

Philip, and her son, Max, back to England in 1961. Dr. (Cohn) Wright remained affiliated with the Wellcome Foundation's Museum of Tropical Medicine until her retirement. Diagnosed with lung cancer in 1968, she died in 1971. Philip Wright died in a motor vehicle accident in 1975; they are survived by their son, Max Wright.

Despite their extraordinary lifelong challenges (or perhaps because of them), some of the International Medical Relief Corps' members and their descendants were to take on leading roles in public health, medical research, politics, journalism, and education. Two of the International Medical Relief Corps' physicians, Drs. Franta Kriegel and Fritz Jensen, had Peace Prizes named after them.[33] Many of the International Medical Relief Corps' members and their descendants would go on to share contributions to the medical literature, the arts, and the social sciences. Finally and perhaps most importantly, they shared the optimism and strength of a collective international conviction: the conviction to fight for the principles of humanity and equality, even when confronted with the worst of circumstances.

12. What Did the International Medical Relief Corps Members Accomplish?

Although they constituted only 10 to 15 percent of the physicians in the Chinese Red Cross/Medical Relief Corps, the International Medical Relief Corps' members included several battle-hardened physicians and military hospital commanders well positioned to aid their Chinese allies. This highly motivated group of young doctors had very strong convictions about continuing the fight against fascism wherever and however they could.

Data from the Guiyang local government shows that the Chinese Red Cross/Medical Relief Corps' doctors conducted operations on more than 200,000 people, treated about 6.5 million outpatients and inpatients, and vaccinated more than 4.6 million people before the team was dismissed in 1945.[1] The International Medical Relief Corps members' medical assistance included sharing the strategies of military medicine and surgical innovations that had proven successful on the battlefields of Spain.

In addition, they documented numerous impromptu and individual efforts to adapt the materials at hand in the fight against malnutrition and infectious disease. Evidence for the impact of these innovations comes from many sources. Dr. Chung, for example, wrote of his medical observations of the International Medical Relief Corps in Guiyang:

> Many of the surgical procedures were refined and adapted from the lessons acquired from the Spanish Civil War, not long ended. In fact, a number of volunteers had arrived recently from Spain to join our ranks as doctors, nurses and laboratory technicians ... early operation on battle wounds and proper transportation to avoid further injury was tested successfully in Spain and adopted by the Chinese Red Cross.[2]

Some of the specific medical lessons that International Medical Relief Corps' members shared with the Chinese Red Cross included the importance of standardization of treatment of typical casualties: "This gave better statistical results than to allow individual doctors to make their own decisions. This led to a scheme to classify casualties and strict rules for the specific treatment."³ The importance of early transportation of casualties and bringing medical units to the front lines was repeatedly emphasized:

> The medical post of the division was a key point.... Its most important task was the sorting out of casualties into different groups and then sending them to specific locations for treatment. The best doctors were out in charge of the station.... Abdominal wounds were operated upon immediately.... It was recognized that the time factor was essential and every effort was made to speed up transportation.⁴

Drs. Heinrich Kent and Fritz Jensen are credited with several additional innovations. These were summarized in the doctors' respective manuscripts, *Concise Comments on Military Surgical Operations and Personal Views on Ways of Improvement* and *Some Features of War Surgery and Army Medical Service During the Spanish Civil War of 1936-1939*.⁵ Dr. Kranzdorf was also well recognized by both the Chinese Red Cross and the Friends Ambulance Units for his ingenious approach to the management of scabies and syphilis in wartime China.

Surgical improvisation with basic supplies was the order of the day. For example, Dr. Bob McClure of the Friends Ambulance Units devised a traction system in which he would pin a bicycle spoke through a broken bone and then attach the traction equipment to the ends of the spoke.⁶ Dr. Chung noted that Dr. McClure's spoke-traction system was not the only orthopedic innovation:

> Fractures of arms and legs were immobilized in special steel frames used with success in the Spanish Civil War and transported to the division field hospital, as were the postoperative patients. The experience gained at the base in Kweiyang [Guiyang] came in handy; I was grateful for that.⁷

Innovations in the construction and modification of delousing and bathing stations by Drs. Freudmann, Iancu, and Kent were important public health contributions to wartime China.

Early recognition, isolation, and management of potentially catastrophic epidemics of infectious diseases were continually on these doctor's minds. Dr. Jensen wrote on January 7, 1940, that "[t]here were two cases of smallpox that were isolated and our doctors succeeded in tracing the origins of smallpox and obtained an order from the Chief director of the division for complete vaccination of the companies concerned."⁸ The impact of this sort of timely diagnosis is incalculable but was clearly of great significance.

In addition to their medical mission, the International Medical Relief Corps succeeded in assimilating with and creating lifelong friendships with many of their Chinese colleagues. Agnes Smedley wrote in 1941 that the Inter-

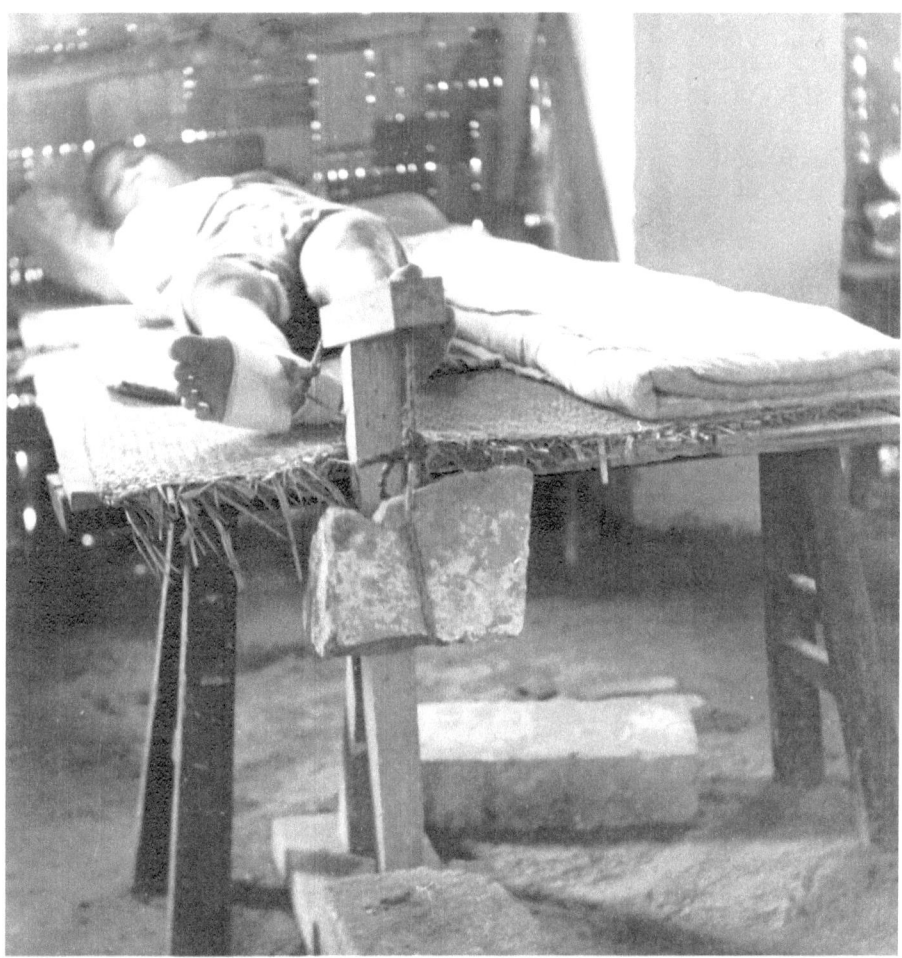

Improvised surgical traction for soldier with left femur fracture (National Archives: 208-FO-OWI-6479).

national Medical Relief Corps "saw all the sanitary and scientific backwardness of China, but they saw these conditions in their proper perspective, and responded by shouldering whatever burdens they could."[9] Further evidence of the International Medical Relief Corps' assimilation into Chinese culture comes from their intermarriage. Although romanticized in theater (*Fremde Erde* [Foreign Soil] (1943) and *Jews in Shanghai* (2012)), Chinese-Jewish intermarriage was a relatively rare event among the tens of thousands of Jews in wartime Shanghai.[10] In contrast, four of the six surviving, single International Medical Relief Corps' physicians who were not sent to Burma (Drs. Kaneti, Kranzdorf, Schön, and Jensen) married Chinese nationals.

The Chinese people have continued to commemorate the International Medical Relief Corps' member's contributions to China's medical needs at the time of her greatest peril (see Appendix B). The legacy of Sino-Western internationalism and cooperation remains an important part of what the International Medical Relief Corps accomplished together with their Chinese Red Cross/Medical Relief Corps' colleagues.

Appendix A: The International Medical Relief Corps Timeline

1936
July 18	General Francisco Franco headed a revolt against Spain's Republican government.
December 12	The Xi´an Incident: Chiang Kai-shek abducted.

1937
April 26	Bombing of Guernica, Spain.
July 7	Marco Polo Bridge incident: The Second Sino-Japanese War begins.
August	Medical Relief Corps founded
September	International Red Cross Committee founded in Wuhan
November	Shanghai falls to Japan
December 13	The Rape of Nanjing

1938
January 28	Dr. Norman Bethune departs for China
January	Ms. Joan Staniforth arrives in Hong Kong
June 6	Yellow River flooded with 1 million deaths
June	Chinese Defence League formed by Madame Sun Yat-sen
September 14	Five Indian physicians arrive in Hong Kong
November	Dr. Theodor and Susanne Wantoch leave England for China
December 28	Dr. Wilhelm Mann leaves from Genoa to Shanghai

1939
February	Chinese Red Cross establishes headquarters in Tuynunguan
April	Dr. Wu removed from the Chinese Red Cross
April 1	Spanish Civil War ends with the Republican's surrender in Madrid
May 20	*Eumaeus* departs Liverpool, England, with Drs. Becker, Jensen, and Kisch

July 27	Drs. Becker, Jensen, and Kisch arrive at Chinese Red Cross Headquarters
August 4	*Aeneas* departs Liverpool, England, with Drs. Baer, Iancu, Kaneti, and Freudmann
August 4	*Jean LaBorde* departs Marseille, France, with Dr. Erich Mamlok
August 12	*Aeneas* stops in Marseille, France
August 23	Nonaggression pact signed by Russia and Germany
August 30	Dr. Mamlok arrives in Hong Kong
September 3	England and France declare war on Germany
September 28	*Aeneas* arrives in Hong Kong
October 7	Dr. Mann arrives at Chinese Red Cross Headquarters
October 16	*Aeneas* Chinese Red Cross volunteers arrive in Tuyunguan
November 12	Dr. Norman Bethune dies of sepsis

1940

June 22	France signs an armistice with Germany
July	Battle of Britain air war begins
July 18	Britain forced to close the Burma Road
July 30	Drs. Kent and Coutelle leave Liverpool, England
August	Dr. Lin summoned to Chiang Kai-shek with communist allegations
September 27	Germany, Italy, and Japan sign the Tripartite Pact

1941

January	New Fourth Army incident ends the Second United Front
February	Dr. Robert Lin's first resignation from the Chinese Red Cross
March	Dr. Robert Lin accepts Dr. Adele Cohn's offer to join the Chinese Red Cross
	Dr. Rosa Coutelle and Maria Rodriquez' ship sank in the Atlantic
May	Dr. Barbara Courtney arrives at Chinese Red Cross Headquarters
June 22	Germany invades Russia (*Operation Barbarossa*)
September	Dr. Adele Cohn arrives in China
	Evert Barger and Philip Wright incident
	International Medical Relief Corps kept inactive in Tuyunguan
December 7	Japanese attack at Pearl Harbor, Hawaii Territory, USA
December 9	China declares war on the Axis powers

1942

	3 million die in Henan famine

	Much of the International Medical Relief Corps kept inactive in Tuyunguan
February	Japanese attack Burma
March	Dr. Barbara Courtney dies
May	General Joseph Stilwell retreats from Burma to India
April 18	Doolittle Raid on Tokyo, Japan
June	Victory at Midway halts Japanese naval advance
August	Dr. Lin resigns again from the Chinese Red Cross Medical Relief Corps
December 9	Dr. Dwarkanath Kotnis dies from epilepsy
December 31	International Medical Relief Corps' physician group arrives in India

1943

January 7	First five International Medical Relief Corps physicians arrive in Ramgarh, India
February 2	Russia defeats Germany in the battle of Stalingrad (Volgograd), Russia
February	Dr. Wu reappointed as director of the Medical Relief Corps
April	Dr. Robert Lin left Chinese Red Cross to join Chinese Expeditionary Force-Y
November	Northern Burma Offensive starts
	Dr. Adele Cohn leaves to Chongqing

1944

March 13	Gisela Kranzdorf dies
April 17	Japanese *Ichigo offensive* begins in China
May	Dr. Robert Lin takes position with American Bureau for Medical Aid to China
May 30	Philip Wright and Dr. Adele Cohn are married in Chongqing
June 6	Allied invasion of Normandy: D-day
June 18	Fall of Changsa, China
August	Japanese defeated in Myitkyina, Burma
October 19	General Joseph Stilwell recalled
October 20	U.S. troops land in the Philippines

1945

February 4	Yalta Conference: Post war Europe formulated
April 12	President Franklin D. Roosevelt dies
April 30	Adolf Hitler commits suicide
May 8	War in Europe ends: VE-Day
August 6	Atomic bomb dropped on Hiroshima
August 9	Russia declares war on Japan

August 15	Japan surrenders
September 5	Dr. Bedřich Kisch returns to Europe
October 24	Six International Medical Relief Corps' members repatriated to Germany
December 12	Dr. Theodor Wantoch dies in Chongqing

Appendix B:
The International Medical Relief Corps' Memorial Dedication
(September 1, 2015, Tuyunguan, China)

The Guizhou People's Association for Friendship with Foreign Countries, the Guiyang People's Association for Friendship with Foreign Countries, and the Friends of the International Medical Relief Corps shared the following dedication in August 2015:

> Owing to historical factors, only twenty-one international volunteers who worked with the Chinese Red Cross Medical Relief Corps and the subordinate units of the Chinese Red Cross were listed on the Monument of Members of the International Aid to China Medical Team that was dedicated in 1985. This year marks the seventieth anniversary of China's victory in the War of Resistance against Japanese Aggression. This name wall is dedicated to reflect our greater and current historic understanding, pay tribute to all of the known international volunteers who worked with the Chinese Red Cross during World War Two, commemorate the contribution of all of the known International Medical Relief Corps' members, and to foster and honor our collective friendship and legacy of working together to overcome the tremendous challenges of the last century. According to the latest historical research from home and abroad, and for the need to preserve the existing monument (which is a Provincial Cultural Relic), the Guizhou People's Association for Friendship with Foreign Countries, the Guiyang People's Association for Friendship with Foreign Countries, and Friends of the International Members of the Medical Relief Corps have worked with great care and camaraderie to create this new legacy to our common heritage.[1]

At the request of the Friends of the International Members of the Medical Relief Corps, the Guizhou People's Association for Friendship with Foreign Countries, and the Guiyang People's Association for Friendship with Foreign Countries continued to separate the experience of the International Medical Relief Corps' members from the equally deserving missionary and other foreign

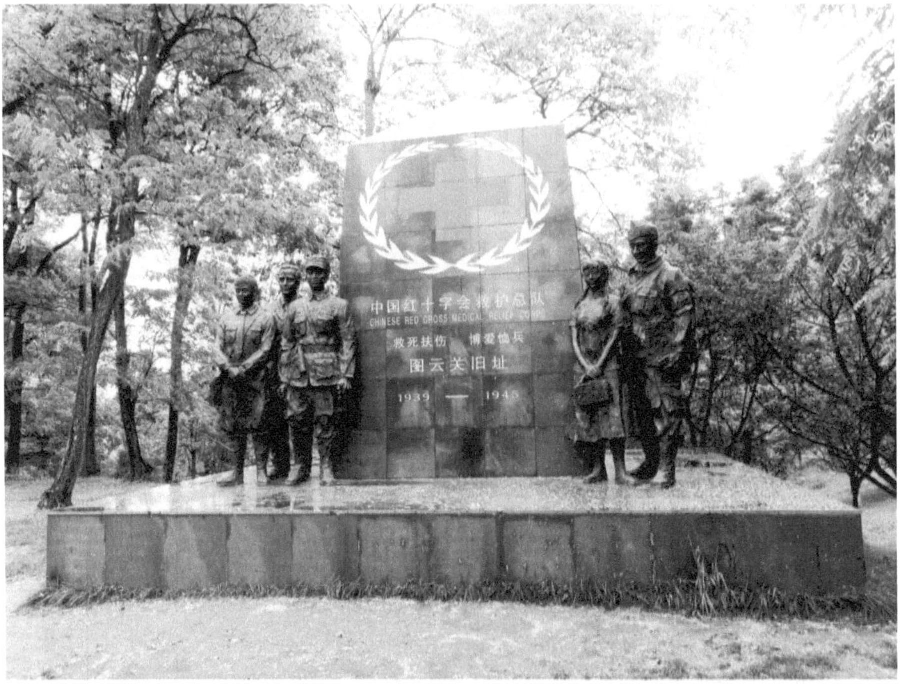

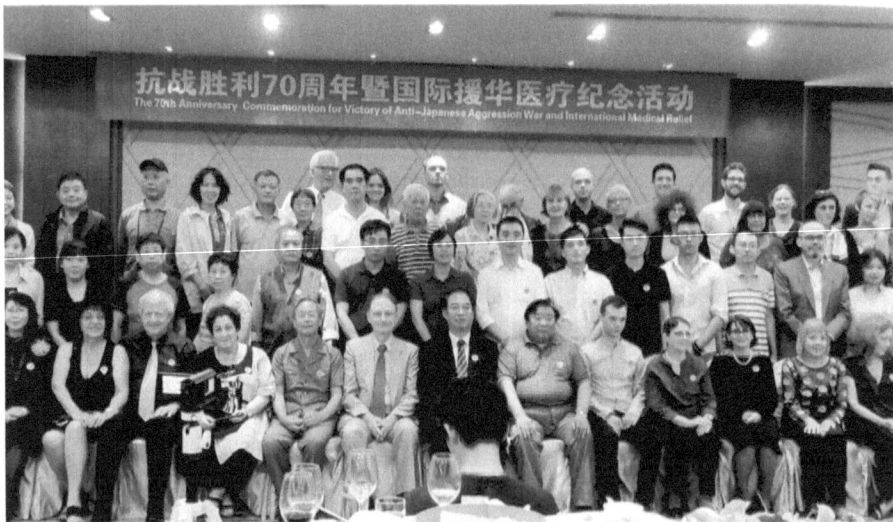

Top: Chinese Red Cross International Medical Relief Corps members memorial in Tuyunguan Park near Guiyang, China, 2015 (author's collection). *Bottom:* International Medical Relief Corps descendants celebrating the 70th anniversary commemoration of the end of the Pacific War with their Chinese hosts in Guiyang, China (author's collection).

volunteer Chinese Red Cross/Medical Relief Corps' members who are separately recognized as the "Other international volunteers of the Chinese Red Cross." The 1985 monument honors twenty-one International Medical Relief Corps' members. All of them were members of different national Communist Parties. Nineteen of the twenty-one were sent to China by the English and Norwegian China Medical Aid Committees. The 2015 monument honors twenty-seven International Medical Relief Corps' members and nineteen "Other international volunteers of the Chinese Red Cross." The six new International Medical Relief Corps members are Drs. Barbara Courtney, Erich Mamlok, Wilhelm Mann, and Adele (Cohn) Wright, Mrs. Joan (Staniforth) Becker, and Mrs. Susanne Wantoch. Of the six new International Medical Relief Corps additions to the 2015 monument, only one, Susanne Wantoch, was then a Communist Party member and only one, Dr. Adele (Cohn) Wright, was supported by a China Medical Aid Committee (American Bureau for Medical Aid to China).

Among the nineteen "Other international volunteers of the Chinese Red Cross" are the five physicians sent by the Indian Government (Drs. Basu, Cholkar, Kotnis, Mukherjee, and Atal), five missionaries (Drs. Ayers (艾逸士), Bryson (贝雅德医生), McClure, and Holm, plus nurse Kathleen Hall (何明清 He Ming Ching), and nine others who served in different healthcare capacities throughout China. Further research is needed to improve our understanding of their contributions and sacrifices.

Appendix C: Other International Volunteers of the Chinese Red Cross

The "other international volunteers of the Chinese Red Cross" included several missionary physicians who remained in China and several physicians who came to China during the Sino-Japanese War. One of the early groups of physicians to interact with the Chinese Red Cross prior to serving the Chinese Communist Party's Eighth Route Army in Yan'an was a group of five physicians sent by the Indian National Party to China.

Agnes Smedley and General Chu Teh (朱德 Zhū Dé)[1] established the first formal contact between the Chinese communists in Yan'an and the Indian Nationalist movement led by Gandhi and Nehru.[2] This group of physicians arrived in Hong Kong on the SS *Fatshan* on September 14, 1938. Dr. M.M. Atal (爱德华) led them. He also had fought in 1936 with the International Brigade in the Spanish Civil War, fleeing to London after the defeat of the Republicans. From England, he formed a medical mission to China that resulted in the formation of a Sino-Indian Committee.[3]

The other four members were Drs. Mohanlal Cholkar (卓克华), the deputy leader; Bijoy Kumar Basu (巴苏华); Debesh Mukherjee (木克华); and Dwarkanath S. Kotnis (柯棣华医生 Ke Di Hua). Dr. Atal would become the second Spanish doctor to reach China, nine months after Dr. Bethune reached Yan'an and nine months before Drs. Kisch, Becker, and Jensen arrived in Hong Kong. Writing from the Lutheran Mission in Wuchang,[4] the group met with Dr. Robert Lin and Agnes Smedley and shared their wish to join the Chinese Communist Party's Eighth Route Army in October 1938.[5]

However, much like the International Medical Relief Corps' physicians were to experience in Tuyunguan, the Indian physicians first endured a period of forced inactivity in Chongqing. Dr. Basu wrote that it was incomprehensible that the Chinese Red Cross would not use qualified doctors while thousands of wounded patients were in dire need of medical assistance. By December 8, 1938, the Indian physicians had become so frustrated by their forced inactivity that they threatened to return home.[6]

In 1938, the prevailing Second United Front between the Chinese Communist Party and the Guomindang Nationalist Party was still strong enough to allow some foreign physicians and medical supplies to reach the Chinese Communist Party's Eighth Route Army. Neither the Chinese Communist Party nor the Guomindang Nationalist Party wanted their supporters or the international press to conclude that they were responsible for the failure of the United Front against Japan.[7]

However, as the Indian physicians would indicate, travel and aid to the Chinese Communist Party–controlled north became increasingly covert, dangerous, and unpredictable: Eventually, they could secure approval to go to Yan'an. They were escorted by the New Zealander Rewi Alley as Zhou Enlai concluded that it was too dangerous to have them led by Chinese Communist Party members such as Wang Bingnam [Ping-nan].[8] The Indian physicians' perseverance prevailed, and they were able to reach the Eighth Route Army medical corps in February 1939.[9]

Although all of these doctors made significant contributions, Dr. Kotnis distinguished himself by his loyal and heroic medical service to the Eighth Route Army. During his three years in China, he joined the Chinese Communist Party and married a Chinese Peking Union Medical College trained nurse, Guo Qinglan (郭庆兰). Much like Dr. Bethune, Kotnis became a medical martyr. He suffered from epilepsy and died from a series of epileptic seizures on December 9, 1942, at the age of thirty-two.[10] The story of Dr. Kotnis' medical service to China continues to be one of the most enduring symbols of Sino-Indian friendship.

Dr. Atal shared many of the experiences of the Chinese Red Cross and International Medical Relief Corps' members. He graduated from the University of Edinburgh Medical School, as had Drs. Lin and McClure.[11] Along with many of the International Medical Relief Corps physicians, Dr. Atal also had served in the International Brigade in Spain, fleeing to London after the defeat of the Republicans. From England, he formed a medical mission to China that resulted in the formation of a Sino-Indian Committee.[12]

Dr. Mukherjee's service in China was limited, as after eleven months he would need to return to India for surgical care for his nephropathy. When he tried to reenter China from Burma with medical supplies, he was arrested by the British and returned to India. Dr. Mukherjee became a social activist and was arrested again in India in 1942 for his involvement in the Quit India Movement (Bhārat Chodo Āndolan).[13]

In addition to the Indian physicians, other doctors with divergent backgrounds and interests continued to trickle into the Chinese Red Cross in the late 1930s to care for Chinese trapped in a critical humanitarian crisis in the wake of the Japanese invasion. Among them was Dr. Harry Talbot, one of three British physicians associated with the 3rd Curative Unit of the Chinese Red Cross/Medical Relief Corps. This unit originated in Hankow in December 1938 under the leadership of Dr. H.L. Chang.

In 1939, Dr. Chang wrote of the contributions of Austrian International Medical Relief Corps physician, Dr. Teddy Wantoch, and two other foreign physicians, Drs. Harrison and Haverson (哈沃森医生).[14] Though reported by the Chinese Red Cross as British, it is more probable that Dr. Harrison was the Canadian Tillson Lever Harrison. Chang noted that Drs. Talbot, Harrison, and Haverson resigned from the 3rd Curative Unit in December 1939, after less than a year of service.

Dr. Talbot, a member of the Chinese Defence League and the Chinese Red Cross, subsequently worked in Europe and North America as a fundraiser for the Chinese Red Cross. He lamented the fact that the Chinese were receiving no aid from the International Relief Committee or the American Red Cross at that time, December 1938, and that all aid was coming from the American Bureau for Medical Aid to China and the China Aid Council. Dr. Talbot and Austrian Dr. Paul Dohan (杜翰医生) helped the Chinese Defence League, in March 1939, with the transport of medical supplies from Hong Kong to Guiyang and then to the northwest.[15] After this, Dr. Dohan left the Chinese Red Cross and became attached to the English Baptist Hospital in Xi'an.[16] He married the physician, Dr. Jean Chiang, who became head of obstetrics with the Eighth Route Army.

Other brief tours of duty of foreign physicians in the Chinese Red Cross in 1938 are noted in the report of the 38th Curative Unit. These physicians included Dr. Stanley C.P. Louie (路易医生), Dr. Tillson Lever Harrison (哈里森医生), and Dr. Frank Aston (阿斯顿医生). Dr. Louie, an American, resigned as the first leader of the 38th Curative Unit on May 16, 1938. Dr. Aston, a British physician, served the 38th Curative Unit from May to September 1938.[17]

By all accounts, the Canadian doctor Tillson Lever Harrison was an adventurer. He had previously served as chief of the medical staff for Poncho Villa in Mexico and traveled extensively in and out of war zones throughout his life. He served in eight armies on five continents and was known as a serial bigamist with four wives.[18]

Dr. Wu, the Secretary General of the Chinese Red Cross, shared with American Bureau for Medical Aid to China a less-than-favorable first impression of some of the few North American volunteers who were appearing in China in the late 1930s:

> We have had rather unfortunate experiences with certain foreign (especially Austrian and 1–2 Canadian and 1 American) so called volunteers who asked to join and then demanded all sorts of terms and behaved as if they had come to save China from ineffi-

ciency—then threatened to make bad publicity for us if we threw them out. God save us from such as these! There are of course some splendid foreign friends who obey discipline and work unostentatiously but it is difficult to know until perhaps too late.[19]

It is not known with certainty if this small group of American and Canadian doctors that Wu spoke of in central China in 1938 were indeed Harrison and Louie or, rather, Parsons, Bethune, and Brown. These are the only two groups of Canadian and American physicians that have been identified when the Chinese Red Cross communicated with Dr. Co-Tui of the American Bureau for Medical Aid to China in January 1939.

Independent of his probably unfavorable initial reception, Dr. Harrison returned to China after the war and worked with the United Nations Relief and Rehabilitation Administration until he died in 1947. The Anglican compound in Kaifeng where he is buried now houses the Dr. Tillson Harrison Memorial School, and the Harrison International Peace Hospital in Hengshui is an active medical center. Dr. Harrison's daughter said that the movie producers George Lucas and Steven Spielberg had interviewed her and that the character Indiana Jones was based on her father's life.[20]

A less flamboyant but equally deserving foreign volunteer physician was the Swedish physician Dr. Ake Holm (科恩医生). Previously, Dr. Holm had been sent to Hong Kong by the Swedish National Chinese Relief Committee to join the International Red Cross Committee as a surgeon and bacteriologist. Prior to his brief service with the Chinese Red Cross Unit 33, he had served with the Swedish Ambulance Service in the Abyssinian war.[21] A February 1939 article in the *Straits Times* noted that Dr. Holm initially might have been assigned to the International Relief Committee but ended up serving in the Chinese Red Cross/Medical Relief Corps.[22] The leader of the Chinese Red Cross/Medical Relief Corps Unit 33 wrote in his June 1940 report: "It was with regret in September 1939 that the Unit had to say goodbye to Dr. Holm ... [After three months] Dr. Holm was recalled to Sweden on the outbreak of the war in Europe."[23]

Some of the politically complex and unfavorable initial interactions between the Chinese Red Cross and foreign physician volunteers may have contributed to the Chinese Red Cross' subsequent reservations about accepting future foreign volunteer physicians. Dr. Lin wrote to the American Bureau for Medical Aid to China in the fall of 1939: "Regarding the 14 Czech doctors associated with Dr. Walter Recht,[24] please assure their personal qualifications. Please note we are not accepting foreign doctors unless American Bureau for Medical Aid to China or other foreign sources can pay for their salary and travel."[25] Dr. Lin expanded on his concerns about recruiting foreign physicians to Co-Tui at the American Bureau for Medical Aid to China:

> Foreign volunteers must know about the primitive conditions here and must live like our own men. Only send men of the best qualifications who are anxious to help. It is

very difficult to find men with this double qualification! The transport must be paid to the Chinese frontier: we can give the Chinese rates of pay, but it would be better to secure their entire support abroad.... There are German Jews here and men who served in Spain are available in Europe, but we have nobody to select them.[26]

The desperate need for more international physicians in wartime China remained unfulfilled as difficult living conditions and divisive politics kept many other medical volunteers from reaching its shores.

Chapter Notes

Chapter 1

1. University of Vienna Archives, Wantoch, Theodor, Nationale Promotion für ordentliche Hörer der Medizinischen Fakultät, 1933, and Jerusalem, Friederich, Nationale Promotion für ordentliche Hörer der Medizinischen Fakultät, 1929, courtesy of the Memorial Book for the Victims of National Socialism at the University of Vienna project, University of Vienna, Austria. Accessed June 20, 2016. http://gedenkbuch.univie.ac.at/index.php?id=435 andno_cache=1andL=2andperson_single_id=22881.

2. Walter Freudmann. *Tschi-Lai!-Erhebet Euch! Erlebnisse eines Arztes in China und Burma 1939–1945* (Linz, Austria: Verlag Neue Zeit, 1947), 9.

3. Correspondence from Fredericka Martin to Wiktor Taubenfligel, Fredericka Martin Papers [ALBA #1 Box, Poland folder]. New York: Tamiment Library and Wagner Labor Archives, New York University. The predominantly Polish Dabrowski Brigade was named for Jaroslaw Dabrowski, a Polish General who died fighting in defense of the Paris Commune in 1871.

4. Correspondence from Dr. Wolf Jungery to Fredericka Martin, January 10, 1979. Oklahoma City, OK, Fredericka Martin Papers [ALBA #1 Box 4, Poland: Wolf Jungery folder]. New York: Tamiment Library and Wagner Labor Archives, New York University.

5. Dr. Stanislaw Flato biographical sketch, Fredericka Martin Papers [ALBA #1 Box 2, Poland folder]. New York: Tamiment Library and Wagner Labor Archives, New York University.

6. Homage to Major Dr. Flato, Fredericka Martin Papers [ALBA #1 Box 4, Poland: Dr. Flato folder]. New York Tamiment Library and Wagner Labor Archives, New York University. The Naftali Botwin Company was part of the Polish Dabrowski (Dombrowski) Battalion. Its flag bore the words "For your freedom and ours" in Yiddish and Polish on one face of the flag and in Spanish on the other.

7. Andy Dugan, "Freedom Fighters or Comintern Army? The International Brigades in Spain," *International Socialism Journal*, Issue, 84, Autumn 1999. Accessed May 12, 2016, http://pubs.socialistreviewindex.org.uk/isj84/durgan.htm.

8. Theodore Bergmann, *Internationalisten an den Antifaschistischen Fronten* (Hamburg, Germany: Verlag, 2009), 29.

9. Dr. Carl Coutelle, In *Personal Memories* (German). Unpublished; in Dr. Charles Coutelle's possession.

10. T. Bergmann. *Internationalisten an den antifaschistischen Fronten*, 72

11. Hans Landauer and Eric Hackl, *Lexikon der Osterreichischen Spanienkämpfer, 1936–1939* (Vienna, Austria: Theodor Kramer Gesellschaft; Auflage 2, 2008), 133.

12. Gabriel Sichon, *Frantisek Kriegel*, l'insoumis, Association pour un judaisme Humaniste et Laique, 2001. Accessed on April 4, 2015. http://www.ajhl.org/plurielles/PL8, 50–51.

13. Communication from Dr. Glaser to the head of the International Brigade Medical Service. August 10, 1938. Vich, Spain, Fredericka Martin Papers [ALBA #1 Box 2, Czechoslovakia physician's folder, Bedřich Kisch]. New York: Tamiment Library and Wagner Labor Archives, New York University.

14. Letter of Erica Wallach to Fredericka Martin, March 19, 1972. Fredericka Martin Papers [ALBA #1 Box 2, Czechoslovakia physician's folder, Bedřich Kisch]. New York: Tamiment Library and Wagner Labor Archives, New York University.

15. Journalist Agnes Smedley would later write on Ruth Domino's behalf to Anna Wang in Chongqing in November 1945. She wrote

that Ruth was living at her literary estate and that she wished to have their divorce finalized.

16. Rolf Becker and M. Strasse. "Fritz Jensen in Memoriam," *The Journal for the Advancement of Medicine*, Vol. No. 13 (July 1, 1955).

17. Correspondence from Dr. Fritz Jensen, December 3, 1938, Barcelona, Spain, Fredericka Martin Papers [ALBA #1, Box 1, Austrian physicians, Dr. Fritz Jensen folder], New York: Tamiment Library and Wagner Labor Archives, New York University.

18. Freudmann, *Tschi-Lai*, 9–10.

19. Correspondence from Edith Kent to Dr. Vazant, July 30, 1940 [Box 3, Edith Kent folder]. New York: Tamiment Library and Wagner Labor Archives, New York University.

20. Correspondence from Moses Ausubel to Fredericka Martin, March 7, 1972, Fredericka Martin Papers [Box 3, Edith Kent folder]. New York: Tamiment Library and Wagner Labor Archives, New York University.

21. Correspondence from Dr. G. Ersler, Guernica, Spain, April 18, 1982, Fredericka Martin Papers [ALBA #1, Box 2, French physicians]. New York: Tamiment Library and Wagner Labor Archives, New York University.

22. Personal communication with Dr. Joseph and Peter Somogyi, February 2016.

23. *Barsky v. Board of Regents of the University of the State of New York,* 347 U.S. 442, S Ct (April 26, 1954).

24. *Activities of the Romanian volunteers of the medical service of the International Brigades,* by David Iancu, Translated by V. Shapiro, October 1981, Fredericka Martin Papers [ALBA #1, Box 4, Romanian physicians, David Iancu folder]. New York: Tamiment Library and Wagner Labor Archives, New York University.

25. Her brother, Max "Coca" Goldstein, was a Romanian anarchist and communist who had organized assassination attempts of Ministers Argetoianu and Greceanu. He died in prison at age twenty-six after a thirty-two-day hunger strike.

26. Lin Yin, *Walking Through Blood and Fire* (Guiyang China: Guizhou People's Publishing House, 2015), 132–135. 林吟著. 在血^火 +穿行. 中国红十字会救护总队抗战救护纪实 1939–1945 (贵州出版集团 贵州人民出版社).

27. J. Kranzdorf, *Luomaniya de Bai quien* (Bukuer Kelieran Yu Zhongguo. di 1 ban. ed. Shanghai: Shanghai ci shu chu ban she, 2009), 16.

28. Ernest Hemingway, *For Whom the Bell Tolls* (New York: Scribner, 1940), 235.

29. Fritz Jensen, *Opfer und Sieger: Nachdichtungen, Gedichte und Berichte* (Berlin, Germany: Dietz Verlag, 1955), 156.

30. David Iancu, *Activities of the Romanian Volunteers of the Medical Service of the International Brigades*, translated by V. Shapiro, October 1981. Fredericka Martin Papers [ALBA #1, Box 4, Romanian physicians, David Iancu folder]. New York: Tamiment Library and Wagner Labor Archives, New York University.

31. Fritz Jensen. "Some Features of War Surgery and army Medical Service During the Spanish Civil War of 1936–1939," *The Chinese Medical Journal*, Vol. 62A (April 1944).

32. Nicholas Coni. "Medicine and the Spanish Civil War," *Journal of the Royal Society of Medicine* (3) 147–150 (March 2002).

33. John Rich (Reich) was an English-born American Quaker who worked for the American Friends Service Committee in Spain from 1937 to 1939 and as the director of public relations for the American Friends Service Committee in China in 1943. John Rich Diary entry, Testimonies in Art and Action: Igniting Pacifism in the Face of Total War. Retrieved October 28, 2015, https://ds-omeka.haverford.edu/peacetestimonies/items/show/154.

Chapter 2

1. Kranzdorf, *Luomaniya de Bai Qiuen*, 17.
2. Sichon, *Frantisek Kriegel*, 50–51.
3. Angela Jackson, *For Us It Was Heaven: The Patience, Grief and Fortitude of Patience Darton* (Brighton, England: Sussex Academic Press, 2012), 120.
4. Jensen, *Opfer und Sieger*, 154–158.
5. The American poet Emma Lazarus coined the expression: "Until we are all free, none of us are free." She is perhaps best known for her 1883 sonnet on the pedestal of the Statue of Liberty in New York City: "Give me your tired, your poor, your huddled masses yearning to breathe free..." This would be a greeting that many of the International Medical Relief Corps members would be happy to see many years later.
6. Kranzdorf, *Luomaniya de Bai Qiuen*, 18.
7. Jensen, *Opfer und Sieger*, 156.
8. Kranzdorf, *Luomaniya de Bai Qiuen*, 20.
9. Dr. Carl Coutelle, In *Personal Memories*.
10. Rolf Becker, "Als Arzt in China," in *Aerzte: Erinnerungen, Erlebnisse Bekenntnisse*, ed. G. Albrecht and W. Hartwig (Berlin, Germany: Buchverlag Der Morgen, 1972), 2.
11. The Kuomintang, or Guomindang Nationalist Party by its Pinyin transliteration, is often translated as the Chinese Nationalist Party or the Nationalist Party of China.
12. Petra Lataser-Czisch, *Eignetlich Rede Ich Nicht Gern Über Mich* (Leipzig, Germany: Gustav Kiepenheuer, 1990), 82.

13. Letter from Edith Kent to Dr. Vazant, Fredericka Martin Papers [ALBA 1, Box 2, Austria, Heinrich Kent file]. New York: Tamiment Library and Wagner Labor Archives, New York University.
14. Ibid.
15. *The Problem of the Chinese Wounded*, by Hilda Selwyn-Clarke, British Relief Funds in China, 1938, Foreign Office Files for China 1938-1940. The National Archives of GB (TNA), FO 371/22141
16. Correspondence from Mrs. Hilda Selwyn-Clarke to Ms. Mildred Price, China Aid Council, January 5, 1940, American Bureau for Medical Aid to China Records [Box 22, Foreign Auxiliary to the Chinese Red Cross folder]. Rare Book and Manuscript Library, Columbia University in the City of New York.
17. Dr. Robert Lin is also referred to as Dr. Bobby Lim, and Dr. Robert Kho-Seng Lim. He is identified in the Chinese literature predominantly as Lin Kesheng, but to ease reading, all references are to Dr. Robert Lin (林可胜).
18. Correspondence from Tor Gjesdahl to Dr. Co-Tui, American Bureau for Medical Aid to China Records [Box 22, Foreign Auxiliary of the National Red Cross of China]. Rare Book and Manuscript Library, Columbia University in the City of New York.
19. Dr. Millais Culpin's taboo love affair with his future wife, Nurse Ethel Bennett, would be broadcast in the BBC television productions, entitled, *Casualty 1907* and *1909*, seventy years later.
20. Arthur Clegg, *Aid China 1937-1939: Memoirs of a Forgotten Campaign* (Beijing, China: Foreign Languages Press, 2003), 103.
21. Fridrich Firsov, *Secret Cables of the Comintern* (New Haven: Yale University Press, 2014), 97.
22. Correspondence to the party committee, Camp Gurs, June 13, 1939 [ALBA VF 001, Box 2, Chinese participation folder 66]. New York: Tamiment Library and Wagner Labor Archives, New York University.
23. Propositions du P. avec accord de comarade Marty: Liste des medecins recommandes pour la Chine, List of physicians recommended for China and prepared for Andre Marty [ALBA VF 001, box 2, Chinese participation folder 66]. New York: Tamiment Library and Wagner Labor Archives, New York University.
24. Ibid.
25. Andre Marty to Harry Pollitt, Paris, 9 May 1939, Moscow Archive, Disc 1/545/6/87, p. 43. As quoted in Jackson, A. *For Us It Was Heaven*, p. 137.
26. Propositions du P. avec accord de comarade Marty: Liste des medecins encore necessaire au camp [ALBA VF 002, Box 2, folder 66]. New York: Tamiment Library and Wagner Labor Archives, New York University.
27. Correspondence from Dr. Glaser about Dr. David Iancu, Fredericka Martin Papers [ALBA # 1, Box 4, Romanian physicians, Dr. David Iancu folder]: New York: Tamiment Library and Wagner Labor Archives, New York University.
28. International Hospital at Vich, Murcia note, Fredericka Martin Papers [ALBA # 1Box 4, Romanian physician, Dr. David Iancu folder]. New York: Tamiment Library and Wagner Labor Archives, New York University.
29. Fredericka Martin Collection [ALBA VF 001, Box 5, Folder 45, Edith Marcus Jungermann]. New York: Tamiment Library and Wagner Labor Archives, New York University.
30. Dr. Len Crome was born Lazar Krom in Dvinsk, Latvia. He became permanent chief of the medical services to the XI Brigade and the XV Brigade. He returned to England became a member of the Communist Party and helped East European veterans escape from France. Dr. Crome later became Chairman of the International Brigade Association.
31. Sichon. *Frantisek Kriegel*, 51.
32. This included Ernst Cohn, Denis Fried, Josef Gardonyl, Andre Kalman, Emeric Mezer, Leon Branchfelb, Michel Perilman, Leon Samet, Iruh Bernstein, Ladislau Schimer, and Adolf Kofler. In addition to Frantisek Kriegel, the physicians absolutely forbidden by Andre Marty from going to China included: Paul Bernstein, Jacob Gluschkim, Fernand Grosfels, Isaak Gutman, Hans Landesberg, Hans Serelman, Max Laufer, Osckar Sigal, and Soltan Davidovitch. Additional physicians not allowed to go to China because they were deemed needed in Gurs were Emmanuel Edel, Hahn Greza, and Tibor Berger [ALBA VF 001, box 2, Chinese participation folder 66], New York: Tamiment Library and Wagner Labor Archives, New York University.
33. Edgar Snow, the American author of *Red Star Over China* (London: Victor Gollanz, Ltd., 1937), chronicled his first-hand accounts with the Eighth Route Army in China in 1937.
34. The seven future International Medical Relief Corps' members who were to leave from England were Drs. Becker, Kisch, and Jensen on the *Eumaeus* and Drs. Baer, Freudmann, Iancu, and Kaneti on the *Aeneas*.
35. Jackson, *For Us It Was Heaven*, 125.
36. Correspondence from Edith Kent to Dr. Vazant, July 30, 1940 [Box 3, Edith Kent folder]. New York: Tamiment Library and Wagner Labor Archives, New York University.
37. Case summary 51a, The National Archives 1938 Nov 07-1946 Feb 27 [KV 2/1013]

38. Personal communication, Bernard Becker, July 2015.
39. Eva Barilich, *Fritz Jensen. Arzt an Vielen Fronten, Biografische Texte zur Geschichte der Österreichischen Arbeiterbewegung* (Vienna, Austria: Globus Verlag, 1991), 78.
40. Herzel Grynspan was a seventeen-year-old Polish Jewish refugee. His assassination of Nazi German diplomat Ernst vom Rath on November 7, 1938, in Paris provided the Nazis with the pretext for the Kristallnacht, the anti-Semitic pogrom of November 9–10, 1938. A trial was not conducted because of the Nazi Party's wish to conceal vom Rath's probable and then illegal homosexuality.
41. Correspondence from Dr. Erich Mamlok to Uncle Robert Hirsch, Dr. Erich Mamlok letters (German). Basel, Switzerland, December 5, 1938. Unpublished in Dr. Robert Mamlok's possession.
42. Walter Lurje, *Ztschr. F. d. ges. Neurol. U. Psychiat.*, 70: 35 (August 9, 1921).
43. Correspondence from Dr. Smets to Dr. Lurje, October 1937 [Registry Files 1937–1940, Classification 50, Folder 31160, Technical Co-operation with China], League of Nations' Archives, Geneva, Switzerland.
44. Stephen Mackinnon, *China Reporting: An Oral History of American Journalism in the 1930s and 1940s* (Berkeley: University of California Press, 1987), 4.
45. Roderick Stewart, *Phoenix: The Life of Norman Bethune* (Montreal, Canada: McGill Queens University Press, 2012); Ted Allan and Sydney Gordon, *The Scalpel and the Sword: The Story of Dr. Norman Bethune* (New York: Monthly Review Press, 1952); Larry Hannant, *The Politics of Passion: Norman Bethune's Writing and Art* (Toronto, Canada: University of Toronto Press, 1998).
46. Dr. Eloesser had returned to Stanford University in Palo Alto, California, where he served as Chief of Surgery. He volunteered to serve with the United Nations Relief and Rehabilitation Association as a specialist in thoracic surgery in China after the war.
47. Allen and Gordon, *The Scalpel and the Sword*, 121–122.
48. Correspondence from Dr. Louis Davidson to Dr. Co-Tui, November 28, 1940, American Bureau for Medical Aid to China Records [Box 30, Dr. Adele Cohn folder], Rare Book and Manuscript Library, Columbia University in the City of New York.
49. Correspondence from Dr. Adele (Cohn) Wright to Jerry Cohn, unpublished, in possession of Max Wright, London, England.
50. Correspondence from Dr. Robert Lim to Dr. Co-Tui, March 16, 1939, American Bureau for Medical Aid to China Records [Box 22, National Red Cross Society of China folder]. Rare Book and Manuscript Library, Columbia University in the City of New York.
51. Correspondence from Dr. Robert Lim to Dr. Adele Cohn, March 24, 1941, American Bureau for Medical Aid to China Records [Box 30, Dr. Adele Cohn folder], Rare Book and Manuscript Library, Columbia University in the City of New York.
52. Correspondence from Helen Stevens to Szeming Sze, October 28, 1944, American Bureau for Medical Aid to China Records [Series II: Box 8, Leo Eloesser folder], Rare Book and Manuscript Library, Columbia University in the City of New York.

Chapter 3

1. After the Japanese had assassinated his father, Zhang Xueliang overcame his opium addiction and fought valiantly against the Japanese occupation of Manchuria. Despite his placement under house arrest for more than fifty years, he remained loyal to the Guomindang Nationalist Party. He died at age 101 in Hawaii.
2. Japanese historians estimate that the death toll ranged from tens of thousands to two hundred thousand.
3. Barbara Tuchman, *Stilwell and the American Experience in China* (New York: Grove Press, 2001), 187.
4. William Withrow, *China and Its People* (New York: W. Briggs, 1894), 23.
5. Sichon, "Les Medecins des deux guerres," 57–64.
6. Diary entries from John F. Rich, April 1941–December 1946, John F. Rich Papers [Box 1, Folder 6], Quaker and Special Collections, Haverford College, Haverford, PA.
7. Bu, Liping. *Public Health and Modernization in China*, 112.
8. Xi Gao, "Foreign Models of Medicine in Twentieth-Century China" in, *Medical Transitions in 20th Century China*, ed. Bridie Andrews and Mary Brown Bullock (Bloomington: Indiana University Press, 2014), 191.
9. Bu Liping. *Public Health and Modernization in China*, 118.
10. Horace W. Davenport, *Robert Kho-Seng Lim: A Biographical Memoir* (Washington, DC: National Academy of Sciences, 1980), 291.
11. "The Situation in China," *The Lancet*, Vol. 231, Issue 5989 (June 11, 1938).
12. Hannant, *The Politics of Passion*, 226.
13. Ka-che Yip, "Disease and the Fighting Men: Nationalist Anti Epidemic Efforts in Wartime China, 1937–1945," in *China and the Anti-Japanese War, 1937–1945, Politics Culture*

and Society, ed. David Barrett and Larry Shyu (New York: Peter Lang Publishing, 2000), 176–177.

14. "Dr. Robert Pollitzer Obituary, March 12, 1968," *UCSF News* (San Francisco, CA: UCSF Press, 1967), 222.

15. Wystan Hugh Auden and Christopher Isherwood, *Journey to a War* (New York: Random House, 1939) 77.

16. Letter #8 from John Rich, April 30, 1943, John F. Rich Papers, Haversford College [Box 1, Folder 1], Quaker and Special Collections, Haverford College, Haverford, PA.

17. Correspondence from Helen Stevens to the American Bureau for Medical Aid to China Board, September 22, 1943, American Bureau for Medical Aid to China Records [Box 38, Miscellaneous letters]. Rare Book and Manuscript Library, Columbia University in the City of New York.

18. Correspondence from Dr. Li Shu-Pui to Dr. Co-Tui, March 19, 1938, American Bureau for Medical Aid to China Records [Box 22, National Red Cross Society of China folder]. Rare Book and Manuscript Library, Columbia University in the City of New York.

19. T. Christopher Jesperson, *American Images of China: 1931–1949* (Stanford, CA: Stanford University Press, 1996), 45–59.

20. John Watt, *Saving Lives in Wartime China: How Medical Reformers Built Modern Healthcare Systems Amid War and Epidemics, 1928–1945* (Leiden: Brill, 2015).

21. C. Pickett, *For More Than Bread* (Boston: Little Brown and Co.), 1953, p. 223.

22. The truck depot in Kutsing, in Yunnan Province, was located 329 miles southwest of Chongqing.

23. Correspondence from John Rich to family, Kutsing, China, April 2, 1943, John F. Rich Papers [Box 1, Folder 1], Quaker and Special Collections, Haverford College, Haverford, PA.

24. Munro Scott, *Bob McClure: The China Years* (New York: Penguin Books, 1977), 295.

25. John Rich diary entries from February 5–September 20th, 1943, Travels in China, John F. Rich Papers [Box 1, Folder 5], Quaker and Special Collections, Haverford College, Haverford, PA.

26. Correspondence from Soong Ching Ling, Chairman Chinese Defence League, July 1938 Newsletter # 1, American Bureau for Medical Aid to China Records [Box 5, China Defence League folder], Rare Book and Manuscript Library, Columbia University in the City of New York.

27. Scott, *Bob McClure*, 116.

28. Correspondence from Dr. Erich Landauer, 1st unit League of Nations, Anti Epidemic Unit, Memorandum of the International Red Cross Committee of China: Activities in Hankow, as published by the China Defence League, September 25, 1938, American Bureau for Medical Aid to China Records [Box 5, China Defence League folder]. Rare Book and Manuscript Library, Columbia University in the City of New York.

29. Freda Utley, *China at War* (London: Faber and Faber, 1939), 141.

30. W.H. Auden and Christopher Isherwood, *Journey to a War* (Paragon House, 1990) 60.

31. Correspondence from Agnes Smedley to the United Aid Council, November 8, 1939, Smedley MacKinnon Collection [Box 1, Folder 4]. Tempe, AZ: Arizona State University Libraries: University Archives.

32. Correspondence from Agnes Smedley to the South China Post: The Japanese in China, April 13, 1940, Smedley MacKinnon Collection [Box 2, Folder 5]. Tempe, AZ: Arizona State University Libraries: University Archives.

33. John Rich diary entries from February 5–September 20th, 1943, Travels in China, John F. Rich Papers [Box 1, Folder 5], Quaker and Special Collections, Haverford College, Haverford, PA.

34. John Rich diary entries, April 1941–December 1946, John F. Rich Papers [Box 1, Folder 6], Quaker and Special Collections, Haverford College, Haverford, PA.

35. F.C. Yang, Director-General, National Health Administration, October 14, 1938, broadcast from Chungking [Chongqing] and published in *People's Tribune*, 1938, American Bureau for Medical Aid to China Records [Box 2, Army Medical College folder]. Rare Book and Manuscript Library, Columbia University in the City of New York.

36. Nichole E. Barnes and John R. Watt, *Medical Transitions in Twentieth Century China* (Bloomington: Indiana University Press, 2014), 230.

37. National Health Administration report (Director Dr. P.Z. King), May 1941, American Bureau for Medical Aid to China Reports [Box 2, Army Medical College folder]. Rare Book and Manuscript Library, Columbia University in the City of New York.

38. Liping Bu. *Public Health and Modernization in China: 1865–2015* (New York: Routledge, 2017), 157.

39. Newsletter # 1, Soong Ching Ling, Chairman Chinese Defence League, July 1938, American Bureau for Medical Aid to China Records [Box 5, China Defence League folder]. Rare Book and Manuscript Library, Columbia University in the City of New York.

40. Ka-che Yip, "Disease and the Fighting Men: National Anti-Epidemic Efforts in

Wartime China, 1937–1945," in *China in the Anti-Japanese War 1937–1945, Politics, Culture and Society*, eds. David Barrett and Larry Shued (New York: Peter Lang), 173.

41. Correspondence from Dr. H. Kent to friends, October 3, 1941, Friedricka Martin Papers, ALBA #1 [Box 3, Dr. Kent folder]. New York: Tamiment Library and Wagner Labor Archives, New York University.

42. John Watt, *Saving Lives in Wartime China*, 117.

43. Winifred (Freda) Utley was an English political activist and journalist who later rejected communism and authored the bestseller, *Japan's Feet of Clay*, which helped initiate the American boycott of Japanese goods.

44. Freda Utley, *China at War*, 122. http://www.fredautley.com/pdffiles/book19.pdf.

45. Dr. Carl Coutelle, in personal memories (German).

46. Chinese Red Cross, Register of the Nym Wales Papers [Box 5, Folder 10], Hoover Institution Archives, Stanford, CA.

47. Relief work in China (folder 4), State of Medicine in the Chinese Army, Correspondence to the British Embassy from Joseph Needham (quoting Dr. Jensen); 1944. The National Archives of the UK (TNA), FO 371-41557.

48. Susanne Wantoch, *Nan Lu: Die Stadt der Verschlungenen Wege* (Vienna, Austria: Globus Verlag, 1948), 58–63.

49. Liping Bu. *Public Health and Modernization in China*, 158.

50. Bullock, *Medical Transitions in 20th Century China*, 193.

51. In November 1944, under the so-called ALPHA plan, General Wedemeyer convinced Chiang Kai-Shek that conscription of all final-year medical students, all medical college graduates from 1942 to 1944, and 30 to 50 percent of all medical practitioners was needed.

52. Arthur Chung, *Of Rats, Sparrows and Flies: A Lifetime in China* (Stockton, CA: Heritage West Books, 1994).

53. John Watt, *Saving Lives in Wartime China*, 125–126.

54. Lin Yin, *Walking Through Blood and Fire*, 120–121.

55. The information office of the Guiyang Municipal Government (2005).

56. Correspondences from Dr. Joseph Needham, British Scientific Mission in China, to Sir Henry Dale, June 24, 1943 [Henry Dale Collection, 93HD, 64.2], The Royal Society Archives, City of London.

57. Utley, *China at War*, 144.

58. Watt, *Saving Lives in Wartime China*, 122.

59. Report on the EMSTS, by Dr. Pao-san Chi, January 1942, American Bureau for Medical Aid to China Records [Box 2, EMSTS folder]. Rare Book and Manuscript Library, Columbia University in the City of New York.

60. May-ling Soong Chiang, *China Shall Rise Again* (New York: Harper and Brothers, 1941), 235–237.

61. Correspondence from Dr. Robert Lim EMSTS, March 3, 1941, American Bureau for Medical Aid to China Records [Box 22, National Red Cross Society of China, Dr. Robert Lim folder]. Rare Book and Manuscript Library, Columbia University in the City of New York.

62. Winfield, *China: The Land and the People*, 142–143.

63. Soong Chiang, *China Shall Rise Again*, 241.

64. Watt, *Saving Lives in Wartime China*, 130–131.

65. Reports of the Curative Units of the Red Cross Medical Relief Corps: 1937–1938, American Bureau for Medical Aid to China Records [Box 23, National Health Administration folder]. Rare Book and Manuscript Library, Columbia University in the City of New York.

66. Correspondence to Dr. Co-Tui, from CY Wu, April 8, 1939, American Bureau for Medical Aid to China Records [Box 22, National Red Cross Society of China, Robert Lim folder]. Rare Book and Manuscript Library, Columbia University in the City of New York.

67. Stewart, *Phoenix*, 246.

68. Jean Ewen, *China Nurse: 1932–1939* (Toronto, Canada: McClelland and Stewart, 1981), 51–2.

69. Stewart, *Phoenix*, 258.

70. Bill Trent, "Dr. Robert McClure: Missionary-Surgeon Extraordinaire," *Canadian Medical Association Journal*, Vol. 132 (February 15, 1985).

71. Mao Tse-Tung, *Selected Works of Mao Tse-Tung* (Honolulu: University Press of the Pacific, 2001), 337.

Chapter 4

1. Fritz Jensen, *China Siegt* (Vienna, Austria: Globus Verlag, 1949), 9.

2. In Greek mythology, Eumaeus was Odyssey's loyal friend and swineherd.

3. Becker, *Als Arzt in China*, 3.

4. Dr. Rolf Becker diary (German), June–July 1939. Unpublished; in possession of Bernard Becker.

5. Dr. Bedřich Kisch vaccination records by Dr. James Scott, the *Eumaeus* physician, July 8, 1939, Correspondence of Dr. Bedřich Kisch, Památník národního písemnictví, Praha, Czech Republic.

6. China Medical Aid Committee report, July 1940, The National Archives of the UK (TNA), FO 371/24667.
7. In Greco-Roman mythology, Aeneas was a Trojan hero and son of Venus. As a descendant of Romulus and Remus, he is considered the first true hero of Rome.
8. David Iancu, 9 Ani Medic Pe Front Spania-China (1937-1945) (Bucharest, Romania: Editura Vitruviu, 2008), 81.
9. According to the alien passenger lists of the Blue Funnel Line, the two Chinese students returning from Scotland to China on the *Aeneas* were Lui-Ling Tai and Hsin Ti Wang.
10. Freudmann, *Tschi-Lai!* 8.
11. Maritime records of the Blue Funnel Lines, "*Aeneas* Vessel, Non Transmigrant Alien Passenger List, Departure, Liverpool, August 5, 1939." Retrieved from http://www.ancestry.com/immigration
12. Freudmann, *Tschi-Lai!* 11.
13. Iancu, *9 Ani Medic Pe Front Spania-China*, 91.
14. Freudmann, *Tschi-Lai!* 18.
15. Iancu, *9 Ani Medic Pe Front Spania-China*, 92.
16. Dr. Ma Haide was a Lebanese-American physician who completed his medical training in 1933 in Geneva, Switzerland, and immigrated to China. He served with the Chinese Communist Party's Eighth Route Army in Yan'an and became a public disease expert.
17. See Appendix IV for a description of Dr. M.M. Atal and the Indian mission to the Chinese Red Cross.
18. B.K. Basu, *Call of Yanan: The Story of the Indian Medical Mission to China* (New Delhi, India: Foreign Language Press, 1986), 180-181.
19. Kranzdorf, *Luomaniya de Bai Qiuen*, 21.
20. Idem., 24.
21. Freudmann, *Tschi-Lai!* 25-26.
22. Wireless to the New York Times, "18 Doctors Who Served in Spain Arrive in China," Chungking [Chongqing], China," October 27, 1939, *New York Times*, 1.
23. Barilich, *Fritz Jensen*, 91.
24. Maritime records, P and O Steamship Line, *Naldera* vessel, Departing London, Destination Yokohama, Japan, January 28, 1938. Retrieved from http://www.ancestry.com/immigration
25. Letters from Miss Joan Staniforth to family, September 1939. Unpublished, in Bernard Becker's possession.
26. Correspondence from Dr. Erich Mamlok to Robert Hirsch (German), Basel, Switzerland, July 1939. Dr. Erich Mamlok letters. Unpublished; in possession of Dr. Robert Mamlok.
27. Ibid.
28. United States Holocaust Memorial Museum Encyclopedia, *Obstacles to Immigration: Emigration from Germany*, Accessed on June 3, 2016, https://www.ushmm.org/wlc/en/article.php?ModuleId=10007455.
29. Correspondence from Harry D. Biele, of the National Committee for Resettlement of Foreign Physicians to Dr. Hans Mamlok, August 28, 1942. In possession of Dr. Robert Mamlok.
30. Barilich, *Fritz Jensen*, 77.
31. Alfred and Frieda Mamlok obtained a visa to immigrate to Montevideo, Uruguay, on the *Cabo de Bueno Esperanza* of the *Ybarra Line* on May 21, 1941.
32. Correspondence from Dr. Erich Mamlok to Uncle Robert Hirsch (German), Basel, Switzerland, July 1939, Dr. Erich Mamlok letters. Unpublished; in possession of Dr. Robert Mamlok.
33. Correspondence from Dr. Alfred and Mrs. Frieda Mamlok to Dr. Erich Mamlok, Grunewald Wallotstrasse 10, Berlin, Germany, August 2, 1939 (German). Unpublished; in possession of Dr. Robert Mamlok.
34. Dr. Carl Coutelle, In personal memories (German). Unpublished, in Dr. Charles Coutelle's possession.
35. Correspondence from Dr. Erich Mamlok to Uncle Robert Hirsch (German), Dr. Erich Mamlok letters (German). Basel, Switzerland, December 5, 1938. Unpublished in Dr. Robert Mamlok's possession.
36. Recommendation letter from Dr. Changyao Wu, Secretary General of the Chinese Red Cross, to Dr. Erich Mamlok, September 2, 1939, Hong Kong (Chinese), Dr. Erich Mamlok letters. In possession of Dr. Robert Mamlok.
37. Scott, *Bob McClure*, 270.
38. Correspondence from Edith Kent to Dr. Vanzant, July 30, 1940, ALBA #1 [Box 3, Dr. Kent folder]. New York: Tamiment Library and Wagner Labor Archives, New York University.
39. Dr. Carl Coutelle, in personal memories (German). Unpublished, in Dr. Charles Coutelle's possession.
40. UK, Outward Passenger Lists, 1890-1960 for Doctor Carl Coutelle. Retrieved from http://search.ancestry.com/cgi-bin/sse.dil?indiv=1anddb=UKOutwardPassengerListsandh=144779726
41. Dr. Carl Coutelle, in personal memories (German). Unpublished, in Dr. Charles Coutelle's possession.
42. Ulricke Unschuld, *You Banfa—Es Findet Sich Immer ein Weg: Wilhelm Manns Erinnerungen an China 1938-1966* (Berlin, Germany:

Hentrich and Hentrich, 2014), 78; The Haffkine Institute originated in Bombay (Mumbai), India, in 1899. It was named after the Jewish Russian zoologist, Dr. Waldemar Mordecai Haffkine, who is credited with inventing the plague vaccine.

43. Erster Bericht Über die Schriftstellerin Susanne Wantoch, In E. Hackl, *In Fester Umarmung: Geschichten und Berichte* (Zurich: Diogenes Verlag, 2003), 297–298.

44. Kranzdorf, *Luomaniya de Bai Qiuen*, 16.

45. Yin, *Walking Through Blood and Fire*, 132–135.

46. *Ibid.*, 135.

47. Correspondence from Ms. Selwyn-Clarke to Dr. Co-Tui, American Bureau for Medical Aid to China Records [Box 13, National Red Cross Society of China: Foreign Auxiliary folder]. Rare Book and Manuscript Library, Columbia University in the City of New York.

48. Becker, *Als Arzt in China*, 3–4.

49. Scott, *Bob McClure*, 300.

50. Becker, *Als Arzt in China*, 13.

51. Iancu, *9 Ani Medic Pe Front Spania-China*, 98–100.

52. Auden, *Journey to a War*, 199.

53. Iancu, *9 Ani Medic Pe Front Spania-China*, 99.

54. Correspondence from Dr. Erich Mamlok to Robert Hirsch, Shanghai, China, September 1939. Dr. Erich Mamlok letters (German). Unpublished; in possession of Dr. Robert Mamlok.

55. Chung, *Of Rats, Sparrows and Flies*, 77.

56. Agnes Smedley Archives, V 28 Gr X-78 35 *China Weekly Review*, May 20, 1939, by Agnes Smedley. Tempe, AZ: Arizona State University Libraries: University Archives.

57. Correspondence from Dr. Erich Mamlok to Robert Hirsch, Lukou, China, January 1940. Dr. Erich Mamlok letters (German). Unpublished; in possession of Dr. Robert Mamlok.

58. Irene Eber, *Wartime Shanghai and the Jewish Refugees from Central Europe* (Berlin, Germany: Walter De Gruyter, 2012), 125.

59. Unschuld, *You Banfa*, 68–9.

60. Correspondence to Dr. Hume from Dr. Adele Cohn, Oct 6, 1941, American Bureau for Medical Aid to China Records [Box 30: Dr. Adele Cohn folder], Rare Book and Manuscript Library, Columbia University in the City of New York.

61. Correspondence to Ms. Hankmeyer from Dr. Adele Cohn, November 17, 1941, American Bureau for Medical Aid to China Records [Box 30: Dr. Adele Cohn folder], Rare Book and Manuscript Library, Columbia University in the City of New York.

Chapter 5

1. Unschuld, *You Banfa*, p. 72.

2. "Tuyunguan" is translated from Mandarin as "the pass where the earth and clouds meet."

3. James Bertram. "From Red Swastika to Red Cross, an Unknown Victory of the China War," *China Defence League Newsletter*, American Bureau for Medical Aid to China Records [Box 5, China Defence League Folder]. New York: Rare Book and Manuscript Library, Columbia University in the City of New York.

4. Freudmann, *Tschi-Lai!* 48.

5. Correspondence from Dr. Adele Cohn, November 17, 1941, American Bureau for Medical Aid to China Records [Box 30, Dr. Adele Cohn folder]. Rare Book and Manuscript Library, Columbia University in the City of New York.

6. The novel, *The Citadel* by A.J. Cronin explored medical ethics through the choices of a young Scottish physician in a Welch mining town. It is credited with helping to develop the National Health Service in England.

7. James Bertram. "From Red Swastika to Red Cross: An unknown victory of the China war," *China Defence League Newsletter* [Series II: Box 5, China Defence League folder]. Rare Book and Manuscript Library, Columbia University in the City of New York.

8. Freudmann, *Tschi-Lai!* 60.

9. Dr. Carl Coutelle, in personal memories (German). Unpublished, in Dr. Charles Coutelle's possession.

10. Unschuld, *You Banfa*, 73.

11. Jensen, *China Seigt*, 99.

12. Correspondence from Dr. Adele Cohn to Dr. Van Slyke, November 17, 1941, American Bureau for Medical Aid to China [Box 30, Dr. Adele Cohn folder]. Rare Book and Manuscript Library, Columbia University in the City of New York.

13. Freda Utley. "If You Could See What I Have Seen," *Asia Magazine*, July 1941. Accessed in: Medical Aid to China 1938–1945, United China Relief Collection [Box 2, folder 12]. New York: New York Public Library.

14. Correspondence from Dr. Robert Lim, Director General Medical Relief Corps to Dr. C.T. Wang, President National Red Cross Society, August 4, 1939, American Bureau for Medical Aid to China Records [Box 8, National Red Cross Society of China Reports folder]. Rare Book and Manuscript Library, Columbia University in the City of New York.

15. Correspondence from Mrs. Hilda Selwyn-Clarke to Ms. Mildred Price, China Aid Council, January 5, 1940, American Bureau for Medical Aid to China Records [Box 22, Foreign Auxiliary to the Chinese Red Cross

folder]. Rare Book and Manuscript Library, Columbia University in the City of New York.
16. Correspondence from Dr. Robert Lim to Dr. C.T. Wang, October 24, 1939, American Bureau for Medical Aid to China Records [Box 23, National Red Cross Society of China reports folder]. Rare Book and Manuscript Library, Columbia University in the City of New York.
17. Correspondence from Dr. Robert Lim to Dr. C.T. Wang, November 5, 1939, American Bureau for Medical Aid to China Records [Box 22, National Red Cross Society of China folder]. Rare Book and Manuscript Library, Columbia University in the City of New York.
18. Correspondence from Dr. Robert Lim to Dr. C.T. Wang, December 14, 1939, American Bureau for Medical Aid to China Records [Box 22, National Red Cross Society of China folder]. Rare Book and Manuscript Library, Columbia University in the City of New York.
19. Jensen, *China Siegt*, 10.
20. Readers interested in the complex relationship between Germany and China from 1937 to 1939 are directed to Wolfram Adolphi and Peter Merker, *Deutschland und China 1937-1949* (Berlin, Germany: Akadamie Verlag GmbH, 1998).
21. Israel Epstein, *My China Eye: Memoirs of a Jew and a Journalist* (San Francisco, CA: Long River Press, 2015).
22. Shalom Wald, *China and the Jewish People, Old Civilizations in a New Era* (Jerusalem, Israel: Gefen Publishing House, 2004), 10-63.
23. Becker, *Als Arzt in China*, 5.
24. Iancu, *9 Ani Medic Pe Front Spania-China*, 103.
25. *Ibid.*, 102-103.
26. Unschuld, *You Banfa*, 77.
27. Iancu, *9 Ani Medic Pe Front Spania-China*, 102-103.
28. Freudmann, *Tschi-Lai!* 55.
29. Interview with Lu Yumming and Zhang Wenjin and the MacKinnons, April 14, 1985, as quoted in MacKinnon, J. and MacKinnon, S., *Agnes Smedley: The Life and Time of an American Radical*, 377.
30. Robert Payne, *Chungking Diaries* (London: William Heinemann Ltd, 1945), 420.
31. Chung, *Of Rats, Sparrows and Flies*, 89.
32. *Ibid.*, 100.
33. Anna Wang, *Ich Kämpfe fur Mao* (Hamburg, Germany: Holsten Verlag, 1973), 261.
34. Communication from Dr. Robert Lim to Dr. Harry Talbot, Changsha September 2, 1938, American Bureau for Medical Aid to China records [Box 26, National Red Cross Society of China, Dr. Robert Lim folder], Rare Book and Manuscript Library, Columbia University in the City of New York.
35. Freudmann, *Tschi-Lai!* 96-97.
36. Becker, *Als Arzt in China*, 9.
37. Dr. Schön Unit 57.3 report to Chinese Red Cross headquarters, October 2, 1941, Guiyang Archives, Guiyang, China.
38. Dr. Carl Coutelle, in personal memories (German). Unpublished, in Dr. Charles Coutelle's possession.
39. Becker, *Als Arzt in China*, 9.
40. Relief work in China (folder 4) (img 10-32); State of Medicine in the Chinese Army, 1944, The National Archives of the UK (TNA), FO 371-41557.
41. Xi Gao, "Foreign Models of Medicine in Twentieth Century China," eds. Bridie Andrews and Mary Brown Bullock, *Medical Transitions in Twentieth Century China* (Bloomington: Indiana University Press, 2014), 192.
42. Correspondence from Dr. Leo Eloesser: The teaching of medicine and the organization of medical services in China, November 4, 1946, American Bureau for Medical Aid to China Records [Series II: Box 8, Leo Eloesser folder]. Rare Book and Manuscript Library, Columbia University in the City of New York.
43. Correspondence from Dr. Leo Eloesser to Ms. Stevens, March 16, 1942, American Bureau for Medical Aid to China Records [Series II: Box 8, Leo Eloesser folder]. Rare Book and Manuscript Library, Columbia University in the City of New York.
44. Watt, *Saving Lives in Wartime China*, 2.
45. Frederic Wakeman, "Occupied Shanghai: The struggle between Chinese and Western Medicine," in *China at War*, eds. Stephen Mackinnon, Diana Lary and Ezra Vogel (Stanford, CA: Stanford University Press, 2007); Volker Scheid and Sean Hsiang-lin Lei, "The Institutionalization of Chinese Medicine" eds. Bridie Andrews and Mary Brown Bullock, *Medical Transitions in Twentieth Century China* (Bloomington: Indiana University Press, 2014), 244-267.
46. Liping Bu, *Public Health and Modernization in China*, 177.
47. Mitchell Cappell, "Profound Long-Term Effects of Nazism on Patient Care in Gastroenterology," *The Israel Medical Association Journal*, Vol. 10: 259-61 (2008).
48. Volker Scheid and Sean Hsiang-lin Lei, "The Institutionalization of Chinese Medicine," eds. Bridie Andrews and Mary Brown Bullock, *Medical Transitions in Twentieth-Century China* (Bloomington: Indiana University Press, 2014), 247
49. E. Manheimer, "Evidence from the Cochrane Collaboration for Traditional Chinese Medicine Therapies," *Journal of Alternative and Complementary Medicine*, Vol. 9: 1001-1014 (2009).

50. Dr. Robert Lim's views on state medicine, American Bureau for Medical Aid to China Records [Box 22, National Red Cross Society of China, Robert Lim folder]. Rare Book and Manuscript Library, Columbia University in the City of New York.

51. Frederick Fu Liu, *A Military History of Modern China* (Princeton, NJ: Princeton University Press, 1956), 160.

52. Becker, *Als Arzt in China*, 10.

53. Drs. Chang Hsien-Lin's wife, Dr. Nieh Chung-En also served with the Chinese Red Cross/Medical Relief Corps and the Emergency Medical Service Training School.

54. Correspondence from Dr. Adele Cohn, November 17, 1941, American Bureau for Medical Aid to China Records [Box 30, Dr. Adele Cohn folder]. Rare Book and Manuscript Library, Columbia University in the City of New York.

55. Barilich, *Fritz Jensen*, 96.

56. Dr. Heinrich Kent letter from October 3, 1941, Friedricka Martin Collection, ALBA #1 [Box 3, Dr. Kent folder]. New York: Tamiment Library and Wagner Labor Archives, New York University.

57. Becker, *Als Arzt in China*, 11.

58. Harold Balme, "The Medical Emergency in China," *Lancet* (April 8, 1939), 836.

59. Dr. Adele (Cohn) Wright diary (English), January 14, 1942 entry. Unpublished; in possession of Max Wright.

60. Correspondence to Alfred Kohlberg from Dr. George Schön [Somogyi] and Dr. Leon Kamieniecki, January 8, 1943, American Bureau for Medical Aid to China Records [Box 38, Alfred Kohlberg file]. Rare Book and Manuscript Library, Columbia University in the City of New York.

Chapter 6

1. Gordon Stifler Seagrave, born in Rangoon, Burma, was the son of Baptist missionaries. He joined the U.S. Army Medical Corps in 1942 and authored the books, *The Burma Surgeon* (New York: W.W. Norton & Co., 1943) and *The Burma Surgeon Returns* (New York: W.W. Norton & Co., 1946).

2. Gordon Seagrave, *The Burma Surgeon Returns* (New York: W.W. Norton & Co., 1946), 30.

3. Report of Red Cross Unit 32, In Lukou, Hunan [China], January 1939-June 1940, American Bureau for Medical Aid to China Records [Box 26, National Red Cross of China, William Hu folder]. Rare Book and Manuscript Library, Columbia University in the City of New York.

4. Register of the Nym Wales Papers, July 1939: [Box 1-46 Box 5/10: Chinese Red Cross], Hoover Institution Archives. Stanford, CA.

5. Erich Landauer, "Recent Changes in the Refugee Situation in China," March 15, 1940, China Defence League Newsletters from the Hong Kong Central Committee of the China Defence League], Hoover Institution Archives, Stanford, CA.

6. John Rich diary entries from February 5 to September 20th, 1943, Travels in China, John F. Rich Papers [Box 1, Folder 5], Quaker and Special Collections, Haverford College, Haverford, PA.

7. Liu, *Military History of Modern China*, 138.

8. Dr. William Wu, Report of Red Cross Unit 1 and 18, January-June 1939, p. 4. American Bureau for Medical Aid to China Records [Series II; Box 22, National Red Cross Society of China folder]. Rare Book and Manuscript Library, Columbia University in the City of New York.

9. C.B. Stephenson. "Vitamin A, Infection, and Immune Function," *Annual Review of Nutrition*, 21:167-92 (2001).

10. Unschuld, *You Banfa*, 82-83.

11. Correspondence from Dr. Robert Lim (EMSTS) to Professor Addis, Chairman of Medicine, Stanford University, December 4, 1940, American Bureau for Medical Aid to China records [Box 22, National Red Cross of Society folder]. Rare Book and Manuscript Library, Columbia University in the City of New York.

12. Chinese Red Cross Reports: August-December 1938, p. 22, American Bureau for Medical Aid to China Records [Box 8, National Red Cross Society of China (Reports) folder]. Rare Book and Manuscript Library, Columbia University in the City of New York.

13. Communication from Dr. Lim (EMSTS), to Professor Addis, Chairman of Medicine, Stanford University, December 4, 1940, American Bureau for Medical Aid to China records [Box 22, National Red Cross of Society folder]. Rare Book and Manuscript Library, Columbia University in the City of New York.

14. Suggestions to improve the rations of the Chinese Army, Nov. 12, 1941, American Bureau for Medical Aid to China Records [National Institute of Health folder: 1940-1]. Rare Book and Manuscript Library, Columbia University in the City of New York.

15. Report to American Bureau for Medical Aid to China and the American Red Cross, June 10, 1941, American Bureau for Medical Aid to China Records [Box 8, National Health Administration, 1940-1941 folder]. Rare Book and Manuscript Library, Columbia University in the City of New York.

16. Correspondence from Dr. Robert McClure to Dr. Hume, 1942, American Bureau for Medical Aid to China Records [Series II, Box XVI, Dr. Robert McClure folder], Rare Book and Manuscript Library, Columbia University in the City of New York.
17. Agnes Smedley, *Battle Hymn of China* (London, England: Victor Gollanz Ltd., 1944), 347.
18. Letter from Dr. Robert Lim to Ms. Stephens, American Bureau for Medical Aid to China, American Bureau for Medical Aid to China Records [Box 22, National Red Cross Society of China, Dr. Robert Lim folder]. Rare Book and Manuscript Library, Columbia University in the City of New York.
19. Report shared on January 8, 1943, from Dr. Bachman to Mr. Kohlberg, American Bureau for Medical Aid to China Records [Series IV, Box 38, Alfred Kohlberg file]. Rare Book and Manuscript Library, Columbia University in the City of New York.
20. Robert Herzstein, *Henry R. Luce, Time and the American Crusade in Asia* (New York: Cambridge University Press, 2005), 65.
21. Correspondence from Arthur Kohlberg, American Bureau for Medical Aid to China Records [Series IV, Box 38, Mr. Alfred Kohlberg folder]. Rare Book and Manuscript Library, Columbia University in the City of New York.
22. Father Patrick J. Scanlon became a chief organizer for the underground food supply to the Weihsien internment camp in Shantung [Shandong] province, earning the nickname of "Friar Tucker" and "chief of the black market."
23. An interview with Father Scanlon, July 15, 1943, American Bureau for Medical Aid to China Records [Series IV, Box 38, Mr. Alfred Kohlberg folder]. Rare Book and Manuscript Library, Columbia University in the City of New York.
24. Correspondence from Major W.S. Flowers, British Red Cross to Dr. Bachman forwarded to American Bureau for Medical Aid to China according to Kohlberg, September 1, 1943, Changsha, American Bureau for Medical Aid to China Records [Series IV, Box 38, Alfred Kohlberg file]. Rare Book and Manuscript Library, Columbia University in the City of New York.
25. The American, Dr. Dwight Edwards spent more than forty years in China and served as the YMCA senior secretary in China prior to taking on the wartime role of Field Director of the United China Relief organization.
26. Gary Alan Fine, *Sticky Reputations: The Politics of Collective Memory in Midcentury America* (New York: Routledge, 2012), 164–5.
27. Correspondence from Major W.S. Flowers, British Red Cross to Dr. Bachman forwarded to American Bureau for Medical Aid to China according to Kohlberg, September 1, 1943, Changsha, American Bureau for Medical Aid to China Records [Series IV, Box 38, Alfred Kohlberg file]. Rare Book and Manuscript Library, Columbia University in the City of New York.
28. Correspondence to Alfred Kohlberg from Dr. George Bachman with approval of Dr. George Schön [Somogyi], September 3, 1943, Report on the living and health conditions of the two group armies on the Ichang front, Jan. 8, 1943, American Bureau for Medical Aid to China Records [Series IV, Box 38, Alfred Kohlberg file]. Rare Book and Manuscript Library, Columbia University in the City of New York.
29. Barbara Tuchman, *Stilwell and the American Experience in China* (New York: Macmillan, 1940), 265.
30. White, *Thunder Out of China*, 163.
31. Communication from British Consulate General to Foreign Office, Situation in Canton [Guangzhou] folder, March 11, 1946, The National Archives of the UK (TNA), FO 371\53598.
32. Hans Van de Ven, *War and Nationalism in China: 1925-1945* (London, England: Routledge Curzon, 2003), 295.
33. Dr. Robert Lim's views on state medicine, American Bureau for Medical Aid to China Records [Box 22, National Red Cross Society of China, Robert Lim folder]. Rare Book and Manuscript Library, Columbia University in the City of New York.
34. Correspondence to Dr. Co-Tui, American Bureau for Medical Aid to China from: Dr. C.Y. Wu, Chinese Red Cross, June 25, 1938, American Bureau for Medical Aid to China Records [Box 22, National Red Cross Society Hong Kong, Dr. Wu folder]. Rare Book and Manuscript Library, Columbia University in the City of New York.
35. National Red Cross Society of China (3rd Report): Aug–Dec 1938, p. 20, American Bureau for Medical Aid to China Records [Box 23, National Red Cross Society of China folder]. Rare Book and Manuscript Library, Columbia University in the City of New York.
36. Robert McClure, "Medical Aspects of the China War," *Public Health Nursing*, vol. 33, 640–645 (1941).
37. Yip, *Disease and the Fighting Men*, 174.
38. Nicole Barnes and James Watt, "The Influence of War on China's Modern Health Systems," *Medical Transitions in 20th Century China*, eds. Andrews, B. and Bullock, M.B., 241.
39. Correspondence to: Dr. Co-Tui, American Bureau for Medical Aid to China from Dr. Robert Lim, July 22, 1940, American Bureau

for Medical Aid to China Records [Box 22, National Red Cross Society of China, Dr. Robert Lim folder]. Rare Book and Manuscript Library, Columbia University in the City of New York.

40. Relief work in China (folder 4) State of Medicine in the Chinese Army, 1944, The National Archives of the UK (TNA), FO 371-41557.

41. Wounded Soldier in China: Abstract of the 4th report of the Chinese Medical Relief Corps, United China Relief Archive [Box 1, folder 6], Epidemics encountered Jan–Jun 1939, 19-25. New York: New York Public Library.

42. National Red Cross Society of China (3rd Report): Aug–Dec 1938, p. 20, American Bureau for Medical Aid to China Records [Box 23, National Red Cross Society of China folder]. Rare Book and Manuscript Library, Columbia University in the City of New York.

43. Ibid.

44. Jensen, *China Siegt*, 100.

45. Chung, *Of Rats, Sparrows and Flies*, 94.

46. "A Medical Service Training School and Hospital in Each War Area Is the Goal of Dr. Robert K.S. Lim." *Time* February 17, 1941: 64-66.

47. American Bureau for Medical Aid to China [Box 2, Army Medical College folder]. Rare Book and Manuscript Library, Columbia University in the City of New York.

48. National Red Cross Society of China (3rd Report), Aug–Dec 1938, American Bureau for Medical Aid to China Records [Box 23, National Red Cross Society of China folder]. Rare Book and Manuscript Library, Columbia University in the City of New York.

49. Wounded Soldier in China: Abstract of the 4th report of the Chinese Medical Relief Corps: Epidemics encountered January–June 1939, United China Relief Archive [Box 1, folder 6]. New York: New York Public Library.

50. Barilich, *Fritz Jensen*, 98.

51. Unschuld, *You Banfa*, 93.

52. Sichon, "Les Medecins des deux guerres," 57-64.

53. Correspondence to Dr. Robert Lim from Dr. Van Slyke, May 16, 1941, American Bureau for Medical Aid to China Records [Box 22, National Red Cross Society of China, Dr. Robert Lim folder]. Rare Book and Manuscript Library, Columbia University in the City of New York.

54. Correspondence from Dr. R. Lim Chinese Red Cross/Medical Relief Corps to Dr. Co-Tui, July 27, 1938, American Bureau for Medical Aid to China Records [Box 22, Red Cross Society of China folder, Robert Lim]. Rare Book and Manuscript Library, Columbia University in the City of New York.

55. Becker, *Als Arzt in China*, 5.

56. Dr. Robert B. McClure. "Dr. Robert Pollitzer, 1885-1968." Unpublished document obtained from Dr. McClure by John Watt. Referenced in Watt, *Saving Lives in Wartime China*, 220.

57. Unschuld, *You Banfa*, 75.

58. McClure, *Medical Aspects of the China War*, 643.

59. John Rich diary entries from February 5–September 20 1943, Travels in China, John F. Rich Papers [Box 1, Folder 5], Quaker and Special Collections, Haverford College, Haverford, PA.

60. American Bureau for Medical Aid to China [Box 21, National Health Administration 1942 folder, The National Health Administration, November 1942]. Rare Book and Manuscript Library, Columbia University in the City of New York.

61. Barilich, *Fritz Jensen*, p. 94.

62. George C. Kohn, *Encyclopedia of Plague and Pestilence: From Ancient Times to the Present* (New York: Infobase Publishing, 2008), 165.

63. May 1941 National Health Administration report from Director Dr. P.Z. King, American Bureau for Medical Aid to China Records [Box 2, Army Medical College folder]. Rare Book and Manuscript Library, Columbia University in the City of New York; National Health Administration, May 1941 report, American Bureau for Medical Aid to China Records [Box 2, Army Medical College folder]. Rare Book and Manuscript Library, Columbia University in the City of New York.

64. China Defense Supplies Collection, Medical, 1941 [Box 17/Folder 9]. Hoover Institution Archives, Stanford University, Stanford, CA.

65. National Health Administration report: May 1940–April 1941, American Bureau for Medical Aid to China Records [Box 2, Army Medical College folder]. Rare Book and Manuscript Library, Columbia University in the City of New York.

66. The information office of the Guiyang Municipal Government (2005), p. 63.

67. Report of Dr. Heinrich Kent, 2nd Group, Taoyan, China, November 1942, Guiyang, China: City of Guiyang Archives.

68. January 1939–June 1940 Report of Red Cross Unit 2, American Bureau for Medical Aid to China Records [Box 22, National Red Cross Society of China, William Hu folder]. Rare Book and Manuscript Library, Columbia University in the City of New York.

69. Ross Terrill, *Mao: A Biography* (Palo Alto, CA: Stanford University Press, 1999), 28.

70. George Hall, "Tuberculosis in China," *The British Journal of Tuberculosis*, Vol. 29, Issue 3, 132-144 (July 1935)

71. Report from P.Z. King, Director General of the National Health Administration Wartime program of Tuberculosis control, 1945, American Bureau for Medical Aid to China Records [Box 2, Army Medical College, PZ King folder]. Rare Book and Manuscript Library, Columbia University in the City of New York.
72. Army Medical Administration report, Dr. Lim., p. 33, American Bureau for Medical Aid to China Records [Box 2, Army Medical College folder]. Rare Book and Manuscript Library, Columbia University in the City of New York.
73. Relief work in China (folder 4) State of Medicine in the Chinese Army, 1944. The National Archives of the UK (TNA), FO 371-41557.
74. "Medical Aid for China." *The Lancet*, Vol. 238, Issue 6149 (July 5, 1941), 24.
75. Correspondence from Dr. Heinrich Kent to Friends, July 1941, Kweiyang [Guiyang], China, Friedricka Martin Collection, ALBA #1 [Box 3, Dr. Kent folder], Tamiment Library and Wagner Labor Archives, New York University.

Chapter 7

1. China Defence League, "A Brief Report of the New Fourth Army Medical Services, 1938–1939," Pam, RA527, Ch., p. 5. Hoover Institution Library.
2. Hannant, *The Politics of Passion*, 204–205.
3. Barilich, *Fritz Jensen*, 84.
4. James Bertram in China Defence League Newsletter, American Bureau for Medical Aid to China Records [Box 5, China Defence League folder]. Rare Book and Manuscript Library, Columbia University in the City of New York.
5. "Help the Northwest. Border Region Orphanage," June 20, 1939, China Defence League Newsletters (from the Hong Kong Central Committee of the China Defence League), DS777.533. R45 C393 [Jul. 1938–Nov. 1941], Hoover Institution Library.
6. Oral interview by Dr. Thomas Ots with Dr. Hans Müller. Personal communication with Michael Ruhland, Dusseldorf, Germany, August 2015 and Dr. Ots, October 2015.
7. Letter from Dr. Mary Gilchrist of the China Medical Aid Committee to Anthony Eden of the British Foreign Office, British and American relief work in china (folder 1), June 29, 1941. National Archives of the UK (TNA), FO 371-27681.
8. MacKinnon, *Agnes Smedley*, 217.
9. Becker, *Als Arzt in China*, 8.
10. Correspondence from Dr. Erich Mamlok to Robert Hirsch, Lukou, Hunan, China, January 18, 1940) (German), unpublished, in possession of Dr. Robert Mamlok.
11. Freudmann, *Tschi-Lai!* 71.
12. Becker, *Als Arzt in China*, 13.
13. Barilich, *Fritz Jensen*, 87.
14. Unschuld, *You Banfa*, 97.
15. Barilich, *Fritz Jensen*, 88.
16. Correspondence from Dr. Fritz Jensen to Dr. Len Crome, September 16, 1939, from Hsiang-Hospital, Changsha, Hunan, China. As quoted in A. Jackson (2012), 139.
17. Yin, *Walking Through Blood and Fire*, 176.
18. China Medical Aid Committee report, July 1940. The National Archives of the UK (TNA), FO 371/24667.
19. Ibid.
20. Freudmann, *Tschi-Lai!* 179.
21. Relief work in China (folder 4), State of medical services in China, 1944, The National Archives of the UK (TNA), FO 371-41557.
22. China Defence League Newsletters, August 1939 (from the Hong Kong Central Committee of the China Defence League) [Box 5, China Defence League Folder]. New York: Rare Book and Manuscript Library, Columbia University in the City of New York.
23. Relief work in China (folder 4), State of medical services in China, 1944, The National Archives of the UK (TNA), FO 371-41557.
24. Freudmann, *Tschi-Lai!* 50.
25. Basu, *Call of Yan-an*, Diary entry of November 14, 1939.
26. Chi, Pao-San, Report on the EMSTS training school, January 1942, AMBAC Records [Box 23, National Red Cross Society of China Reports]. New York: Rare Book and Manuscript Library, Columbia University in the City of New York.
27. Speech of Robert Lim, China Defence Supplies record: 1941–1943 [Box 17, Folder: 9 Medical], Hoover Institution Archives.
28. E. Landauer, "Field Report: Recent Changes in the Refugee Situation in China," March 15, 1940, China Defence League Newsletters (from the Hong Kong Central Committee of the China Defence League), DS777.533. R45 C393 [Jul. 1938–Nov. 1941], Hoover Institution Library.
29. Iancu, *9 Ani Medic Pe Front Spania-China*, 128.
30. Correspondence from Dr. Carl Coutelle to Dr. Rosa Coutelle, 1940, in personal memories (German). Unpublished, in Dr. Charles Coutelle's possession.
31. Correspondence from Dr. Erich Mamlok to Robert Hirsch, Lukou, Hunan, China, January 17, 1940 (German), Dr. Erich Mamlok

letters. Unpublished; in possession of Dr. Robert Mamlok.
32. Barilich, *Fritz Jensen*, 89.
33. Freudmann, *Tschi-Lai!* 91.
34. Relief work in China (folder 4), State of medical services in China, 1944, The National Archives of the UK (TNA), FO 371/41557.
35. Tuchman, *Stilwell and the American Experience in China*, 363.
36. Dr. Rolf Becker diary (German), June 18–20. Unpublished; in possession of Bernard Becker.
37. Graham Peck was an American author who witnessed and reported first-hand on the Japanese war in China. He joined the Office of War Information in Chongqing after Pearl Harbor and detailed their journey in his book, *Two Kinds of Time*, in 1950.
38. Graham Peck, *Two Kinds of Time* (Seattle: University of Washington Press, 2008), 11–20.
39. *Ibid.*, 31.
40. National Red Cross Society of China (3rd Report): Aug–Dec 1938, p. 20, American Bureau for Medical Aid to China Records [Box 22, Robert Lim Folder]. Rare Book and Manuscript Library Columbia University in the City of New York.
41. Report of Red Cross Unit 49, January 1939–June 1940, American Bureau for Medical Aid to China Records [Box 22, National Red Cross Society of China, William Hu folder]. Rare Book and Manuscript Library, Columbia University in the City of New York.
42. Iancu, *9 Ani Medic Pe Front Spania-China*, 114.
43. Smedley, *Battle Hymn of China*, 351.
44. The information office of the Guiyang Municipal Government (2005), 63.
45. Correspondence to Mrs. Hilda Selwyn-Clarke from Dr. Co-Tui, October 28, 1940, American Bureau for Medical Aid to China Records [Box 22, Foreign Auxiliary to the Chinese Red Cross folder]. Rare Book and Manuscript Library, Columbia University in the City of New York.
46. Correspondence to Dr. Co-Tui from Mrs. Hilda Selwyn-Clarke, November 13, 1940, American Bureau for Medical Aid to China Records [Box 22, Foreign Auxiliary to the Chinese Red Cross folder]. Rare Book and Manuscript Library, Columbia University in the City of New York.
47. Dr. Carl Coutelle, in personal memories (German). Unpublished, in Dr. Charles Coutelle's possession.
48. *Ibid.*
49. Watt, *Saving Lives in Wartime China*, 245.
50. Liping, *Public Health and Modernization in China*, 191.

Chapter 8

1. Frederic Wakeman, "Occupied Shanghai: The Struggle Between Chinese and Western Medicine," *China at War*, eds. Stephen Mackinnon, Diana Lary and Ezra F. Vogel (Stanford, CA: Stanford University Press, 2007), 269.
2. Ilona Ralf Sues, *Shark's Fins and Millet* (Boston: Little, Brown and Company, 1944), 89–90.
3. Watt. *Saving Lives in Wartime China*, 147–149.
4. Israel Epstein. *The Unfinished Revolution in China* (Boston: Little Brown and Co., 1947), 133.
5. Correspondence from Dr. Mary Gilchrist of the China Medical Aid Committee to Anthony Eden of the British Foreign Office, June 29, 1941, British and American Relief work in China (folder 1), The National Archives of the UK (TNA), FO 371-27681.
6. Anthony Eden was a close confident of Winston Churchill in the Foreign Office and became the leader of the House of Commons in 1942 and Prime Minister of the United Kingdom from 1955–1957.
7. Correspondence from Anthony Eden of the British Foreign Office to Dr. Mary Gilchrist of the China Medical Aid Committee, July 8, 1941, British and American Relief work in China (folder 1), The National Archives of the UK (TNA), FO 371-27681.
8. Correspondence from Dr. Robert McClure to Ms. Selwyn-Clarke. September 23, 1941, Red Cross activities in China folder, The National Archives of the UK (TNA), FO 676/301.
9. For a detailed account of this battle between the Guomindang Nationalist Party and the Chinese Communist Party forces see: G. Benton, New Fourth Army: *Communist Resistance Along the Yangtze and the Huai, 1938–1941* (Berkeley: University of California Press, 1999).
10. Epstein, *The Unfinished Revolution in China*, 134.
11. Correspondence from Dr. Erich Mamlok to Robert Hirsch, March 6, 1941 (German), Dr. Erich Mamlok letters. Unpublished; in possession of Dr. Robert Mamlok.
12. Correspondence from Hilda Selwyn-Clarke, Foreign Auxiliary of the National Red Cross Society of China to Archibald Clark Kerr, Red Cross Activities in China, July 8, 1941, The National Archives of the UK (TNA), FO 676/301.
13. Interview with Lu Yumming and Zhang Wenjin and the MacKinnons, April 14, 1985, as quoted in MacKinnon, J. and MacKinnon, S.,

The Life and Times of an American Radical, 377.
14. Watt, *Saving Lives in Wartime China*, 149.
15. MacKinnon, *The Life and Times of an American Radical*, 217.
16. Dr. Carl Coutelle, in personal memories (German). Unpublished, in Dr. Charles Coutelle's possession.
17. Chung, *Of Rats, Sparrows and Flies*, 90.
18. Letter from Dr. Kaneti to Dr. Lim at the Chinese Red Cross Medical Relief Corps Headquarters, June 18, 1941. Guiyang and Guizhou Archives, Guiyang, China.
19. Ms. Chon, nursing supervisor of the Chinese Red Cross, Chinese Red Cross folder, City of Guiyang and Province of Guizhou Archives, Guiyang, China.
20. Medical Aid to China 1938–1945, Dr. Robert Lim, Medical Relief Corps: Interview with *Central News* at Hong Kong meeting of the National Red Cross Society, February 28, 1941, United China Relief Collection [Box 2 folder 12]. New York: New York Public Library.
21. Dr. Robert Lim outlines medical relief work, China Information Committee daily bulletin, No 66, June 21, 1941, American Bureau for Medical Aid to China Archives [Box 23, Robert Lim folder]. Rare Book and Manuscript Library, Columbia University in the City of New York.
22. McClure, *Medical Aspects of the China War*, 644–645.
23. Watt, *Saving Lives in Wartime China*, 160.
24. The China Defense Supply Company was the organization established by the U.S. Government to oversee transport of lend-lease goods in the China-Burma-India Theater. Estimates are that the United States supplied China with lend-lease military supplies that amounted to less than 2 percent of all U.S. annual lend-lease aid to its allies during World War II.
25. Correspondence from Dr. Co-Tui, China Defense Supplies to Dr. Robert Lim, July 14, 1941, American Bureau for Medical Aid to China Records [Box 22, National Red Cross Society of China folder]. Rare Book and Manuscript Library, Columbia University in the City of New York.
26. Medical Aid to China 1938–1945, United China Relief Collection [Box 2 folder 12]. New York: New York Public Library.
27. Edward Hume, a missionary doctor, founded the Xiangya School of Medicine in association with the Yale-China Association. He led the Christian Medical Council for Overseas Work in China throughout the war.
28. Correspondence from Dr. Robert McClure c/o International Relief Committee, Guiyang, to Dr. Ed Hume, Christian Medical Council, Sept. 15, 1941, American Bureau for Medical Aid to China Records [Box 18, Dr. Robert McClure folder]. Rare Book and Manuscript Library, Columbia University in the City of New York.
29. John Rich diary entries from February 5–September 20th, 1943, Travels in China, John F. Rich Papers [Box 1, Folder 5], Quaker and Special Collections, Haverford College, Haverford, PA.
30. Communication from Evert Barger, B.G. Courtney, LRCM, Medical Relief Corps, DTM, Michael Sullivan and Phillip Wright to the British Secretary of State for Foreign Affairs, Medical and Red Cross Relief Folder, 1942, The National Archives of the UK (TNA), FO 676-456.
31. Alex Danchev and Shelagh Vainker, Michael Sullivan Obituary, *The Guardian (U.S. Edition)*, October 25, 2013.
32. Correspondence from Dr. Robert Lim to Dr. Co-Tui, December 12, 1941, American Bureau for Medical Aid to China Records [Box 22, National Red Cross Society of China folder]. Rare Book and Manuscript Library, Columbia University in the City of New York.
33. Correspondence to Ms. Stevens from Dr. Robert Lim M.R.C., American Bureau for Medical Aid to China Records [Box 22, National Red Cross Society of China folder]. Rare Book and Manuscript Library, Columbia University in the City of New York.
34. Iancu, *9 Ani Medic Pe Front Spania-China*, 119.
35. Freudmann, *Tschi-Lai!* 141.
36. This probably refers to Kanchou City, an older English name of Ganzhou, in Jiangxi, China. The Ganzhou airport originally was known as Kanchow (Kan Hsien) Airfield. It was used by the U.S. Army's 14th Air Force.
37. Barilich, *Fritz Jensen*, 94.
38. Letter from Dr. Carl Coutelle to Dr. Rosa Coutelle, August 10, 1942, Tuyunguan, China, Dr. Carl Coutelle, in personal memories (German). Unpublished, in Dr. Charles Coutelle's possession.
39. Distribution of Red Cross Medical Relief Corps Medical Service Units, December 10, 1942, American Bureau for Medical Aid to China Records [Box 23, National Red Cross Society of China Reports folder]. Rare Book and Manuscript Library, Columbia University in the City of New York.
40. Clifford Matthews and Donald Cheung, *Dispersal and Renewal: Hong Kong University During the War Years* (Hong Kong: Hong Kong University Press, 1998), 299.
41. Letter from the Spanish Doctors to the

China Medical Aid Committee, Message of Goodwill for China Folder, 1942, The National Archives of the UK (TNA), FO 371/35714.
42. Letter from January 3, 1942, in personal memories (German), Unpublished, in Dr. Charles Coutelle's possession. Email October 29, 2014.
43. Sichon, *Frantisek Kriegel*, 53.
44. Yin, *Walking Through Blood and Fire*, 159.
45. Dr. Carl Coutelle, in personal memories (German). Unpublished, in Dr. Charles Coutelle's possession. October 29, 2014.
46. Payne, *Chungking Diaries*, 415.
47. Letter from June 10, 1942, Dr. Carl Coutelle, in personal memories (German). Unpublished, in Dr. Charles Coutelle's possession.
48. Epstein, *The Unfinished Revolution in China*, 131.
49. Correspondence from Alfred Kohlberg, Chairman, Executive Committee, American Bureau for Medical Aid to China Records [Series IV: Box 38, Alfred Kohlberg folder]. Rare Book and Manuscript Library, Columbia University in the City of New York.
50. Correspondence from Alfred Kohlberg, August 1, 1943, American Bureau for Medical Aid to China Records [Series IV: Box 38, Alfred Kohlberg folder]. Rare Book and Manuscript Library, Columbia University in the City of New York.
51. Monthly report for August 1942 by Dr. Heinrich Kent, 2nd Group, Taoynan, Guiyang and Guizhou Archives, Guiyang, China.
52. Correspondence from Dr. Robert McClure to Paul Cadbury, March 1943, Pi Sheh Chai, Mengtze, Yunnan, China [Temp MSS 876, Box 13, Chinese Red Cross, 1943], Library of the Society of Friends, London.
53. Watt, *Saving Lives in Wartime China*, 154–164.

Chapter 9

1. Dr. Carl Coutelle, in personal memories (German). Unpublished, in Dr. Charles Coutelle's possession.
2. The Information Office of the Guiyang Municipal Government, *The International Medical Team in Guiyang*, 81.
3. *Ibid.*, 86.
4. Correspondence to Dr. Erich Mamlok, Dr. Erich Mamlok letters (German). Unpublished; in possession of Dr. Robert Mamlok.
5. Sichon, "Les Medecins des deux guerres," 57–64.
6. Iancu, *9 Ani Medic Pe Front Spania-China*, 150.
7. Joan Staniforth letter to her mother, February 17, 1943. Unpublished, in Bernard Becker's possession.
8. Freudmann, *Tschi-Lai!* 184.
9. Letter from Dr. Carl Coutelle to his wife, Dr. Rosa Coutelle, November 11, 1942, Tuyunguan, China, Dr. Carl Coutelle, in personal memories (German). Unpublished in Dr. Charles Coutelle's possession.
10. Iancu, *9 Ani Medic Pe Front Spania-China*, 152.
11. Dr. Carl Coutelle, in personal memories (German). Unpublished, in Dr. Charles Coutelle's possession. August 31, 2015.
12. Iancu, *9 Ani Medic Pe Front Spania-China*, 178.
13. The information office of the Guiyang municipal government, *The International Medical Team in Guiyang*, 89.
14. Freudmann, *Tschi-Lai!* 188.
15. Foreign refugee doctors in India 1943, Correspondence of February 8, 1943, From the Government of India to the British Embassy in Chungking [Chongqing], The National Archives of the UK (TNA), FO 371/35820.
16. Foreign refugee doctors in India 1943, February 6, 1943. The National Archives of the UK (TNA), FO 371/35820.
17. Foreign refugee doctors in India 1943, Correspondence from Horace James Seymour in Chungking [Chongqing] to the Foreign Office, February 16, 1943, The National Archives of the UK (TNA), FO 371/35820.
18. Foreign refugee doctors in India 1943, Correspondence to Mr. Silver in the India Office in Britain from the government of India home department, New Delhi, April 13, 1943, The National Archives of the UK (TNA), FO 371/35820.
19. The information office of the Guiyang municipal government, *The International Medical Team in Guiyang*, 87.
20. The Lend-Lease policy was a program under which the United States supplied the Allied nations with supplies between 1941 and August 1945.
21. Tuchman, *Stilwell and the American Experience in China*, 315.
22. Seagrave, *Burma Surgeon Returns*, 36–37.
23. Conference between Generals Joseph Stilwell and Ho Ying-ch'in, January 22, 1943, Microfilm reel #0202, Folder 3, TV Soong Collection, Hoover Institution Archives, published with the permission of the Soong family representative.
24. Tohmatsu Haruo, "The Strategic Correlation Between the Sino-Japanese and Pacific Wars," *The Battle for China: Essays on the Military History of the Sino-Japanese War of 1937–1945*, eds. Mark Peattie, Edward Drea and Hans

Van de Ven (Stanford, CA: Stanford University Press, 2011), 431.
25. Correspondence to General Marshall from TV Soong August 17, 1943, Microfilm reel #0204–205, Folder 3, TV Soong Collection, Hoover Institution Archives.
26. Dr. Carl Coutelle, in personal memories (German). Unpublished, in Dr. Charles Coutelle's possession.
27. Correspondence from General W.E. Bergen to Dr. Erich Mamlok, March 1, 1944, Dr. Erich Mamlok letters (German). Unpublished, in possession of Dr. Robert Mamlok.
28. Correspondence from General Boatner to Dr. Bedřich Kisch, HQ (Prov) 5303rd Area Command, Chinese Army in India, May 13, 1944, Památník národního písemnictví, Praha, Czech Republic.
29. Dr. Carl Coutelle, in personal memories (German). Unpublished, in Dr. Charles Coutelle's possession. June 15, 2014.
30. John Sweeney (1942–1945), *Ramgarh, Now It Can Be Told* (Senior Instructor, Chinese Training and Combat Command), John Sweeney Papers: [Box 1, Folder 1], Hoover Institution Archives, copyright Stanford University.
31. Lt. Col. E.M. Rice. "Medical Mother Goose," *CBI Roundup*, Vol. 1, No 11 (November 26, 1942).
32. Idem. Retrieved from http://www.dtic.mil/dtic/tr/fulltext/u2/a286774.pdf.
33. Iancu, *9 Ani Medic Pe Front Spania-China*, 27.
34. Ibid., 157–158.
35. Freudmann, *Tschi-Lai!* 193.
36. General Correspondence, Entry # UD-UP 7, Container 9, ARC #6317867, Record Group 0493, U.S. Forces in the C-B-I theaters of operations, India–Burma theater of operations, U.S. Army/Historical Section National Archives at College Park, College Park, MD.
37. Tuchman, *Stilwell and the American Experience in China*, 329.
38. Historical records 1941–1946, North Burma Campaign Reports to Mountbatten, ARC #565374, Entry # UD-UP 105, Container 652, U.S. Forces in the C-B-I theaters of operations, India-Burma theater of operations, U.S. Army/Historical Section, Record Group 0493, National Archives at College Park, College Park, MD.
39. W. Ruifu, "After Flying Over the Hump: An Army Interpreters Report," in J. Pei, *Under the Same Flag: Recollections of the Veterans of World War II* (Beijing, China: China Intercontinental Press, 2005), 236–237.
40. *Burma Surgeon* was rated in December 1943 as the second best-selling book by the *New York Times*.

41. Seagrave, *Burma Surgeon Returns*, 61.
42. Zang Yunhu, "Chinese Operations in Yunnan and Central Burma," *The Battle for China: Essays on the Military History of the Sino-Japanese War of 1937–1945*, eds. Mark Peattie, Edward Drea and Hans Van de Ven (Stanford, CA: Stanford University Press, 2011), 390.
43. Hukwang Valley in the state of Kachin in northern Burma is ringed by steep mountains on the north, east, and west. It is known as the world's largest tiger preserve.
44. Correspondence to Dr. Van Slyke from Colonel Haueh Ying Kwei, Surgeon, A Peking University Medical College and EMSTS graduate assigned to the 38th Division and then promoted to the 1st Chinese Army in India, American Bureau for Medical Aid to China Records [Box AMA, Robert Lim Reports 11–16 folder]. Rare Book and Manuscript Library, Columbia University in the City of New York.
45. T. Durdin. "Best Care of Chinese In History," *CBI Roundup*, Vol. II, Issue No. 25, Delhi, India (March 2, 1944).
46. Sichon, *Frantisek Kriegel*, 54.
47. Seagrave, *Burma Surgeon Returns*, 105.
48. Correspondence from Lt. Col. V. Slater to Dr. Bedřich Kisch, Chinese Army in India, March 30, 1944, Dr. Bedřich Kisch Archives, Památník národního písemnictví, Prague, Czech Republic.
49. Incoming messages 1942–45, Records of the Chinese Army in India, Entry #UD-UP 216, Container #33, ARC #6741020, Record Group 0493 U.S. Forces in the C-B-I theaters of operations, India-Burma theater of operations National Archives at College Park, College Park, MD.
50. Relief work in China, Repatriation folder, 1945, The National Archives of the UK (TNA), FO 371/46158.
51. Historical records 1941–1946, North Burma Campaign Reports to Mountbatten, ARC #565374, Entry # UD-UP 105, Container 652, U.S. Forces in the C-B-I theaters of operations, India-Burma theater of operations, U.S. Army/Historical Section, Record Group 0493, National Archives at College Park, College Park, MD.
52. Dr. Erich Mamlok, personal communication with Dr. Robert Mamlok.
53. Edward J. Drea and Hans Van de Ven, "An Overview of Major Military Campaigns During the Sino Japanese War: 1937–1945," *The Battle for China: Essays on the Military History of the Sino-Japanese War of 1937–1945*, eds. Mark Peattie, Edward Drea and Hans Van de Ven (Stanford, CA: Stanford University Press, 2011), 46.
54. Order from Colonel Breidster to Dr.

Walter Freudmann and Dr. Erich Mamlok. Unpublished; in possession of Dr. Robert Mamlok.

55. Lui, *A Military History of Modern China*, 215.

56. Correspondence from Lt. Colonel L.J. Bullis to the Commanding General (July 12, 1945). Unpublished; in possession of Dr. Robert Mamlok.

57. Dr. Erich Mamlok letters, Award of the emblem of meritorious civilian service (October 25, 1945). Unpublished; in possession of Dr. Robert Mamlok.

58. Correspondence from Lt. Colonel LJ Bullis to the Commanding General, July 12, 1945, Dr. Bedřich Kisch Archives, Památník národniho pisemnictvi, Praha, Czech Republic.

59. Anonymous correspondent, "Surgeon praises Chinese courage," *CBI Roundup*, April 13, 1944. Vol. II, Issue No. 31, Delhi, India.

60. General Correspondence, Records of the Chinese Army in India, Entry # UD-UP 215: Decimal Files 1943–5, Container 28, ARC #6780874, RG 0493 U.S. Forces in the C-B-I theaters of operations, India-Burma theater of operations, National Archives at College Park, College Park, MD.

61. Iancu, *9 Ani Medic Pe Front Spania-China*, 246.

62. Correspondence to Dr. Erich Mamlok, Dr. Erich Mamlok letters (German). Unpublished; in possession of Dr. Robert Mamlok.

63. Sichon, *Frantisek Kriegel*, 52.

Chapter 10

1. The Burma Road was not the only civil engineering marvel of the time. When the Japanese were sighted in the Aleutian Islands in June 1942, the Army Corps of Engineers began frantic construction of the Alaska Highway and completed their work in the fall of 1942.

2. Lyle Powell, *A Surgeon in Wartime China* (Lawrence: University of Kansas Press, 1946), 21.

3. John Rich diary entries from February 5–September 20, 1943, Travels in China, John F. Rich Papers [Box 1, Folder 5], Quaker and Special Collections, Haverford College, Haverford, PA.

4. Correspondence quoted from Dr. Robert McClure in Kenneth Bennett's, *Memorandum on Minute Seven* [Temp MSS 876, Box 13 Chinese Red Cross, 1943], Library of the Society of Friends, London.

5. Davies, *Friends Ambulance Unit*, 272.

6. Scott, *Bob McClure*, 308.

7. In 1910, Paul Ehrlich, a Jewish-German chemist, announced a combination of arsenic with other drugs that he claimed would destroy the spirochetes without killing the patient. Ehrlich continued his experiments until he performed 914, giving us the effective antibiotic neo-salvarsan, which he named "914." He received the Nobel Prize for this work. A street in Germany was named for him in 1910 but was renamed during the Third Reich, but after the war, Ehrlich's name was restored to the street. Mercury bichloride was used to treat syphilis in the pre-antibiotic era, though its toxicity limited its utility. The treatment of syphilis with mercury bichloride became popular in wartime China. Subsequent, "preliminary" reports of its value would continue to appear several years after the war.

8. Correspondence from Dr. Robert McClure to Michael Harris, July 8, 1942, Pi Sheh Chai, Mengtze, Yunnan, China, Temp MSS 876 [Box 13, Chinese Red Cross, 1943], Library of the Society of Friends, London.

9. Correspondence from Dr. Robert McClure, June 9, 1943, Temp MSS 876 [Box 13, Chinese Red Cross, 1943], Library of the Society of Friends, London.

10. Becker, *Als Arzt in China*, 15.

11. Barilich, *Fritz Jensen*, 117.

12. Joan (Staniforth) Becker, Letter to her mother, February 17, 1943. Unpublished; in possession of Mr. Bernard Becker.

13. Unschuld, *You Banfa*, 125.

14. Confidential report on the EMSTS and the Medical Relief Corps, April 1943, American Bureau for Medical Aid to China Records [Series IV: Box 38, Alfred Kohlberg]. Rare Book and Manuscript Library, Columbia University in the City of New York.

15. John Rich diary entries from February 5–September 20th, 1943, Travels in China, John F. Rich Papers [Box 1, Folder 5], Quaker and Special Collections, Haverford College, Haverford, PA.

16. Correspondence from Dr. Adele Cohn, February 5, 1943, American Bureau for Medical Aid to China Records [Box 30, Dr. Adele Cohn folder]. Rare Book and Manuscript Library, Columbia University in the City of New York.

17. Correspondence from Helen Stevens to the American Bureau for Medical Aid to China Board, September 22nd, 1943, American Bureau for Medical Aid to China Records [Box 38, Miscellaneous letters], Rare Book and Manuscript Library, Columbia University in the City of New York.

18. Correspondence from Dr. McClure to Dr. Van Slyke, Feb 16, 1943, American Bureau for Medical Aid to China Records [Box 18, Dr. Robert McClure Folder]. Rare Book and Man-

uscript Library, Columbia University in the City of New York.

19. John Rich diary entries from March 29–April 3, 1943, John F. Rich Papers [Box 1, Folder 5], Quaker and Special Collections, Haverford College, Haverford, PA.

20. Medical Units of the National Red Cross of China, July 1943, American Bureau for Medical Aid to China Records [Box 22, Foreign Auxiliary to the Chinese Red Cross, Dr. Robert Lim folder]. Rare Book and Manuscript Library, Columbia University in the City of New York.

21. Becker, *Als Arzt in China*, 74.

22. Ni Dandan, "The Norman Bethune of Romania," *Global Times*, December 30, 2014, http://www.globaltimes.cn/content/899285.shtml.

23. Rebecca Ewing Peterson, Find a grave: Bucur Clejan, Accessed on June 21, 2016, http://www.findagrave.com/cgi-bin/fg.cgi?page=grandGRid=116231592andref=acom.

24. Correspondence from Dr. Bob McClure to the unit M.O. in Kutsing from Hsiakwan, Yunnan, July 27, 1944 [Temp MSS 876, Box 13, Chinese Red Cross, 1943], Library of the Society of Friends, London.

25. Correspondence to Dr. Van Slyke from Dr. Cohn, November 29, 1943, American Bureau for Medical Aid to China Records [Box 30: Dr. Adele Cohn folder]. Rare Book and Manuscript Library, Columbia University in the City of New York.

26. Letter from Dr. Lurje to Dr. Jung, Guiyang City and Guizhou Province Archives, Guiyang, China.

27. Michael Harris' report on visits to hospitals, March 28, 1944 [Temp MSS 876, Box 13, Chinese Red Cross, 1943], Library of the Society of Friends, London.

28. *Ibid.*

29. Jay Taylor. *The Generalissimo: Chiang kai Shek and the Struggle for Modern China* (Cambridge, MA: Belknap Press, 2011), 276.

30. Correspondence to Dr. Van Slyke from Dr. Adele Cohn, June 11, 1944, American Bureau for Medical Aid to China Records [Box 30, Dr. Adele Cohn folder]. Rare Book and Manuscript Library, Columbia University in the City of New York.

31. Agnes Smedley Collection, V 18 Group 5, 72–9, James Burke Hospital Reports, September 1944. Tempe, AZ: Arizona State University Libraries: University Archives.

32. *Ibid.*

33. Agnes Smedley Collection, V 18, Group 5, May 1945 newsletter. Tempe, AZ: Arizona State University Libraries: University Archives.

34. Some argue that T.V. Song rather than Chiang Kai-Shek had pressed for General Stilwell's recall, but his dismissal was initially opposed by Song Meiling and Song Ailing, who viewed TV as a potential threat to their respective husbands, Chiang Kai-Shek and H.H. Kung.

35. Dean Atchison, "The Chinese Crisis," *New York Times* (November 1, 1944).

36. Jesperson. *American Images of China*, 120–121.

37. Correspondence from Madame Sun Yat-sen to Mildred Price, December 1944, Register of the Nym Wales Papers [Box 5/34: Mildred Price], Hoover Institution Archives.

38. Dr. Carl Coutelle, in personal memories (German). Unpublished, in Dr. Charles Coutelle's possession. August 3, 2014.

39. Personal communication from Dr. Erich Mamlok to Dr. Robert Mamlok, ca. 1971.

40. "Japanese drive to Guiyang." *New York Times* (November 30, 1944).

41. Correspondence from Dr. Robert Lim to Dr. Van Slyke, December 19, 1944, American Bureau for Medical Aid to China Records [Box 2, Army Medical Administration (Robert Lim reports 1–10) folder]. Rare Book and Manuscript Library, Columbia University in the City of New York.

42. Correspondence to Dr. Van Slyke from: Dr. Robert Lim, Dec 22, 1944, American Bureau for Medical Aid to China Records [Box 2, Army Medical Administration (Robert Lim reports 1–10) folder]. Rare Book and Manuscript Library, Columbia University in the City of New York.

43. Correspondence from Dr. Adele Cohn, February 5, 1943, American Bureau for Medical Aid to China Records [Box 30: Dr. Adele Cohn folder]. Rare Book and Manuscript Library, Columbia University in the City of New York.

44. Unschuld, *You Banfa*, 91.

45. Correspondence from Dr. Adele (Cohn) Wright, January 25, 1945, American Bureau for Medical Aid to China Records [Box 30: Dr. Adele Cohn folder]. Rare Book and Manuscript Library, Rare Book and Manuscript Library, Columbia University in the City of New York.

46. Correspondence to Dr. Van Slyke from Dr. Adele Cohn, April 2, 1945, American Bureau for Medical Aid to China Records [Box 30: Dr. Adele Cohn folder]. Rare Book and Manuscript Library, Columbia University in the City of New York.

47. Correspondence from Dr. Adele (Cohn) Wright, September 4, 1945, American Bureau for Medical Aid to China Records [Box 30: Dr. Adele Cohn folder]. Rare Book and Manuscript Library, Columbia University in the City of New York.

48. Barilich, *Fritz Jensen*, 116.

49. Joan Staniforth Becker letter, May 8, 1945. Unpublished; in possession of Bernard Becker.
50. Correspondence from Dr. Robert Lim, American Bureau for Medical Aid to China Records [Box 13, Robert Lim folder]. Rare Book and Manuscript Library, Columbia University in the City of New York.
51. Correspondence from Dr. Robert Lim to Dr. Van Slyke, June 17, 1945, American Bureau for Medical Aid to China Records [Box 2, Army Medical Administration, Robert Lim Reports 17–22 folder). Rare Book and Manuscript Library, Columbia University in the City of New York.
52. Ibid.
53. The nine British-sponsored physicians who left England were Drs. Becker, Jensen, Kisch, Iancu, Baer, Kaneti, Freudmann, Coutelle, and Kent. The ten Norwegian-sponsored healthcare providers were the physicians Drs. Taubenfligel, Kriegel, Volokhine, Schon, Kranzdorf, Kamieniecki, Jungermann, Flato, and the radiology technician Mania Kamieniecki and medical student Edith Marens (Marcus Jungermann).
54. Relief work in China, Repatriation folder (image 361-8), 1945, from Dr. Mary Gilchrist of the China Medical Aid Committee to the Chinese Embassy, April 6, 1945, The National Archives of the UK (TNA), FO 371/46158.
55. Foreign refugee doctors in India 1943 folder, The Foreign Service of the United States to the UK Foreign Service, June 8, 1945, The National Archives of the UK (TNA), FO 371/35820.
56. Ibid.
57. Foreign refugee doctors in India 1943 folder, From the External Affairs office of the Government of India to Great Britain, August 8, 1945, The National Archives of the UK (TNA), FO 371/35820.
58. Dr. Erich Mamlok letters, Communication from General Boatner, Chief of staff to Dr. Erich Mamlok, Headquarters of the China Combat Command, U.S. Forces, Kunming, China, June 6, 1945. Unpublished; in possession of Dr. Robert Mamlok.
59. Barilich, *Fritz Jensen*, 126.
60. Dr. Erich Mamlok letters, Correspondence from Paul Elza, Acting United Nations Relief and Rehabilitation Administration personnel officer to Dr. Erich Mamlok, September 24, 1945. Unpublished; in possession of Dr. Robert Mamlok.
61. Dr. Adele Cohn Diary, June 6, 1943, p. 8.
62. Dr. Carl Coutelle, in personal memories (German). Unpublished, in Dr. Charles Coutelle's possession. October 5, 2014.
63. USAAF Air Transport Command receipt of Dr. Kisch, Correspondence of Dr. Bedřich Kisch, Památník národniho písemnictví, Praha, Czech Republic.
64. Sichon, *Frantisek Kriegel*, 53.
65. Iancu, *9 Ani Medic Pe Front Spania-China*, 160.
66. Hackl, *In Fester Umarmung*, 300.
67. Relief work in China, 1945, The National Archives of the UK (TNA), FO 371/46160.
68. Maritime records, Aberdeen and Commonwealth Line, Largs Bay vessel, Departing Bombay to London, November 11, 1946. Retrieved from http://www.ancestry.com/immigration.
69. Becker, *Als Arzt in China*, p. 18.
70. United Nations Archives, S-0399-0001-02. United Nations Relief and Rehabilitation Administration fonds. [AG-18-001 China Office File [Box: S-0528-0547 Regional Offices Liuchow, Folder: Reports—from Kent, Dr.—S-1159-0000-0037], Correspondence from H. Kent, Acting Regional Medical Director to Dr. R. Borcic, Chief medical Officer, United Nations Relief and Rehabilitation Administration, May 6, 1946.
71. United Nations Archives, S-0399-0001-02. United Nations Relief and Rehabilitation Administration fonds. [AG-18-001 China Office File, Box: S-0528-0144, Administration—Central Registry, Folder: Medical Division] Correspondence from Ira Hirschsy, Chief Medical Officer, United Nations Relief and Rehabilitation Administration, January 8, 1948.
72. United Nations Archives, S-0399-0001-02. United Nations Relief and Rehabilitation Administration fonds. [AG-18-001 China Office File, Box: S0528-0136, Administration Registry, Folder: Health Division, Tsingtao], Correspondence form Grank Harrington, Medical Officer United Nations Relief and Rehabilitation Administration to Stanley Leland, Chief Medical Officer, United Nations Relief and Rehabilitation Administration, May 27, 1947.
73. United Nations Archives, S-0399-0001-02. United Nations Relief and Rehabilitation Administration fonds. [AG-18-001 China Office File, Box: S-0528-0488, Kamieniecki folder], Correspondence from Dr. Kamieniecki to Clay Hansen, Acting Chief Regional Representative United Nations Relief and Rehabilitation Administration, Hengyang, January 15, 1947.
74. From a correspondent, "Medical Aid to China," British Medical Journal, March 16, 1946, p. 400.

Chapter 11

1. Correspondence from Dr. Wolf Jungery to Fredericka Martin, January 10, 1979. Okla-

homa City, OK, Fredericka Martin Papers [ALBA #1 Box 4, Poland: Wolf Jungery folder]. New York: Tamiment Library and Wagner Labor Archives, New York University.

2. Personal communication with Karin (nee Jungery) Kleiner, 2016.

3. Dr. Wolf Jungery obituary, The Oklahoman, October 5, 1989.

4. Rodriguez MH, Jungery M. A protein on Plasmodium falciparum-infected erythrocytes functions as a transferring receptor. Nature 1986 Nov 27–Dec 3;324 (6095):388–91.

5. Personal communication with Adam Taubenfligel in Guiyang, China, September 1, 2015.

6. Filip Kubicz-Andryszak, Azja-Pacifyk: Spoleczenstwo, polityka, kultura (Warsaw, Poland: Rocznik, 2005), 39–42.

7. Retrieved from http://www.holocaust.cz/en/database-of-victims/victim/23403-hugo-mamlok and http://www.holocaust.cz/en/database-of-victims/victim/27962-selma-proskauer/

8. Correspondence from Dr. Pfabel, State Board of Health, City of Berlin to Dr. Erich Mamlok, January 9, 1948, Dr. Mamlok letters. Unpublished; in possession of Dr. Robert Mamlok.

9. Robitzek, E, Selikoff, I.J., Mamlok E., "Isoniazid and Its Isopropyl Derivative in the Therapy of Tuberculosis in Humans," Chest, 23(1): 1–15 (1953).

10. Readers interested in the wartime story of the Jewish Hospital of Berlin are directed to D.B. Silver, Refuge in Hell (New York: Houghton Mifflin Company, 2003).

11. Correspondence from Agnes Smedley to Anna Wang, August 31, 1946, Agnes Smedley Collection [Box 1, folder 9]. Tempe, AZ: Arizona State University.

12. Dr. Walter Lurje Presents Short Concert, TPEA, The Rusk Cherokeean (Rusk, Tex.), Vol. 105, No. 7, Ed. 1 Thursday, August 14, 1952. Accessed on July 2, 2016, http://texashistory.unt.edu/ark:/67531/metapth326324/m1/4/.

13. Personal communication with Bernard Becker, 2016.

14. Personal communication with Dr. Charles Coutelle, 2017.

15. Unschuld, You Banfa, 77.

16. Yin, Walking Through Blood and Fire, 357.

17. The information office of the Guiyang municipal government, The International Medical Team (2005), 114.

18. H. Domeinski, 40 Jahre Landambulatorium "Dr. Herbert Baer" Golssen—Sozialistische Gesundheitspolitik auf dem Lande: Beiträge des Kolloquiums Anlässlich des 40. Jahrestages der Gründung des Ersten Landambulatoriums am 25. November 1988 in Golssen (Akad. für Ärztliche Fortbildung, Arbeitsgruppe Geschichte des Gesundheitswesens, 1989).

19. R. Becker and M. Strasse, "Fritz Jensen in Memoriam," The Journal for the Advancement of Medicine, Volume No. 13 (July 1, 1955).

20. Correspondence from Dr. Ausubel to Fredericka Martin, Fredericka Martin Papers [Box 3, Dr. Edith Kent Folder]. New York: Tamiment Library and Wagner Labor Archives, New York University.

21. Landauer, Lexikon der Osterreichischen Spanienkämpfer, 133.

22. Hackl, In Fester Umarmung, 301.

23. L. Tauber, Preserving Jewish Memory. Accessed on June 20, 2016, http://www.centropa.org/biography/lilli-tauber

24. Walter Freudmann, Qi lái! (Arise!): A Physician's Adventures in China and Burma, 1939–1945, Katzenschwanz Edition (Los Gatos, CA: Smashwords, 2012), 9.

25. Clegg, Aid China 1937–1939, 103.

26. Karel Pacner, Osudove okamziky Ceskoslovenska (Prague, Czech Republic: Albatros, 1997), 455–6.

27. Sichon, Frantisek Kriegel, 57.

28. Bergmann, Internationalisten an den Antifaschistischen Fronten, 70.

29. Personal communication with Dr. Joseph and Peter Somogyi. 2017.

30. List of Hungarian participants, Fredericka Martin Papers [ALBA #1, Box 2, Hungary folder]. New York: Tamiment Library and Wagner Labor Archives, New York University.

31. Personal communication with Peter and Dr. Joseph Somogyi, Brussels, Belgium, December 2, 2016.

32. Idem.

33. The Frantisek Kriegel Award, founded in 1987, is awarded annually to a person who has fought for human rights. The Fritz Jensen Prize was awarded annually from 1960–65.

Chapter 12

1. Foreign doctors honored for aiding China during World War II, Accessed on September 6, 2015. Retrieved from http://newscontent.cctv.com/NewJsp/news.jsp?fileId=314938.

2. Chung, Of Rats, Sparrows and Flies, 89.

3. Jensen, Some Features of War Surgery, 95.

4. Ibid., 98–100.

5. The information office of the Guiyang municipal government, The International Medical Team, 63; Fritz Jensen, Some Features of War Surgery, 7.

6. Scott, Bob McClure, 120.

7. Chung, Of Rats, Sparrows and Flies, 98.

8. China Medical Aid Committee report, July 1940, The National Archives of the UK (TNA), FO 371/24667.
9. Agnes Smedley, *Battle Hymn of China* (London: Victor Gollanz Ltd., 1944), 347.
10. Jonathan Goldstein, "Shanghai as a mosaic and microcosm of Eurasian Jewish identities, 1850–1950" in *Religions and Christianity in Today's China*, Vol. 3, No. 2 (2013) p 38.

Appendix B

1. Inscription shared with the International Medical Relief Corps' Memorial in Tuyunguan Park unveiling, Guiyang, China, August 2015.

Appendix C

1. A close affiliate of Chairman Mao Zedong and survivor of the Long March, Chu Teh became Commander in Chief of the Red Army.
2. Janice MacKinnon and Stephen MacKinnon, *Agnes Smedley: The Life and Times of an American Radical* (Los Angeles: University of California Press, 1988), 199.
3. Deepak, *My Life with Kotnis,* 365.
4. Wuchang is part of the urban core of Wuhan, the capital of Hupeh [Hubei] province.
5. Basu, *Call of Yanan,* 36–37.
6. Idem., 68.
7. Rana Mitter, *Forgotten Ally: China's World War II, 1937–1945* (New York: Houghton Mifflin Harcourt Publishing, 2013), 223.
8. Wang Bingnam (Ping-nan) was the husband of German journalist Anneliese "Anna" (Maertens) Wang, a future friend of the International Medical Relief Corps' physicians and they became close confidents of Zhou Enlai in the Chinese Communist Party.
9. Basu, *Call of Yanan,* 82.
10. B.R. Deepak, *My Life with Kotnis* (Beijing, China: Manak Publications, 2006), 362.
11. The University of Edinburgh Medical School holds the distinction of offering the first Chinese student, Wang Fun, the opportunity of graduating from a Western medical school in 1855.
12. Deepak, *My Life with Kotnis,* 365.
13. Idem., 376.
14. Reports of the Curative Units of the Red Cross Medical Relief Corps, Report of the 3rd curative unit. December 1937–December 1938, American Bureau for Medical Aid to China Records [Box 8, National Health Administration, Dr. P.Z. King folder]. Rare Book and Manuscript Library, Columbia University in the City of New York.

15. "New 4th Army Medical Services," April 1, 1939, China Defence League Newsletters (from the Hong Kong Central Committee of the China Defence League), DS777.533. R45 C393 [Jul 1938–Nov. 1941], Hoover Institution Library.
16. Correspondence from the British Embassy to the Foreign Office, March 15, 1943, Messages of goodwill for China, Folder 7, 1943, The National Archives of the UK (TNA), FO 371-35717.
17. Report of the 38th Curative unit, February 1938–November 1938, American Bureau for Medical Aid to China Records [Box 8, National Health Administration, Dr. P.Z. King folder]. Rare Book and Manuscript Library, Columbia University in the City of New York.
18. Allan Levine, "'I Dare Do All...': The Saga of Dr. Tillson Lever Harrison," *Canadian Medical Association Journal,* 177 (10): 1237–1239 (November 6, 2007).
19. Correspondence from Dr. Wu of the Chinese Red Cross to Dr. Co-Tui, January 7, 1939, American Bureau for Medical Aid to China Records [Box 22, National Red Cross Society folder], Rare Book and Manuscript Library, Columbia University in the City of New York.
20. Levine, *I Dare Do All,* 1238.
21. Viveca Haldin Norberg, *Swedes in Haile Selassie's Africa: 1924–1952* (Uppsala, Sweden: Scandinavian Institute of African Studies, 1977).
22. "Help for Victims of China War," *The Straits Times* (February 23, 1939).
23. Report of Curative Unit 33, 1940, American Bureau for Medical Aid to China Records [Box 22, National Red Cross Society of China: Dr. William Hu folder]. Rare Book and Manuscript Library, Columbia University in the City of New York.
24. Dr. Walter Karl Recht (1904–89) was a Czech orthopedist who immigrated to the United Kingdom in 1939 and served with the Royal Army Medical Corps in the Middle East. He returned to Prague in 1945 and worked in the Ministry of Health. In 1947, shortly before the Communist takeover in Czechoslovakia, he returned to Britain.
25. Correspondence from Dr. Robert Lim to Dr. Co-Tui, August 24, 1939, AMBAC Records [Box 22, National Red Cross of China, Robert K. Lim, 1939 folder]. New York: Rare Book and Manuscript Library, Columbia University in the City of New York.
26. Correspondence from Dr. Robert Lim to Dr. Co-Tui, August 24, 1939, ABMAC Records [Box 22, National Red Cross of China, Robert K. Lim, 1939 folder]. Rare Book and Manuscript Library, Columbia University in the City of New York.

Bibliography

Administrative Office of the Mausoleum of Song Qing Ling, Commemorative album of Kranzdorf, J. *Luomaniya de Bai Qiuen: Bukuer Kelieran Yu Zhongguo. di 1 ban.* ed. Shanghai, China: Shanghai ci shu chu ban she, 2009.
Allan, T., and S. Gordon. *The Scalpel and the Sword: The Story of Dr. Norman Bethune.* New York: Monthly Review Press, 1952.
Andrews, B., and M.B. Bullock. *Medical Transitions in 20th Century China.* Bloomington: Indiana University Press, 2014.
Auden, W.H., and C. Isherwood. *Journey to a War.* New York: Random House, 1939.
Balme, H. "Medical Help for China," Lancet, 1939, pp. 300–317.
Barilich, A. *Fritz Jensen. Arzt an Vielen Fronten, Biografische Texte zur Geschichte der Österreichischen Arbeiterbewegung,* Vienna, Austria: Globus Verlag, 1991.
Basu, B.K. *Call of Yanan: The Story of the Indian Medical Mission to China.* New Delhi, India: Foreign Language Press, 1986.
Becker, R. "Als Arzt in China," in G. Albrecht and W. Hartwig, *Aerzte: Erinnerungen, Erlebnisse Bekenntnisse.* Berlin: Buchverlag Der Morgen, 1972.
Becker, R., and M. Strasse. "Fritz Jensen in Memoriam." *The Journal for the Advancement of Medicine,* July 1, 1955, Vol. 13.
Bergmann, T. *Internationalisten an den antifaschistischen Fronten.* Hamburg, Germany: Verlag, 2009.
Bullock, M.B. *An American Transplant.* Berkeley: University of California Press, 1980.
Christensen, E. *In War and Famine: Missionaries in China's Honan Province in the 1940s.* Montreal, Canada: McGill–Queens University Press, 2005.
Chung, A.W. *Of Rats, Sparrows, and Flies: A Lifetime in China.* Stockton, CA: Heritage West Books, 1994.
Clegg, A. *Aid China 1937-1939: Memoirs of a Forgotten Campaign.* Beijing, China: Foreign Languages Press, 2003.
Davenport, H.W. *Robert Kho-Seng Lim: A Biographical Memoir.* Washington, D.C.: National Academy of Sciences, 1980.
Davies, T. *Friends Ambulance Unit: The Story of the F.A.U. in the Second World War, 1939-1946.* London: George Allen and Unwin, 1947.
Deepak, B.R. *My Life with Kotnis.* Beijing, China: Manak Publications, 2006.
Eber, I. *Wartime Shanghai and the Jewish Refugees from Central Europe.* Berlin: Walter De Gruyter, 2012.
Epstein, I. *My China Eye.* San Francisco: Long River Press, 2005.
Epstein, I. "On Being a Jew in China: A Personal Memoir," in A. Goldstein, *The Jews of China.* New York: M.E. Sharpe, 2000.
Ewen, J. *China Nurse: 1932-1939.* Toronto, Canada: McClelland & Stewart, 1981.

Flowers, W. *A Surgeon in China: Extracts from Letters from Dr. W.S. Flowers*. London: The Carey Press, 1946.
Freudmann, W. *Tschi-Lai!-Erhebet Euch! Erlebnisse eines Arztes in China und Burma, 1939–45*. Linz, Austria: Verlag Neue Zeit, 1947.
Grabman, R. *Bosques' War: How a Mexican Diplomat Saved 40,000 from the Nazis*. Mazatlan, Mexico: Editorial Mazatlan, 2011.
Griffith, S.B. *The Chinese People's Liberation Army*. New York: McGraw-Hill, 1967.
Gulick, E.V. "Peter Parker and the Opening of China," *Journal of the American Oriental Society*, Vol. 95, No. 3, July 1975.
Hackl, E. *In Fester Umarmung: Geschichten und Berichte, Erster Bericht über die Schriftstellerin Susanne Wantoch*. Zurich, Switzerland: Diogenes, 2000.
Hannant, L. *The Politics of Passion: Norman Bethune's Writing and Art*. Toronto: University of Toronto Press, 1998.
Hauser, E. *Shanghai: City for Sale*. Beijing: Chinese American Publishing Company, Inc., 1940.
Iancu, D. *9 Ani Medic Pe Front Spania–China (1937–1945)*. Bucuresti, Romania: Editura Vitruviu, 2008.
The Information Office of the Guiyang Municipal Government, *International Medical Team in Guiyang*. Guiyang, China: China Intercontinental Press, 2005.
Jackson, A. *For Us It Was Heaven: The Patience, Grief, and Fortitude of Patience Darton*. Brighton, England: Sussex Academic Press, 2012.
Jensen, F. *China Siegt*. Vienna, Austria: Globus Verlag, 1949.
Jensen, F. *Opfer und Sieger: Nachdichtungen, Gedichte und Berichte*. Berlin: Dietz Verlag, 1955.
Jensen, F. "Some Features of War Surgery and Army Medical Service During the Spanish Civil War of 1936–1939," *The Chinese Medical Journal*. Vol. 62A, April 1944, 95–100.
Keene, J. "Snow Boots in Sunny Spain: White Russians in Nationalist Spain," *Fighting for Franco: International Volunteers in Nationalist Spain During the Spanish Civil War, 1936–1939*. Leicester, England: Leicester University Press, 2001.
Kohn, G.C. *Encyclopedia of Plague and Pestilence: From Ancient Times to the Present*. New York: Infobase Publishing, 2008.
Landauer, H. *Lexikon der Osterreichischen Spanienkämpfer, 1936–1939*, 2d ed. Vienna, Austria: Theodor Kramer Gesellschaft, 2008.
Lataster-Czisch, P. *Eignetlich Rede Ich Nicht Gern über Mich*. Leipzig, Germany: Gustav Kiepenheuer, 1990.
Levine, A. "I Dare Do All: The Saga of Dr. Tillson Lever Harrison," *Canadian Medical Association Journal*, 177(10): 1237–1239, November 6, 2007.
Liu, F.F. *A Military History of Modern China*. Princeton, N.J.: Princeton University Press, 1956.
MacKinnon, J., and S. MacKinnon. *Agnes Smedley: The Life and Times of an American Radical*. Berkeley: University of California Press, 1988.
MacKinnon, J., and S. MacKinnon. *China Reporting: An Oral History of American Journalism in the 1930s and 1940s*. Berkeley: University of California Press, 1987.
Mitter, R. *Forgotten Ally: China's World War II, 1937–1945*. Boston: Houghton Mifflin Harcourt, 2013.
Norberg, V.H. *Swedes in Haile Selassie's Africa: 1924–1952*. Upssula, Sweden: Scandinavian Institute of African Studies, 1977.
Palmier, J.M. *Weimar in Exile: The Anti-Fascist Migration in Europe*. London, England: Verso Publishers, 2006.
Peck, G. *Two Kinds of Time*. Seattle: University of Washington Press, 2008.
Powell, L. *A Surgeon in Wartime China*. Lawrence: University of Kansas Press, 1946.
Romanus, C.F., and R. Sutherland. *U.S. Army in World War II: The China Burma India Theater*. Washington, D.C.: U.S. Department of the Army, 1959.
Ruifu, W. "After Flying Over the Hump: An Army Interpreters Report," in J. Pei, *Under the Same Flag: Recollections of the Veterans of World War II*. Beijing, China: China Intercontinental Press, 2005.
Scott, M. *Bob McClure: The China Years*. New York: Penguin, 1977.

Seagrave, G.S. *Burma Surgeon Returns*. New York: W.W. Norton & Co., 1946.
Seagrave, S. *The Soong Dynasty*. New York: Harper & Row, 1985.
Sichon, G.E. *Frantisek Kriegel, l'insoumis Plurielles numero 8—Les Juifs et l'engagement politique* (Frantisek Kriegel Biography), 1979.
Sichon, G.E. "Les Medecins des deux guerres: Espagna 1936–1939, Chine 1939–1945," in *Materiaux pour l'histoire de Nôtre Temps*. 1990, No. 19: *Materiaux pour une nouvelle lecture de l'histoire de l'Europe Centrale et Orientale*.
Smedley, A. *Battle Hymn of China*. London: Victor Gollanz, Ltd., 1944.
Soong Chiang, M. *China Shall Rise Again*. New York: Harper and Brothers, 1941.
Stephenson, C.B. "Vitamin A, Infection, and Immune Function," *Annual Review of Nutrition*, 2001; 21:167–192.
Stewart, R. *Phoenix: The Life of Norman Bethune*. Montreal, Canada: McGill–Queens University Press, 2012.
Stilwell, J.W., and T.H. White. *The Stilwell Papers*. New York: Da Capo Press, 1991.
Sues, I.R. *Shark's Fins and Millet*. Boston: Little, Brown and Company, 1944.
Taylor, J. *The Generalissimo: Chiang Kai Shek and the Struggle for Modern China*. Cambridge, MA: Belknap Press, 2011.
Terrill, R. *Mao: A Biography*. Palo Alto, CA: Stanford University Press, 1999.
Trent, Dr. R. "Robert Mcclure: Missionary–Surgeon Extraordinaire," *Canadian Medical Association Journal*, Vol. 132, February 15, 1985.
Tuchman, B. *Stilwell and the American Experience in China*. New York: The Macmillan Co., 1940.
Unschuld, U. *You Banfa—Es Findet Sich Immer Ein Weg: Wilhelm Manns Erinnerungen an China 1938–1966*. Berlin: Hentrich & Hentrich, 2014.
Utley, F. *China at War*. London: Faber & Faber, 1939.
Van de Ven, H. *War and Nationalism in China: 1925–1945*. London: Routledge Curzon, 2003.
Wang, A. *Ich Kämpfe Für Mao*. Hamburg, Germany: Holsten Verlag, 1973.
Wantoch, S. *Nan Lu: Die Stadt Der Verschlungenen Wege*. Vienna, Austria: Globus Verlag, 1948.
Watt, J. *Saving Lives in Wartime China: How Medical Reformers Built a Modern Healthcare System Amid War and Epidemics, 1928–1945*. Leiden: Brill, 2014.
White, T. *Thunder Out of China*. New York: DeCapo Press, 1946.
Winfield, J. *China: The Land and the People*. New York: William Sloane Associates, 1948.
Yin, Lin. *Walking Through Blood and Fire*. Guiyang, China: Guizhou People's Publishing House, 2015.
Yip, K. "Disease and the Fighting Men: Nationalist Anti-Epidemic Efforts in Wartime China, 1937–1945," in D.R. Barrett and L.N. Shyu, *China and the Anti-Japanese War, 1937–1945, Politics Culture and Society*. New York: Peter Lang, 2000.
Yuxiang, Y. "Reminisce the Past," in J. Pei, *Under the Same Army Flag*. Beijing China: Intercontinental Press, 2005.

Index

Aaquist, Robert 27
Aeneas 62-64, 66, 75-76, 84, 198; *see also* the Blue Funnel Lines
Alley, Rewi 137, 205; *see also* Chinese Industrial Cooperatives (Indusco)
American Bureau for Medical Aid to China 34, 53, 105, 199, 206-207; need for physicians in China 56, 102-103, 135, 137, 176; relations with other relief organizations 42-43, 47, 91, 115, 126; and Wright (Cohn), Adele 32-33, 73, 101, 171-173, 179, 203;
American Friends Service Committee 39, 108, 172, 210; relations with other relief organizations 42-43, 47, 136, 167; *see also* The Society of Friends
Anchang, Lui 54
Anhui Province, China 185
anti-Semitism 30; absence in China 88, 116; in Europe 11-12, 14, 67, 186-187, 212
Argeles, France 21
Army Medical Corps, China 49-52, 127, 169, 205; inadequacy of 53, 55, 95-96
Army Medical Corps, United States 154-155
atabrine 158
Atal, M.M. 63, 203-205, 215
Atkinson, Brooks 176
Auden, W.H. 17, 76; on McClure, Robert 41; on Smedley, Agnes 47
Ausubel, Moses 17, 189

Bachman, George 102
Baer, Herbert (贝尔医生 Beier) 33, 63, 67, 80, 118, 188; in Burma-India 149-152, 180, 182; enemy alien status 64-65, 75, 87; in England 28, 60-62; forced inactivity 137, 140
Balme, Harold (巴慕德 Ba Mude) 25, 96-97
Barcelona 16-19, 22
Barger, Evert 130-131, 136, 198
Barnett, Robert 47
Barsky, Edward 18, 157
Basu, Bijoy Kumar (巴苏华) 63, 118, 203-204

The Battle Hymn of China 147; *see also* Smedley, Agnes
Battle of Britain 126, 128, 198
Battle of Hong Kong 138
Battle of the Bulge 177
Becker (Staniforth), Joan (唐莉华) 4, 66-67, 149, 184, 188, 197, 203; with the Medical Relief Corps 123, 170-171, 179
Becker, Rolf (白乐夫医生 Bai Lefu) 2-4, 61, 69, 74-75, 80, 84, 86, 88, 91-92, 95-96, 107, 113-119, 122-123, 126, 149-150, 187-188, 191, 197-198, 203-204; in England 27-30; in Spain 14-18; with UNRRA 184; in Yunnan, China 170-171, 173
Beijing 8-9, 36, 52, 88, 184, 189
beriberi 100, 156, 169
Bertram, James "Jack" 58-59, 84, 113
Bethune, Norman (白求恩 Baiqiuen) 16, 31, 40, 46, 58-59, 80, 85, 112-114, 130, 184, 197-198, 204-205, 207
Bethune International Peace Hospital 46, 176
Bingnam, Wang 205
biomedicine 9, 97; conflict with Chinese medicine 92-94, 96, 135
Blue Funnel Line 61-62, 72; *see also* the *Aeneas*; the *Eumaeus*
Boatner, Haydon Lemaire 151, 154-155, 181
Botwin Company 14
Breidster, Waldemar 162
British Friends Service Council 42-43; *see also* The Society of Friends
British Fund for the Relief of Distress in China *see* Lord Mayor Fund
British Red Cross 47, 102-103, 167; *see also* Flowers, Wilfred
Brown, Richard 46, 113, 207
Brown, Rothwell 164
Bullis, Harry 162, 164
Burma Road 29, 43-44, 57-58, 74, 77, 124, 127, 140, 157, 162, 167, 198
Burma Surgeon *see* Seagrave, Gordon

C. Pan *see* Pan Ji
The California 73
Camp Gurs *see* Gurs, France
Camp Ramgarh *see* Ramgarh, India
Canton, China *see* Guangzhou, China
Capa, Robert 17
Casablanca Agreement 152
Cassidy, Maurice Allen 25
Changjiang River *see* Yangzi River
Changsha 63, 96, 115–117, 133, 161, 177
Chiang Ching-kuo (蔣經國 Jiǎnfēng) 96, 137
Chiang Kai-shek 9, 24, 35–36, 39, 42, 45, 50–51, 87, 96, 130, 137, 140, 149, 197, 214; and conflict with the Chinese Communist Party 8, 35, 153, 175–176; and Lin, Robert 56, 115, 130, 132–133, 198
Chiang Kai-shek, Madame (宋美齡 Song, Mei-ling) 24, 45, 51, 56, 115, 118, 131, 170, 197
China Aid Council 24, 42, 58, 86, 206
China Convoy 43; *see also* Friends Ambulance Unit
China Defense Supplies 135
China Medical Aid Committee of London 25, 27–29, 60–61, 63, 70, 72, 114, 117, 122, 126, 130, 133, 139, 148, 151, 161, 180, 185; *see also* Gilchrist, Mary
China Medical Aid Committee of Norway 29, 126, 128
China Medical Board 39
Chinese Academy of Sciences 185, 188
Chinese Army in India 148, 155, 157–158, 160, 164–165, 180
Chinese Communist Party 9, 10, 24, 66, 75, 115, 131–133, 149, 176; armies 31, 46, 59, 63, 79–80, 88, 109, 113–114, 118, 145, 147, 184, 204; conflict with Guomintang 35–36, 48–49, 89–90, 93, 112, 119, 134, 153, 205
Chinese Convalescent Hospital 161–162
Chinese Defence League 45, 61, 131, 206; Mme Sun Yat-sen 115, 130, 138, 170, 192; Spanish doctors 24, 63, 65
Chinese Expeditionary Force 5, 140, 142, 144, 166, 168
Chinese Expeditionary Force-X 147, 148, 153, 167, 182
Chinese Expeditionary Force-Y 167, 169, 170–171, 173, 199
Chinese Industrial Cooperatives (Indusco) 42; *see also* Alley, Rewi
Chinese medicine 129, 135–136; conflict with biomedicine 93–96
Chinese National Relief and Rehabilitation Administration 184
Chinese Red Cross Medical Relief Corps Headquarters *see* Tuyunguan, China
cholera 40–41, 94, 104, 107–109
Cholkar, Mohanlal (卓克华) 203–204
Chongqing 9, 31, 36, 44, 47–49, 133, 138, 140, 144, 151, 175, 179, 204, 209; Guomintang 35, 176; Lin, Robert 130, 132, 171, 179; Spanish doctors 75, 80, 87, 89, 113, 119, 131, 149, 170, 180, 187, 189, 200; Wright (Cohn), Adele 73, 80–81, 90, 173, 175, 178, 199
Chu Teh (朱德 Zhū Dé) 119, 204
Chung, A.W. 52, 78; and Spanish doctors 90, 106, 193–194
Chungking *see* Chongqing
The Citadel 84
Ciudad de Barcelona 18
Clejan, Bucur *see* Kranzdorf, Iacob
Clejan, Nelly *see* Jingpu, Zhao
Co-Tui, Frank 42–43, 56, 73, 135, 207; *see also* American Bureau of Medical Aid to China
Cohn, Adele *see* Wright (Cohn), Adele
Comintern 8–9, 13–15, 21–25, 27, 70, 89
conscription in China: of physicians 52; of soldiers 103, 121–122
corruption 49, 104, 176; in Army Medical Corps 9, 100; Atkinson, Brooks on 176; international medical relief corps on 5, 90–92; Kohlberg, Arthur on 102–103; Lin, Robert on 54, 129; Wantoch, Susanna on 51–52; Wright (Cohn), Adele on 171
Courtney, Barbara (高田宜医生 Gao Tianyi) 2, 4, 30, 66, 73–74, 132, 136–137, 184, 198, 203; death 109, 141–143, 199
Coutelle, Carl (顾泰尔医生 Gu Taier) 2–4, 12, 18–19, 50, 60, 66, 69–70, 80, 86–88, 90, 92, 107, 119, 126, 133–134, 137, 140–142, 188; in Burma-India 149–153, 155–156, 161, 177, 180, 182; in England 27–28, 72; in Spain 14–15, 17; why China? 22–23
Coutelle, (Sussman) Rosa 127–128, 133, 141–142, 148, 188, 198; in England 27–28, 60, 70–72; in Spain 19, 22–23
Crome, Len 27, 116
Cronin, A.J. 84
Csu Te Lin, Éva 190–191
Culpin, Millais 25, 211

Damau, Peng 54
dams 36
Darton, Patience 22–23, 27–29, 121, 141
Davidson, Louis 32, 58
Delin Zhu *see* Csu Te Lin Éva
delousing and bathing stations 41, 106–107, 124–127, 173, 194
Deucalion 70–72, 80
diphtheria 94, 108
Dohan, Paul 206
Dutch East Indies 57–58, 115
dysentery 22, 47, 98, 104, 106–107, 141, 169, 174

Eden, Anthony 130, 222
Edwards, Dwight 102–103, 221
Eighth Route Army 9, 79–80, 88, 109, 114, 130, 176, 204, 215; and Bethune, Norman

31, 40, 46, 59, 112–113; and Indian physicians 63, 118, 205–206; and Spanish doctors 88, 113–114, 116, 118–119, 131
Eisenberger (Kohn), Elizabeth 73; *see also* Kent, Heinrich
Eloesser, Leo 31, 93–94, 118, 212
Emblem of Meritorious Civilian Services 163, 166
Emergency Medical Service Training Schools 54–56, 119, 127, 135, 144, 173–174
The Empress of Asia 58
enemy aliens 68, 72, 88, 185; in Hong Kong 64, 70; in India 138, 151–152
Enlai, Zhou 35, 58, 133, 179, 189, 205; and the Spanish doctors 89, 113, 115, 119, 131, 149, 187
Epstein, Israel 143
Ersler, Gabriel: on Kriegel, Frantisek 16; on Volokhine, Alexander 17
Eumaeus 61–62; *see also* the *Blue Funnel Lines*
Evans, Ernest 43
Ewen, Jeanne 58, 113

famine 103
Flato, Stanislaw (柯理格医生 Fu Ladu) 117, 119, 137, 141, 149–152, 166, 187; in Spain 2–4, 14, 16, 26–27
Flowers, Wilfred 47, 102
For Whom the Bell Tolls 19
Foreign Auxiliary-Chinese Red Cross 24, 61, 63, 65, 73, 86, 133, 180; *see also* Selwyn-Clarke, Hilda
Franco, Francisco 7, 13, 14, 16–18, 40, 197
fraxine 105
French, Norman 138
French Communist Party 13–15, 25–29
Freudmann, Walter (富华德医生 Fu Huade) 60–67, 75, 79–80, 84–85, 87, 89, 91–92, 115, 117–118, 122, 137, 140, 149; in Burma-India 150–152, 157, 160, 162, 180, 182, 188–189, 194, 198; in England 27–29; in Spain 13, 16–18
Frey, Richard (Fu Lai) 79–80
Friedrich-Wilhelms Universität zu Berlin see University of Berlin
Friends Ambulance Unit 43–44, 46–47, 70, 73–74, 131–136, 144, 169, 172, 174, 194; *see also* Society of Friends (Quakers)
Friends of the International Members of the Medical Relief Corps 201

Gellhorn, Martha 17
Gilchrist, Mary 28–29, 63, 72, 130, 148, 161, 180; *see also* China Medical Aid Committee of London
Gjesdahl, Tor 24
Glaser, Wilhelm 16, 26
Goldstein, Gisela *see* Kranzdorf, Gisela
Grynspan, Herzel 29–30

Guangxi 80, 120, 122, 170
Guangzhou 36, 75, 108
Guernica, Spain 9, 24, 197
Guilin 122, 153, 177
Guiyang 4, 9, 70, 83, 86–87, 89 100, 107–110, 114–116, 122–123, 131–133, 136, 138, 141, 148–149, 174–175, 177–180; Chinese Red Cross HQ 56, 61, 67, 71, 73; prison 174; travel to 74–79; *see also* Tuyunguan
Guizhou 4, 12, 83, 109–110, 114–115, 119, 125, 153, 200
Guomindang 9, 23, 50, 53, 66, 88, 92, 100, 103–104, 113–114, 123, 127, 138, 149, 176–177; and the Chinese Communist Party 24, 35–36, 89, 93, 112, 133–134; healthcare policy 10, 49, 130–132, 145; second united front 36, 75, 129, 131, 198, 205
Gurs, France 21–23, 25, 27, 62

Hai-teh, Ma (马海德马海德 Ma Haide) 63
Hall, Kathleen 203
Hall, Ronald 24
Hankou 47, 58, 75, 117; *see also* Wuhan, China
Han-yuan, Li 50
Harris, Michael 174; *see also* Friends Ambulance Unit
Harrison, Tillson Lever 206
Harvard University 48, 186
Hastings, Somerville 29
Hatem, George *see* Hai-teh, Ma
Hemingway, Ernest 19
Henan 54, 104; famine 103, 198; mission hospitals 39, 46–47
Hengyang 161, 185
herbal medicine *see* Chinese medicine
Hiroshima 182, 199
Hodam, Max 25
Holm, Ake (科恩医生) 203, 207
Hong Kong 52, 72, 80, 108, 113, 124, 126, 133–135, 142, 204, 206–207; battle of 138; and Becker (Staniforth), Joan 66, 123, 197; China Defence League 24, 126, 130; and Courtney, Barbara 136; and Mamlok, Erich 66–68, 70–71, 152; and the Spanish doctors 61–66, 76, 78, 122–123; University 54, 96; and Wright (Cohn), Adele 73–75, 179
Hsien-Lin, Chang 96
Huanghe River *see* Yellow River
Hubei 47, 102, 120
Hucheng, Yang 35
Humboldt University, Berlin 188
Hume, Edward 136
Hunan 58, 138, 152; Kent, Heinrich 159; Kohlberg, Arthur 149; Mamlok, Erich 144, 177; Schöen, George 252; Spanish doctors 124, 170

Iancu, David (杨固医生 Yang Gu) 3–4, 63–64, 76, 88, 92, 124, 137, 183, 190, 194, 198; in

Burma-India 150–152, 157, 161, 180, 182; in England 28–29, 60–62; with Enlai, Zhou 89, 119, 149; in Spain 16, 18–19, 26
imperialism 11; Japanese 13, 31, 39
inflation 76, 148, 207
International Brigade 8, 13, 37, 66, 90, 132, 144, 171; Atal, M.M. 204–205; Bethune, Norman 31; Coutelle, Rosa 28, 72; Crome, Len 27; Eloesser, Leo 31, 93; Spanish doctors 13–22, 25–27, 28–29, 62; Tudor-Hart, Alex 28–29
International Red Cross 53, 148
International Red Cross Committee 41–42, 45, 141, 197; and Holm, Ake 207; and Landauer, Eric 45; and Sullivan, Michael 136
International Relief Committee see International Red Cross Committee

Jean Laborde 66, 69, 198
Jensen, Fritz (严斐德医生 Yan Feide) 3–4, 11–12, 51, 68, 74–75, 79–80, 84–87, 92, 96, 103, 114–118, 121–122, 126, 137, 150, 188–189, 192, 194–195, 197; biomedicine 93, 95; in Chongqing 170, 179; diphtheria 108; dysentery 106; in England 28–29, 60–61; and Enlai, Zhou 113, 119; eulogy 3; in Hong Kong 66, 204; in Spain 16–17, 19–20, 22, 26–27; UNRRA 181, 184; why China? 16, 23
Jerusalem, Friederich see Jensen, Fritz
Jerusalem, Ruth Domino 16
Jettmar, Heinrich 40; see also League of Nations Health Organization
Jewish Hospital of Berlin 94, 187
Jiangsu 87, 182
Jiangxi 78, 96, 115, 117, 120, 137
Jin Baoshan (金宝善) 48–49, 109, 123
Jingpu, Zhao 190; see also Kranzdorf, Iacob
Jung, T.S. (荣独山 Rong Dushan) 174
Jungermann, Edith see Marens, Edith
Jungermann, Wladislav (戎格曼医生 Rong) 2–5, 12, 62, 64–65, 150; in Spain 13–15, 19, 25–26; with UNRRA 184, 186; in Yunnan 173
Jungery, Wolf see Jungermann, Wladislav

Kaifeng 207
Kaixi, Wang 54
Kamieniecki, Leon (甘理安医生 Gan Lian) 3, 62, 64, 67, 117, 137, 144, 173, 191; on nutrition 101–102; in Spain 14, 19, 26; with UNRRA 184–185
Kamieniecka, Mania (甘曼妮 Gan Manni) 62–64, 67, 84, 121, 141–142, 173, 191; in Spain 14, 19; UNRRA 184–185
Kaneti, Ianto (甘扬道医生 Gan Yangdao) 3–4, 67, 84, 117, 134, 137, 141–142, 171, 173, 190; in England 28, 60–62; in Spain 27
Kent, Edith see Marens, Edith
Kent, Heinrich (肯德医生 Kende) 3–4, 12, 16, 49–50, 60, 66, 68, 80, 96, 110, 119, 125–126, 140, 144, 150, 188–189, 194; in England 27–29, 70, 72; and the plague 109; in Spain 17, 23; with UNRRA 184; in Yunnan 170, 173
Kent, Maria see Rodriquez Gonzales, Maria
Kerr, Archibald 133
Kho-Seng Lim see Lin, Robert
King, P.Z. see Jin Baoshan
Kisch, Bedřich (纪瑞德医生 Ji Ruide) 4–5, 33, 74–75, 80, 84, 86, 107, 113, 115–119, 137, 149–150, 189–190, 204, 214; Bethune, Norman 31, 113–114; in Burma-India 151, 154, 158, 164, 171, 180, 182; in England 27, 61; in Spain 15–16, 22, 28; why China 23
Kisch, Edith see Marens, Edith,
Kjesdal, Tor 126
Kohlberg, Arthur 102, 103, 173; see also American Bureau for Medical Aid to China
Kohn, Elizabeth see Eisenberger, Elisabeth
Kohn, Heinrich see Kent, Heinrich
Kotnis, Dwarkanath (柯棣华医生 Ke Di Hua) 184, 199, 203–205
Kranzdorf, Gisela 2, 4, 19, 66, 73, 134, 173, 184
Kranzdorf, Iacob (柯让道医生 Ke Rangdao) 2–3, 12, 18–19, 62, 64, 66–67, 190, 194–195; in Gurs 21–22; in Spain 19, 26; with UNRRA 184; in Yunnan 169, 173
Kriegel, Frantisek (柯理格医生 Ke Lige) 4, 38, 44, 62, 64–65, 134, 141, 189–190, 192; in Burma-India 149–151, 161, 164–166, 180, 182–183; in Gurs 21, 27; in Spain 15–16, 26
Kung, H.H. (孔祥熙 Kung Hsiang-hsi or Kong Xiangxi) 45; and Wright (Cohn), Adele 175
Kung, H.H., Madame (宋蔼龄 Song Ailing) 45
Kunming 36, 44, 148–153, 167, 184
Kuomintang see Guomintang
Kwangsi see Guangxi, China
Kweiyang see Guiyang, China

Landauer, Erich 40–41, 99, 119; on the International Red Cross Committee 45–46; and Mann, Wilhelm 79; see also League of Nations Health Organization
Lanset, A. 40; see also League of Nations Health Organization
Largs Bay 184; see also Wantoch, Susanne
Lazarus, Emma 2
League of Nations Health Organization 38, 40–41, 53, 104; and Brown, Richard 46; and Landauer, Erich 45, 79; and Lurje, Walter 30; and Mooser, Hermann 70, 79; and Pollitzer, Robert 41, 108
Lin, Robert (Lin Kesheng, Bobby Lim, 林可胜) 4, 24, 39, 46, 53–56, 58–59, 91–94, 96, 104–105, 107, 109, 118–119, 127, 134, 136–137, 140, 147, 150, 167, 170, 175, 179, 204–

205, 207; and Bethune, Norman 85, 112; and bioscience 95; and the Guomintang–Chinese Communist Party conflict 9, 88, 112, 115, 129–133, 142–145; and Mamlok, Erich 70–71, 132; and Mann, Wilhelm 86; and McClure, Robert 41, 135, 172; and Spanish doctors 84–88, 92, 97, 113, 117, 126, 180; Wright (Cohn) Adele 32–33, 80–81, 101, 171, 173
Liu, J. Heng see Ruiheng, Liu
London School of Medicine for Women 30
Loo, Chih-teh (卢致德 Lu Zhide Loo) 51, 54, 167
Lord Mayor Fund 55, 61–62
Louderbough, Henry 44; see also The Society of Friends
Luce, Henry 42, 135, 176
Luo Shengte see Rosenfeld, Jacob
Lurje, Walter (罗益医生 Luo Yi) 30, 132, 140, 174, 187

Ma, Thomas 54
Madrid 16, 31, 144, 197
malaria 47, 50, 94–95, 104–107, 109, 119, 158, 169, 173–174, 176; and Becker, Rolf 29; and Jungery, Michelle 186–187; and Lin, Robert 105
malnutrition 66, 98, 103, 110, 112, 120, 153–4, 156, 193
Mamlok, Erich (孟乐克医生 Meng Leke) 1–3, 66–71, 76–80, 87, 99, 102, 115, 120–121, 132, 140–141, 148, 187–188, 203; on anti-Semitisim in Europe 11–12, 29, 50; in Burma-India 150–152, 155, 161–163, 165–166, 177, 180–183
Manchurian Plague Prevention Service 40
Mann, Wilhelm (孟威廉医生 Meng Weilan) 3–5, 66, 83, 89, 100, 107–108, 150, 170, 174, 177, 185, 188, 203; on anti-Semitism 30, 116; in Europe 29, 79; on Lim, Robert 86
Marcus, Edith see Marens, Edith
Marens, Edith (马绮迪 Ma Kusi) 4, 62, 64–65, 84, 150, 171, 173, 188–189; in Spain 14–15, 19, 26; with UNRRA 184
Marshall, George 153
Martens, Anneliese see Wang, Anna
Marty, Andre 25–26
McClure, Robert 41, 44–45, 51, 99, 105, 107, 131, 136, 194, 203, 205; and Becker, Rolf 170; and Bethune, Norman 46, 59; and Bryson, Arthur 101; and Friends Ambulance Unit 44, 70, 74; and Kent, Heinrich 170; and Kranzdorf, Iacob 169–170; and Lin, Robert 41, 135, 144, 167–169, 172; and Schön, George 174
Mexico 23, 28, 34, 206
mission hospitals 38–39, 44–47, 50–51, 108; Canadian mission hospital in Chongqing 184; Catholic Mission in Hunan 185; International Red Cross Committee 41–42, 141;

Lutheran Mission in Wuchang 49; Methodist Union Mission in Koloshan 173
Mogaung Valley, Myanmar 139, 158, 161
Mooser, Hermann 40–41, 46, 70, 79; see also League of Nations Health Organization
Mukden (Manchurian or Shenyang) Incident 35
Mukherjee, Debesh (木克华) 203–205
Müller, Hans (汉斯·米勒博士 Hansi Mileboshiì) 67, 88, 99, 102, 113–114, 119, 176

Nanchang 112
Nanjing 36, 55; rape of 9, 24, 58, 197
National Health Administration (China) 38, 48–49, 53, 55, 94, 100–101, 107, 109, 127, 129, 144
National Institute of Health (China) 49, 100, 102
Nationalist Party see Guomindang
Needham, Joseph (李约瑟 Li Yue se) 54, 179
New Fourth Army 9, 59, 79, 88, 109, 112, 130, 176; incident 131, 198
New York Times 66, 147, 158, 176

Onufrio, Eduardo d' 21
Operation Barbarossa 177, 198
Operation Ichigo 119, 175, 177
opium 118
overseas Chinese 52–58, 78, 90, 115, 134

Pan Ji, (潘骥 C. Pan) 129, 131, 142–144
Pang, Kohlhaus 55
Paris, France 14, 16, 22–23, 28, 72, 80, 189
Parker, Peter 38
Parsons, Charles Edward 58, 207
Payne, Robert 89
Pearl Harbor, Hawaii 138, 198
Peck, Graham 123, 222
Peking University Medical College 39, 46, 48, 52–55, 93, 96, 205
Pinner, Max 32
plague 40–41, 104, 108–109, 141
Price, Mildred 24
Pyrenees Mountains 15, 17, 19–21

Quakers see Society of Friends

Rajchman, Ludwik 40; see also League of Nations Health Organization
Ramgarh, India 148, 153, 156, 167; international medical relief corps physicians 151–152, 160, 170, 199
Rangoon 72, 74, 80, 138, 140
Rape of Nanjing, China see Nanjing, China
Recht, Walter 207
Red Book 31, 59
Red Star Over China 28
relapsing fever 47, 106–107, 124–125, 174
rice 74, 78, 80, 92, 100, 102, 116, 122
Rich, John 17, 20, 39, 210; and British Red

Cross 47; and international medical relief corps physicians 170–171; and Lin, Robert 167; and McClure, Robert 41, 44, 99–100; *see also* American Friends Service Committee
Robertson, R.C. 40; *see also* League of Nations Health Organization
Rockefeller, John D. III 42
Rockefeller Foundation 38- 39, 41
Rodriquez Gonzales, Maria 23, 28; in England 27, 60, 127–128; in Spain 17, 19
Rosenfeld, Jacob (羅生特 / 罗生特 General Luo, or Luo Shengte) 79–80, 88
Ruifu, Wang 157
Ruiheng, Liu (刘瑞恒 Liu, J. Heng) 48, 53, 129; *see also* National Health Administration
Russian Civil War 17

St. Cyprien, France 21
Salween Gorge 168–169
scabies 109–110, 124; and Kranzdorf, Iacob 194; and Lin, Robert 109; and McClure, Robert 169; and Smedley, Agnes 125–126; *see also* delousing and bathing stations
Scanlon, Patrick 102, 219
Schön, George (沈恩医生 Shen En) 5, 12, 62, 67, 91, 97, 101–102, 107, 119, 144, 150, 170, 178, 190–191, 195; Guiyang prison 174; in Spain 18, 26; with UNRRA 184–185
Scott, A.L. 161
Seagrave, Gordon 98, 158–160
Second United Front 36, 75, 119, 129, 131, 205
Selwyn-Clarke, Hilda 115, 131; and Courtney, Barbara 136, 141; and international medical relief corps physicians 24, 63–65, 70, 73–74, 113, 126, 180; and Lin, Robert 86, 133; and Staniforth, Joan 66, 123; *see also* Foreign Auxiliary-Chinese Red Cross
Selwyn-Clarke, Percy 24
Shandong 96, 184
Shanghai, China 68, 129, 182, 190–191, 195; and Becker, Rolf 184; Jewish refugees 79–81; and Mamlok, Erich 76–78; and Mann, Wilhelm 79, 188; St. Johns College 96
Shanxi 114
Sheng, C.C. 176
Shoukai, Zhou 54
Shu-Pui, Li 42
Siao, Ping 164
Sichon, Gabriel *see* Ersler, Gabriel
Sichuan 36, 127
Sing, Sze Tsung 54
Singapore 63, 72, 124, 138; and Lin, Robert 53–54, 57
Smedley, Agnes 46, 51, 58, 78, 125, 187, 204, 209–210; and the international medical relief corps physicians 3, 101, 115, 147, 194–195; and Lin, Robert 130, 133; and mission hospitals 47

Smets, Charles 30
Society of Friends 41–43; *see also* the American Friends Service Committee; the British Friends Service Committee
Somogyi, György *see* Schön, George
Song, Ailing *see* Kung, H.H., Madame
Song, Mei-ling *see* Chiang Kai-shek, Madame
Song, Qingling *see* Sun Yat-sen, Madame
Song, Tse-Vung (宋子文 T.V. Soong) 200
Song, Ziwen *see* Song, Tse-Vung
Soviet Occupation Zone, Berlin 188
Soviet Union 15, 35–36, 69, 177, 189, 191; and enemy aliens 138; and the Spanish Civil War 7, 17
Staffordshire 127–128
Stalin, Joseph 35
Staniforth, Joan *see* Becker (Staniforth), Joan
Stein, Richard *see* Frey, Richard
Stevens, Helen 171, 173; *see also* American Bureau of Medical Aid to China
Stilwell, Joseph 56, 141, 144, 175; and international medical relief corps physicians 147–148, 151–154, 156, 160, 163; recall 176–177
Sues, Ilona Ralf 129
Sullivan, Michael (苏立文) 136–137
Sun Yat-sen, Madame (宋庆龄 Song Qingling) 24, 56, 138, 170, 176–177; and the international medical relief corps physicians 65–66, 113, 115 on medical care 45, 49, 130–132
Sunfen, Zhang 190
Sussman, Rosa *see* Coutelle (Sussman), Rosa
Sweeney, John 156

Tah-moi, Peng 54
Talbot, Henry 206
Taubenfligel, Wiktor (陶维德医生 Tao Weide) 3–4, 62, 67, 141, 183, 187; in Burma-India 149–151, 158, 160–161, 165–166, 180, 182; in Spain 13–14, 16, 26
Tembien 78
Time magazine 135
trachoma 100, 110, 169
traditional Chinese medicine *see* Chinese medicine
Tsuyung 170
tuberculosis 94, 109–110, 113; and Kent, Heinrich 17; and Mamlok, Erich 187; and Wantoch, Theodore 184; and Wright (Cohn), Adele 32, 73, 171, 173, 175, 179, 191
Tuchman, Barbara 122
Tudor-Hart, Alex 28, 29, 72
Tung, Eva Ho 54
Tuyunguan 1–2, 54, 61, 81, 89–90, 101, 107; Courtney, Barbara tomb 142–143; and forced inactivity 133–134, 137, 141, 144, 161, 204; Spanish doctors arrival 75, 83–84, 119

Index

typhoid fever 22, 94, 104, 107–108, 110
typhus 40, 46, 106–108, 124–125, 169, 174

United China Relief 42–43, 47, 102–103, 176, 179; *see also* Luce, Henry
United Nations 179
United Nations Relief and Rehabilitation Administration 40, 181–182, 184–185, 190, 207
University of Belgrade, Serbia 13
University of Berlin, Germany 11, 12, 50
University of Frankfurt, Germany 30
University of Halle, Germany 188
University of Iasi, Romania 18
University of Padua, Italy 13
University of Paris (Sorbonne), France 14
University of Parma, Italy 18
University of Prague, Czech Republic 15
University of Vienna, Austria 11, 17, 28, 73, 79
Utley, Freda on Lin, Robert 55, 86; on physician shortage in China 135

Van Slyke, Donald 172; *see also* American Bureau of Medical Aid to China
Vazant, Francis 28; *see also* Kent, Heinrich
VE day 179
Vitamin A deficiency 100
Vitamin B1 (thiamine) deficiency *see* beriberi
Volokhine, Alexander (何乐经医生 He Lejing) 3, 62, 64, 67, 69; in Burma-India 150, 161, 180, 191; in Spain 16–18, 26
Vouzeron, France 23

Wang, Anna (王安娜; Anneliese Martens) 90, 187
Wang, Hsin Ti 62
Wang, Kai Hsi 96
Wang, Wu-An 179, 189
Wang, Zhengting (王正廷; Wáng Zhèngtíng) 86–87, 118, 129, 131, 143
Wantoch, Susanne (Wang Daodi) 51–52, 66, 68, 73, 184, 189, 203

Wantoch, Theodor (王道医生 Wang Dao) 2, 4, 66, 70, 73, 79, 87, 184, 206; in Europe 11, 29–30
warlords 9, 36
Wedemeyer, Albert 177, 212
White, Theodore 103–104, 118
White Russia 17, 69; *see also* Volokhine, Alexander
Wilkie, Wendell 42
Wright (Cohn), Adele (科恩医生) 4, 66, 73–74, 80, 84, 96–97, 101, 110, 132, 136, 150 171, 174–175, 178, 191, 203; and ABMAC 32, 171–173, 179; in America 32–34, 58; and Lin, Robert 33, 81, 86, 137
Wright, Philip 130–131, 136, 175, 191–192
Wu, William 99–100, 104
Wuhan 36, 41, 58, 106

Xi'an 35, 40, 116, 118, 130, 137, 206
Xueliang, Zhang 35, 212

Yale University 38, 49
Yan'an 9, 35, 59, 63, 113, 118, 130, 176, 204–205
Yangzi (Yangtze) River 148, 152, 154, 214
Yellow River 105, 114, 130, 137
Yen, F.C. 48; *see also* National Health Administration
Ying Kwei, Haueh 158
Yingcan, Wu 57
Ying-ch'in, Ho 153
Yuesheng, Du 129
Yunnan 76–77, 80, 148–149, 173; Chinese Expeditionary Force-Y 167, 169–172; infectious diseases 105, 109–110; McClure, Robert 144
Yuxiang, Feng 125

Zedong, Mao 8–9, 35, 109; and Atal, M.M. 63; and Bethune, Norman 31, 59; and international medical relief corps physicians 28, 149
Zhang, D.C. 89, 133
Zhengzhou 36

www.ingramcontent.com/pod-product-compliance
Lightning Source LLC
Chambersburg PA
CBHW021352300426
44114CB00012B/1189